Crisis Management in
Anesthesiology

SECOND EDITION

Crisis Management in Anesthesiology

DAVID M. GABA, MD
Associate Dean for Immersive and Simulation-based Learning
Professor
Department of Anesthesiology, Perioperative and Pain Medicine
Stanford University School of Medicine
Stanford, California
Staff Anesthesiologist
Veterans Affairs Palo Alto Health Care System
Palo Alto, California

KEVIN J. FISH, MSC, MB CHB
Professor Emeritus
Department of Anesthesiology, Perioperative and Pain Medicine
Stanford University School of Medicine
Stanford, California
Per Diem Staff Anesthesiologist
Anesthesiology and Perioperative Care Service
Veterans Affairs Palo Alto Health Care System
Palo Alto, California

STEVEN K. HOWARD, MD
Associate Professor
Department of Anesthesiology, Perioperative and Pain Medicine
Stanford University School of Medicine
Stanford, California
Staff Anesthesiologist
Anesthesiology and Perioperative Care Service
Veterans Affairs Palo Alto Health Care System
Palo Alto, California

AMANDA R. BURDEN, MD
Associate Professor of Anesthesiology
Director, Simulation Program
Cooper Medical School of Rowan University
Cooper University Hospital
Camden, New Jersey

ELSEVIER
SAUNDERS

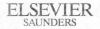

1600 John F. Kennedy Blvd.
Ste. 1800
Philadelphia, PA 19103-2899

CRISIS MANAGEMENT IN ANESTHESIOLOGY, SECOND EDITION ISBN: 978-0-443-06537-8

Library of Congress Cataloging-in-Publication Data
Crisis management in anesthesiology / [edited by] David M. Gaba, Kevin J. Fish, Steven K. Howard, Amanda R. Burden. – Second edition.
    p. ; cm.
    Preceded by Crisis management in anesthesiology / David M. Gaba, Kevin J. Fish, Steven K. Howard ; with contributions by Emily Ratner, Robert S. Holzman. 1994.
    Includes bibliographical references and index.
    ISBN 978-0-443-06537-8 (pbk. : alk. paper)
    I. Gaba, David M., editor. II. Fish, Kevin J., editor. III. Howard, Steven K., editor. IV. Burden, Amanda R., editor. V. Gaba, David M. Crisis management in anesthesiology. Preceded by (work):
    [DNLM: 1. Anesthesiology–methods. 2. Anesthesia–adverse effects. 3. Decision Making. 4. Emergencies. WO 200]
    RD82.5
    617.9'6041–dc23

                                                                                            2014027627

Executive Content Strategist: William R. Schmitt
Content Development Specialist: Angela Rufino
Publishing Services Manager: Anne Altepeter
Project Manager: Louise King
Designer: Ellen Zanolle

Printed in India

Last digit is the print number: 9

Working together
to grow libraries in
developing countries

www.elsevier.com • www.bookaid.org

Contributors

Gregory H. Botz, MD, FCCM
Distinguished Teaching Professor
Professor of Anesthesiology and Critical
  Care
The University of Texas MD Anderson
  Cancer Center
Houston, Texas
Adjunct Clinical Associate Professor
Department of Anesthesiology,
  Perioperative and Pain Medicine
Stanford University School of Medicine
Stanford, California

Amanda R. Burden, MD
Associate Professor of Anesthesiology
Director, Simulation Program
Cooper Medical School of Rowan University
Cooper University Hospital
Camden, New Jersey

Johannes Dorfling, MB ChB
Assistant Professor
Department of Anesthesiology
University of Kentucky College of Medicine
Lexington, Kentucky

Jeremy S. Dority, MD
Assistant Professor
Department of Anesthesiology
University of Kentucky College of Medicine
Lexington, Kentucky

Jan Ehrenwerth, MD
Professor of Anesthesiology
Yale University School of Medicine
Attending Anesthesiologist
Yale – New Haven Hospital
New Haven, Connecticut

James B. Eisenkraft, MD
Professor of Anesthesiology
Icahn School of Medicine at Mount Sinai
New York, New York

Ruth M. Fanning, MB, MRCPI, FFARCSI
Clinical Assistant Professor
Co-Director, Evolve Simulation Program
Department of Anesthesiology,
  Perioperative and Pain Medicine
Stanford University School of Medicine
Stanford, California

Kevin J. Fish, MSc, MB ChB
Professor Emeritus
Department of Anesthesiology, Perioperative
  and Pain Medicine
Stanford University School of Medicine
Stanford, California
Per Diem Staff Anesthesiologist
Anesthesiology and Perioperative Care
  Service
Veterans Affairs Palo Alto Health Care
  System
Palo Alto, California

David M. Gaba, MD
Associate Dean for Immersive and
  Simulation-based Learning
Professor
Department of Anesthesiology, Perioperative
  and Pain Medicine
Stanford University School of Medicine
Stanford, California
Staff Anesthesiologist
Veterans Affairs Palo Alto Health Care
  System
Palo Alto, California

Sara Goldhaber-Fiebert, MD
Clinical Assistant Professor
Co-Director, Evolve Simulation Program
Department of Anesthesiology,
  Perioperative and Pain Medicine
Stanford University School of Medicine
Stanford, California

T. Kyle Harrison, MD
Staff Physician
Anesthesiology and Perioperative Care
   Service
Veterans Affairs Palo Alto Health Care
   System
Palo Alto, California
Clinical Associate Professor
Department of Anesthesiology,
   Perioperative and Pain Medicine
Stanford University School of Medicine
Stanford, California

Gillian Hilton, MB ChB, FRCA
Clinical Assistant Professor
Department of Anesthesiology,
   Perioperative and Pain Medicine
Stanford University School of Medicine
Stanford, California

Steven K. Howard, MD
Associate Professor
Department of Anesthesiology, Perioperative
   and Pain Medicine
Stanford University School of Medicine
Stanford, California
Staff Anesthesiologist
Anesthesiology and Perioperative Care Service
Veterans Affairs Palo Alto Health Care System
Palo Alto, California

Calvin Kuan, MD, FAAP
Clinical Associate Professor
Pediatric Cardiac Anesthesia
Lucile Packard Children's Hospital
Department of Anesthesiology,
   Perioperative and Pain Medicine
Stanford University School of Medicine
Stanford, California
Attending Physician
Pediatric Intensive Care Unit
Children's Hospital and Research Center
   Oakland
Oakland, California

Geoffrey K. Lighthall, MD, PhD
Associate Professor
Department of Anesthesiology,
   Perioperative and Pain Medicine
Stanford University School of Medicine
Stanford, California
Staff Anesthesiologist and Intensivist
Anesthesiology and Perioperative Care Service
Veterans Affairs Palo Alto Health Care System
Palo Alto, California

Erin White Pukenas, MD, FAAP
Assistant Professor of Anesthesiology
Associate Director
Division of Pediatric Anesthesiology
Director, Elizabeth Blackwell Advisory
   College
Cooper Medical School of Rowan
   University
Cooper University Hospital
Camden, New Jersey

Johannes Steyn, MD
Department of Anesthesiology
University of Kentucky College of
   Medicine
Lexington, Kentucky

Ankeet Udani, MD
Clinical Instructor
Department of Anesthesiology, Perioperative
   and Pain Medicine
Stanford University School of Medicine
Stanford, California
Assistant Professor of Anesthesiology
Duke University School of Medicine
Durham, North Carolina

When we wrote the Foreword to the first edition of this book, I didn't know that it would become a classic. It is still widely read in the anesthesiology and simulation communities. I also didn't know that it would take more than 20 years to update it to a second edition. To the credit of the authors, there was so much novel, excellent material in the first edition that much of the original work has held up well through the ensuing years. Thus what was written in the Foreword to the first edition still holds true. Unfortunately, I'm writing this second Foreword alone; our friend and patient safety visionary, Ellison (Jeep) C. Pierce, Jr., MD, passed away in 2011. Jeep set us on a great course. It is universally acknowledged that the profession of anesthesiology has made huge strides in reducing adverse events and risk.

But the battle is far from over; in fact, it's never over. That's why this second edition is as important as the first. We are reminded in many ways that anesthesia safety improvements are always under siege, both in the moment and in general; there are so many ways that things can go wrong. Some readers will be reminded while others will learn, perhaps for the first time, about the kinds of things that have to be done to achieve the vision of the Anesthesia Patient Safety Foundation: "that no patient is harmed by anesthesia."

Many things have changed in the past 20 years that make a new edition of this pioneering text necessary. Some of the concepts first presented in this book are accepted but still not well practiced (e.g., the importance of good hand-offs). Other ideas aren't adequately understood or implemented (e.g., debriefing following simulation scenarios). I'll come back to this later, because I believe it's the most essential teaching approach to make simulation effective. Finally, after 20 years, the compilation of information about the original 80-plus anesthesia crises needs some updating. There are 99 in this edition; all of the old ones, some under new names, and several new ones for situations that weren't recognized or appreciated 20 years ago (perioperative visual loss) or responses that weren't available (treatment for local anesthetic systemic toxicity). For more detail on what's new in this edition, see the Preface.

Patient safety in anesthesia and all of health care has changed dramatically in 20 years. I can't even begin to document all that encompasses here. This book introduced some of the most important concepts and interventions, including Crisis Resource Management (CRM), which the Stanford University anesthesia team adapted from aviation, and the rest of health care soon emulated. The acronym is now commonly heard in patient safety conversations. But CRM is not only a better approach in managing a crisis. It's a new way of thinking—giving teamwork a higher priority over the individual team member and focusing on what's best for the patient. Although CRM and teamwork principles are now widely taught, they are still not sufficiently practiced. I have confidence that will come in time.

One reason for my confidence is that the use of simulation for training in CRM in anesthesia has also caught on. It also was initially introduced by those who wrote the first edition of this book. And simulation, like CRM in general, has since been adopted in various ways throughout the health care industry, primarily as an educational tool and specifically as a highly effective patient safety enhancer. All anesthesiologists certified after 2000 are required to enroll in Maintenance of Certification in Anesthesiology (MOCA), to remain board certified. One of the most innovative, challenging, and probably effective elements is the requirement that all anesthesiologists first certified after 2007 attend 1 day of simulation-based CRM training. I suspect that as anesthesiologists come to understand the value of the simulation experience they will gladly accept even more frequent training, whether required or not. Given what I've witnessed over 20 years in simulation, I hope they do. Simulation-based training of complete operating room teams is just starting to catch on as well.

I also feel positive about the continuing improvements in patient safety to which CRM and simulation principles contribute. There is now a robust patient safety movement. People talk about safety as if it were second nature. Anesthesiology is heralded as *the* safety-conscious specialty. And it is. It got the ball rolling and others have taken safety in new directions. Anesthesia is safer. The training, personnel selection, technology, drugs, and most important, better attitudes, have made that so.

It is also worth noting that all these patient safety elements are now understood to be part of the larger concept of high reliability organizations (HRO). HRO is another idea introduced into anesthesia and health care by David M. Gaba and his colleagues in the late 1980s. HRO wasn't fully developed when the first edition of this book was published. It is now more fully appreciated and applied. Likewise, the term "production pressure" wasn't widely used 20 years ago but is now frequently mentioned in discussions about anesthesia practice and adverse events. These are concepts adapted to anesthesia and health care by the authors of this book. We also learn more in this edition about the influence of fatigue and other performance-shaping factors, all of which have been studied more intensely since the first edition. The concept of cognitive aids for managing crises more effectively is also new in the past 20 years. Soon that concept will surely be widely introduced in the form of emergency manuals that will be as routine for use in anesthesia emergencies as they are in aviation, the field from which the idea is adapted.

From my perspective (perhaps a biased one), simulation (and its manifestations) is the single most important new concept that has been expanded upon in this edition. The idea of practicing for emergencies seems obvious, although some are likely still waiting for the randomized controlled trials and detailed cost benefit analysis. Aviation, wisely and fortunately for its passengers, did not bother to wait to achieve the impossible before it embraced the training approach as a fundamental aspect of its overall approach to safety. That decision surely accounts for the remarkable safety record of commercial aviation.

Simulation was a nascent concept in 1994. The field of anesthesia pioneered its adoption. The use of simulation is now embedded in anesthesia training. Its use will continue to grow as a vital part of CRM training and in all aspects of anesthesia care. For that to be done well and for simulation to contribute to the more fundamental culture change that has yet to transpire in perioperative care, truly effective methods of debriefing must be widely adopted. Many forms of debriefing are now described in what for me is the most critical new chapter of this book. What isn't yet completely understood or accepted is that the use of simulation with effective debriefing will do more than improve CRM, especially when used with intact perioperative teams. Simulation has the potential to improve the often dysfunctional relationships among those teams, relationships that are "latent errors" in the chain that leads to critical events. Those relationships and interactions can be greatly improved by better understanding of cross-disciplinary needs, by open discussion of each person's contribution to adverse events, and most important, to greater and more transparent self-reflection on personal behavior and team interaction. This can only come about via debriefings that are conducted with mutual respect between teacher and students, or facilitators and participants, and creating a safe environment in which to conduct those conversations.

Creating a psychologically safe environment and truly effective debriefings is easier said than done, but it is more important than some would think. Although learning is often seen as a cognitive task, it also involves matters of identity (Will I be a good doctor? Am I a good nurse?) and emotion (Do I feel threatened? Do I feel included?).

Concepts addressed in the debriefing chapter help to illustrate how that can happen. Not all of those concepts are founded in identified pedagogy; that is one area where simulation and all of patient safety still can improve by borrowing from the theory and research of the social sciences. Where that has been done most for debriefing science is in the application of concepts from action science, the work of Argyris and others, and that leads to the idea of "debriefing with good judgment." (Admittedly I am biased since the derivative work was developed by our simulation group at Massachusetts General Hospital.) The principle is relatively simple but powerful—foster in teacher and learner a true spirit of curiosity, inquiry, and then self-reflection about the reasons for their actions. Most importantly, debriefing helps develop in us a respect for all individuals with whom we work, to assume they are doing their best. When they err or are less than perfect, we give them the benefit of the doubt and work to understand the reasons for their actions. It is by fostering this spirit of respect and inquiry that simulation can have its greatest impact on patient safety.

Every anesthesia provider needs to study, not just read, this new edition, even if you read the first edition. Also, distilled instructions of key elements of the cases covered in this book need to be included in manuals made available for emergencies (although that, too, needs further study on how best to use them). If I were your patient, I would ask if you had studied these principles. If you hadn't, I might ask for another health care provider into whose hands I would want to entrust my life.

Jeffrey B. Cooper, PhD
Professor of Anaesthesia
Harvard Medical School
Executive Director, Center for Medical Simulation
Department of Anesthesia, Critical Care and Pain Medicine
Massachusetts General Hospital
Boston, Massachusetts

Foreword to the First Edition

Managing critical events is one of the most challenging and important tasks required of the anesthetist. So, why is it that, until now, no one has written a book about the basic principles of how to do it? To be sure, there are plenty of books, articles, refresher course syllabuses, and audio and video tapes about how to perform every conceivable anesthesia task safely and about what is medically correct to do in response to a critical event. The operative word is *medically*. Plenty of advice is available about what is or is not medically sound, but almost no educational material, grounded in theory, is available that discusses the human aspects of crisis intervention. What are the general principles for managing such events? What is the generic approach, a "mental model," for thinking about and for responding to those rare situations that all anesthetists hope will never happen to them? These may be rare events, yet they are the reason anesthetists must train so long before being allowed to stand at the head of the table alone. Now there is a textbook that captures the essence of what it is hoped will become instinctive during that training. What is described in this innovative text should be required reading for anyone who administers anesthesia.

Why is this material so important? Anesthesia continues to be a unique speciality that demands of its practitioners something approaching perfection. The training is essentially an apprenticeship, during which it is expected that there will be enough challenges to practice, under close supervision, the management of problems that arise unexpectedly. But, of course, not all problems will be seen; in reality, very few will be experienced. In addition, there will probably not be too many really "exciting" opportunities to practice crisis management skills. When an event does happen, learning certainly occurs, but it does so without the benefit of a theoretical basis for teaching the general skills that will apply to the next event. It is unlikely that one event will have the same specific attributes as the last one, or probably any previous event experienced by that individual. That is why a general approach to crisis management, which takes skills that are common to management of many events, should be an important new component of anesthesia training.

The roots of *Crisis Management in Anesthesiology* derive from disciplines that are foreign to anesthesia and that are on the "soft" side of the research spectrum. Such interdisciplinary work is the hardest kind of research for an investigator to attempt because it carries the risk of not being recognized in any of the disciplines to which it relates. Journal reviewers get confused because this is not something with which they are familiar. It does not seem like the "science" they usually consider. The authors should be commended for taking the risk. It has been worth it.

It is not enough to read about crisis management. Reading provides only the foundation; practice is the teacher. This is one of the roles for courses using simulators of various kinds. *Crisis Management in Anesthesiology* is the textbook that should accompany such a course. Only time will tell whether the use of simulators and other similar technology will achieve a place in medical education. Even if medical economics constrains the use of such technology, this book will still stand by itself as a source for education and training about what none but the most thrill-seeking anesthetist *wants* to experience, but which every anesthetist *will* experience. This book, and the theoretical ground it lays in medicine, should make the probability of successful experiences much more likely.

Jeffrey B. Cooper, PhD
Associate Professor
Department of Anaesthesia
Harvard Medical School and Harvard–MIT Division of
Health Sciences and Technology
Director
Biomedical Engineering and Anesthesia Technology
Massachusetts General Hospital
Boston, Massachusetts

Ellison C. Pierce, Jr., MD
Associate Clinical Professor
Department of Anaesthesia
Harvard Medical School
Chairman
Department of Anaesthesia
New England Deaconess Hospital
Boston, Massachusetts

Preface

WHO THIS BOOK IS FOR

This book is written primarily for everyone who administers anesthesia, although it may also be useful to other health care professionals. A central tenet of our teaching is that whoever is present with the patient during administration of the anesthetic needs to be highly skilled at responding to crises, both as an individual and in concert with other members of the patient care team. However, we strongly emphasize that optimum management of crises requires coordinated input from *all* team members. In this book we use the generic term "anesthesia professional" to refer to anesthesiologists, certified registered nurse anesthetists, or anesthesia assistants.

Crisis Management in Anesthesiology is aimed at both experienced practitioners and trainees. We contend that the concepts we present in this edition have not been adequately taught to anesthesia professionals in the past, nor are they easily learned during everyday clinical work. Novices will want to learn them early to make them a part of their routine practices. Experts will need to constantly review and reinforce existing routines, just as pilots must continually train and practice their crisis management skills, regardless of their years of flying experience.

WHAT THIS BOOK IS ABOUT

Crisis Management in Anesthesiology focuses on different issues than those found in traditional medical or anesthesia textbooks. Whereas other books about anesthesia primarily deal with the patient's normal or abnormal physiology, or with the technical and clinical characteristics of drugs and equipment, this book focuses primarily on the *mind* of the anesthesia professional. Just as pharmacologists attempt to synthesize the "perfect" anesthetic drug, and as engineers aim to build "fail-safe" devices, we strive to help anesthesia professionals optimize their own performance because that is the most crucial link in the chain of safe patient care.

This book is a guide to crisis management in anesthesia. The first section covers the theory and practice of Anesthesia Crisis Resource Management (ACRM)—our adaptation of concepts that originated in commercial aviation's Cockpit (now Crew) Resource Management training paradigm. The ideal anesthesia professional uses a repeated process of observation, decision, and action under the adaptive control of an "internal supervisor." Besides managing his or her own activities, the expert must manage those of a team of individuals working together on the patient's behalf. Chapter 1 covers the theory of patient safety in dynamic situations, while Chapter 2 provides guidance on the specific skills and practices of ACRM. Chapters 3 and 4 are new to this edition and provide overviews of how to train anesthesia professionals in ACRM and how to conduct debriefings—either of simulation scenarios or of real cases. This first section of the book may be particularly useful for health care professionals in fields other than anesthesia, as these principles and techniques are widely applicable in all domains and disciplines of health care.

The second section, Catalog of Critical Events in Anesthesiology, is designed to assist anesthesia professionals in implementing another strategy used in aviation. The Catalog is a systematic compilation of emergency procedures for the kinds of crises encountered in clinical practice. Just as all pilots must learn to recognize and respond to a variety of emergency situations, we believe that health care professionals should do the same. The Catalog presents events of interest to anesthesia professionals in a uniform, concise fashion designed to improve their recognition of and response to crises. It can be used as a study guide to allow anesthesia professionals to prepare in advance to recognize and manage crisis situations, as well as during the debriefing after a crisis as a reminder of information that might have been considered or actions that could have been performed. Finally, it can be used as a tool for interactive training in anesthesia crisis management using verbal simulation, role-playing, or high-fidelity simulation.

Although the events in the Catalog are described in the context of anesthesia management, many of them will present very similarly in other settings, such as in the intensive care unit, in the emergency department, or in surgical or medical ward settings. Health care professionals in these or other areas are likely to find value in the Catalog, even though the descriptions and guidance there may need to be adapted for nonperioperative settings.

WHAT THIS BOOK IS NOT ABOUT

Although crisis management in anesthesia is built on the foundation of a sound knowledge base and adequate technical skills, this edition of *Crisis Management in Anesthesiology* assumes that the reader is either already familiar with, or in the process of learning, the medical knowledge and technical skills necessary to practice anesthesia. It is not meant to be a reference text on anesthesia practice, nor is it a text on the pathophysiology of perioperative patients or their specific preoperative or postoperative evaluation and treatment. These topics are covered thoroughly in numerous other textbooks and reference works.

Perhaps most important, this book is *not* a "cookbook" of anesthesia. You will not find recipes for perfect anesthetics. The Catalog of Critical Events in Anesthesiology is a guidebook only. The Management section of each entry in the Catalog is purposefully *not* in the format of a decision tree or algorithm. We believe that patient care in the anesthesia environment is too complicated to use simple decision trees with distinct branch points. Such algorithms are also difficult to remember because of their branching structure. Therefore our management guides are written as a hierarchical list of what to check or to do, roughly in the order that an experienced practitioner might do them.

In particular, we make no claim that following the management guide for any listed event will guarantee the resolution of a clinical problem or will forestall an adverse outcome for the patient. The material is intended only for the education of health care professionals. We have tried to be comprehensive, but we make no claim to be exhaustive. The lists of manifestations for each event contain those signs that we believe to be most important; they do not include every possible sign. Similarly, no management guide can take into account every combination of patient status and atypical circumstance.

NOTE: We strongly encourage all health care professionals to deviate from the responses listed in the management sections of the Catalog entries *whenever* and *however* necessary to deal with a specific situation. We also strongly encourage health care professionals to adapt this Catalog to their own practices, based on their experiences with different drugs and techniques.

WHAT IS DIFFERENT ABOUT THE SECOND EDITION?

After nearly 20 years, a number of things have stayed the same about ACRM, but we have developed new ideas about it and about how to teach it and how to apply it in real life. Chapters 1 and 2 on dynamic decision making and CRM have been updated and honed. New material was added about cognitive aids (e.g., checklists and emergency manuals). This idea, which was introduced in the health care setting in the first edition, has undergone a new emphasis in the past few years, triggered by the success of the Catalog of Critical Events in the first edition, and the need to convert some of that material to forms more usable during actual patient care. Chapters 3 and 4 are completely new. They were added because many readers of the first edition have a strong interest in teaching these principles and skills to others, with or without the use of simulation, and they told us that material about these issues would be valuable. The ACRM simulation course has gone from being a rarity when the first edition of this book was published to being commonplace around the world. Thousands of anesthesia professionals have already undergone such training. Many things that we have learned directly from teaching such courses, and some things that we have learned from our colleagues around the world, are incorporated in this updated edition.

The Catalog of Critical Events in Anesthesiology has been completely overhauled and updated. New events have been added; some from the first edition have been removed or combined with others. Clinical information has been modernized, consistent with literature available in 2014. In some cases clinical practice has, perhaps surprisingly, changed little since 1994. For example, we know much more about the basic science of malignant hyperthermia, but the fundamental management is unchanged. In other cases, advances in the field have markedly altered the approach to patient care. The management of the septic patient, for example, has undergone significant change in 20 years and we have tried to capture that with a new event that describes a management approach to this complex condition.

In 1994 the notion of applying Cockpit or Crew Resource Management in health care was very new. The use of simulation in health care was also in its infancy. Now, 20 years later, both of these ideas are commonplace, even if neither has penetrated fully into the fabric of health care. Thus for the first edition it went without saying that the first two chapters as well as the Catalog of Critical Events were largely a description of the authors' opinions and practices, abetted by their knowledge of the literature. Now, for the second edition, we need to say this explicitly. This is a textbook that focuses on the work, opinions, and practices of the authors and contributors as informed by their extensive reviews of recent literature. To be a usable textbook it cannot be, and does not claim to be, an exhaustive review of all the work in the field (published or unpublished) related to the topics presented. We have tried to cite and/or present some of the work that we think is relevant, but we recognize that much useful work goes unmentioned in this text. For the Catalog of Critical Events in this edition, there are references to many reviews that were published in the 5 years preceding the summer of 2013.

WHO ARE THE AUTHORS

In nearly 20 years a few things have changed about the authors. First, and most important, we added a major author. Amanda Burden, MD, is associate professor of Anesthesiology and director of the Simulation Program at Cooper Medical School of Rowan University and Cooper University Hospital. She is an active clinician and educator and serves on the Simulation Editorial Board of the American Society of Anesthesiologists. She, and many of her colleagues who have contributed to the new Catalog of Critical Events, represent a new generation of anesthesiologists working on patient safety, crisis resource management, and simulation. Dr. Burden and many of the new contributors to the Catalog also represent clinical practices different from those at Stanford University School of Medicine and Veterans Affairs Palo Alto Health Care System (VAPAHCS). In the first edition, most of the book was written by individuals from only those two institutions. Having material from, or reviewed by, individuals affiliated with different institutions is valuable, both in representing alternate viewpoints, and in helping to check that the material in the book is widely applicable and not limited to the Stanford and VAPAHCS sites.

David Gaba, MD, is now the associate dean for Immersive and Simulation-based Learning, and a tenured professor at Stanford University School of Medicine. He holds one of a handful of decanal positions in the United States dedicated to simulation. He directs the 28,000-square-foot

Immersive Learning Center at Stanford. He also is the founding co-director of the Simulation Center at VAPAHCS. He is currently not practicing clinical anesthesia—at least on real patients. He is a former private pilot (single engine land), rock climber, and scuba diver—all pursuits that exercised his crisis management skills. Both Dr. Howard and Dr. Gaba are heavily involved in instructor training for CRM-oriented simulation activities. They conduct many instructor courses for the VA's national simulation program SimLEARN as well as for non-VA instructor groups. Dr. Gaba is the founding and current editor-in-chief of the only indexed, peer-reviewed journal on simulation in health care—aptly titled *Simulation in Healthcare*—which in 2014 is in Volume 9 of publication.

Kevin Fish, MSc, MB ChB, has retired after more than 30 years of full-time practice and 12 years as chief of the Anesthesia and Perioperative Care Service at VAPAHCS, but still practices anesthesia on a per diem basis at that institution. He is now professor emeritus of the Department of Anesthesiology, Perioperative and Pain Medicine at Stanford. He remains a role model for current trainees and for many others who trained under him in Canada and the United States. His years of experience have been put to good use in updating the Catalog of Critical Events.

Steve Howard, MD, is now an associate professor with the Department of Anesthesiology, Perioperative and Pain Medicine at Stanford. He is clinically active, doing both general and cardiac anesthesia. He is the co-director of the Simulation Center at VAPAHCS and chairs the Scientific Evaluation Committee (i.e., "study section") of the Anesthesia Patient Safety Foundation.

The authors of this book are responsible for the writing of Chapters 1 through 4 and the Catalog of Critical Events. Several colleagues contributed to either Chapter 4 or the Catalog and they are listed on the Contents and Contributors pages. Primary drafts in the Catalog were written by the section contributors and then iteratively edited by the authors and contributors.

GENERAL ACKNOWLEDGMENTS

The first edition of *Crisis Management in Anesthesiology* would never have been published without the support of the Anesthesia Patient Safety Foundation (APSF). We are grateful to the APSF, whose grants funded the development of the simulator and the creation of the ACRM curriculum, and sustained the program when all hope seemed lost.

We owe a debt to the many residents of the Stanford University School of Medicine who, as part of their training, wrote the earliest drafts of some of the entries in the first edition of the Catalog. Collectively, their efforts gave us a place to start in the compilation of the Catalog and their grist for our editorial mill made the job considerably easier.

We acknowledge that our ability to produce both editions of this book was aided immensely by a close-knit band of colleagues dedicated to research and education in the Anesthesiology and Perioperative Care Service of the VAPAHCS, a close affiliate of the Department of Anesthesiology, Perioperative and Pain Medicine at Stanford. In particular, although he was not involved in writing the second edition, we would like to acknowledge the assistance in the early stages of the development of the Catalog of Critical Events and the ACRM simulation course of Frank Sarnquist, MD, now professor emeritus at Stanford.

We are indebted to the Department of Veterans Affairs for providing the environment and the time in which to write this book. We also acknowledge the contribution and support of Michael E. Goldberg, MD, professor and chair of Anesthesiology, Cooper Medical School of Rowan University and Cooper University Hospital, in completing the second edition of this work.

David M. Gaba
Kevin J. Fish
Steven K. Howard
Amanda R. Burden

Acknowledgments

I would like to acknowledge my wife, Deanna Mann, who was there and involved even before the ideas and experiences referred to in this book were a gleam in my eye. In the early days of ACRM, when there were no simulation staff, Deanna helped us with a variety of tasks in conducting courses, in working long hours, and in fighting the tide of disbelief and belittlement about our efforts; her support to me and to the group has continued unabated for nearly 30 years. I would like to thank our clinical mentors, Kevin Fish and Frank Sarnquist, who were the prototype anesthesia crisis managers upon whom this teaching is based. I thank my closest friend and colleague, Steve Howard, for "drinking the Kool Aid"; what a long, strange, and wonderful trip it's been. I would also like to acknowledge Richard Mazze, the former chief of Anesthesia and then chief of staff at Veterans Affairs Palo Alto Health Care System (VAPAHCS). Dick created the academic environment at VAPAHCS that enabled crazy ideas like patient safety, ACRM, and simulation to flourish. He also was instrumental in providing the space for the simulation centers that were and are home to three of the authors. I would also like to acknowledge my mentor, Jeff Cooper, who has been an inspiration scientifically, academically, and ethically, and who first allowed us to spread the concepts and simulation-based teaching methods described in the book outside the Stanford cocoon.

David Gaba

I acknowledge the many people for their contributions to my career in anesthesia. The most important person I thank is Pamela, my wife of more than 40 years, who had no idea when we married that I would move her to Canada and then the United States to fulfill my ambitions of an academic career. She has been my strength and soul mate through some very challenging times. My thanks go also to my family, a source of inspiration and support in so many ways. I learned so much from all my teachers in England and Canada: from Richard Mazze, my mentor, and from my colleagues at Stanford and VAPAHCS, who all made my career so interesting. I am thankful to David Gaba and Steve Howard for the opportunity to contribute to their endeavors. Two other groups I must include are (1) the residents of Stanford's Department of Anesthesiology, Perioperative and Pain Medicine, a talented and enthusiastic group of physicians who have been a pleasure to teach, and (2) the veterans who have given so much to their country and now are the most amazingly supportive patients to our residents in training. It has been a privilege to care for them throughout most of my career.

Kevin Fish

I thank my teachers David Gaba and Kevin Fish for bringing me into their practice and for teaching me about the profession and so much more. David, you are a great friend and mentor and I hope you know how much your friendship means to me. Kevin, the best part about writing the second edition of this book was that we had to spend time together hashing things out. Thank you to my parents, who encouraged all of my efforts, and to my sister for always believing in me. Most important, I would like to thank my wife, Jenifer, and daughter, Rachel, for their constant love and support. Life is good because you are in it. I know I am the lucky one!

Steven Howard

I thank David, Kevin, and Steve very much for inviting me to join their group and for welcoming, teaching, and inspiring me. David, I am truly grateful to learn from and work with you, and I treasure your friendship. I would like to also acknowledge my family, friends, and the mentors in whose steps I walk—some who are here and some who are no longer here—whose sacrifices and support greatly helped me and my career. Thank you especially to my husband, Guy, for his love, support, and terrific advice—and for making sure that life is full of fun and possibilities.

Amanda Burden

Contents

Chapter 9
Neurologic Events
JEREMY S. DORITY

Chapter 10
Equipment Events
JAN EHRENWERTH and JAMES B. EISENKRAFT

Chapter 11
Cardiac Anesthesia Events
ANKEET UDANI

Chapter 12
Obstetric Events
GILLIAN HILTON

Chapter 13
Pediatric Events
CALVIN KUAN and ERIN WHITE PUKENAS

Basic Principles of Crisis Management in Anesthesiology

Section I

Basic Principles of Crisis Management in Anesthesiology

"Hours of boredom, moments of terror." For most clinicians outside of anesthesia, this saying captures the essence of the work experience of anesthesia professionals. It is largely the occasional moments of terror, not the routine hours of boredom, that define our role in the operating room (OR) and the mental attitudes required to perform our job successfully. This is one aspect of anesthesia that sets our field (and a few related ones such as intensive care and emergency medicine) apart from most other branches of health care, certainly apart from primary or chronic care. Another aspect is the direct physical involvement of the anesthesia professional in the tasks of patient care. This includes the performance of invasive procedures; the administration of rapidly acting, potentially lethal medications; and the operation of increasingly complex devices. In all likelihood, the emphasis on direct action and the aura of danger lurking just below the surface are key factors that attracted many of us to this line of work.

Surprisingly, beyond the American Society of Anesthesiologists' enshrined motto of "Vigilance," little attention has been paid to how anesthesia professionals go about, or should go about, working in a setting in which moments of terror do in fact occur. The practice of anesthesia is a complicated collection of mental and physical activities attuned more to the *efficient* care of routine cases than it is to the handling of life-threatening crises. What constitutes "expertise" in anesthesia has only recently been explored. How newcomers to anesthesia become skilled practitioners is still not very well known. The traditional systems of educating and training anesthesia professionals assumed that merely by selecting intelligent and motivated individuals to undergo training in anesthesia, they *guaranteed* that trainees would be able to transform their own mental abilities into those of the ideal anesthesia professional, solely on the basis of abstract scientific lessons and performing the routine daily tasks of the OR. They assumed that crisis prevention and crisis management skills would emerge naturally through learning the basic science of anesthesia, pharmacology, and physiology or through repeated exposure to clinical experiences (by "osmosis"). These modalities were supplemented by a smattering of morbidity and mortality conferences and occasional continuing medical education lectures.

The standard assumption that every anesthesia professional who has successfully completed a training program is a capable crisis manager has been challenged over the last 25 years. We discovered that the initial training and continuing education of anesthesia professionals often leaves substantial gaps in the ability of anesthesia professionals to deal with crises. When a crisis does present itself—a patient suffers an unexpected cardiac arrest or a surgical catastrophe occurs—it is obvious to everyone who works in an OR that some anesthesia professionals cope better than others. These individuals take more steps to prevent a crisis, and they are better prepared when they occur. They are the ones who can bring order from chaos. They take command, know what to do, and how to ensure that work gets done. They are the people who most of us would choose to administer "our" anesthetic if we needed it. The skills that distinguish these expert crisis managers go beyond the traditional aspects of medical, scientific, and technical knowledge. Why are some anesthesia professionals seemingly better suited than others to manage the "moments of terror" that are so much a part of our world? Is it strictly an unlearnable aspect of the individual's personality? Conversely, if some are not well suited to handle crises, where does the fault lie?

In this book we contend that crisis management involves skills that can be identified and taught. Although it has gained ground considerably in the last 20 years, why was the anesthesia community slow to realize this fact? Medicine, in general, has been attached to a view of the physician as a pensive provider of healing arts based on careful applications of personal skill and, in the last 100 years, scientific knowledge. This view worked well enough for relatively static branches of health care in which careful reflection and an extended clinician-patient relationship are the dominant aspects of care. Yet we believe that this view has prevented the training process of anesthesia professionals from addressing the real dominant aspects of our work: dynamism, time pressure, intensity, complexity, uncertainty, and risk. In our opinion, to understand the anesthesia professional better we must turn away from research on learning and decision making in medicine and look at the experience of other human activities that share the key aspects of our domain.

Dynamism, time pressure, complexity, uncertainty, and risk are seen in such activities as aviation, spaceflight, process control (nuclear power and chemical manufacturing), shipping, military command, and firefighting. Aviation offers considerable parallels with anesthesia, and in fact pilots share our aphorism, "hours of boredom, moments of terror." Especially in aviation, cognitive psychologists and human factor engineers have been actively trying to pinpoint the elements of optimal performance and to design work routines and training strategies to improve the abilities of both new and existing personnel. Over the last 25 years several successful strategies to improve air crew performance and safety in aviation have begun to be adopted for anesthesia safety. They include the following:

1. Use of written checklists to help prevent crises from occurring
2. Use of established procedures (both memorized and written) in responding to crises
3. Training in decision making and crew coordination for anesthesia professionals and perioperative teams, including systematic practice in the handling of crisis situations in various types of simulations

Although the use of these strategies is not yet uniform in perioperative settings, they now appear to be here to stay and their dissemination and implementation into the fabric of health care seems only a matter of time.

Finally, we would like to share with you our philosophy of anesthesia practice, which underlies this book. *Each of us* is responsible for giving the best possible care to his or her patients. Although perfect performance is unachievable, we should strive to approach it. Honing the understanding of medicine, physiology, and anesthesia technology is an essential step. Sharpening diagnostic and technical skills is another. Each of us must realize, however, that the real world in which we work will make it difficult to translate these skills into optimal patient care. Experience alone will not guarantee good performance, nor can it make us immune to the types of errors that plague all humans in complex, dynamic domains. Production pressures, distractions, and the intensity of cases will challenge the best intentions. An important beginning is to admit that crises *will* occur in spite of, or even because of, our own best efforts. Approach each case as if it is a disaster waiting to happen, and plan as well as possible to prevent it. Make explicit provisions for the failure of elements in the anesthetic or surgical plans. Prepare to recognize and manage *all* the crises that could occur regardless of how they might be triggered. Utilize the local institution's quality management programs to adapt practice as required, based on individual experiences and the collective wisdom of the community. As we review our own performance and that of our colleagues, we should try to avoid becoming fixated solely on the medical and technical aspects of how a crisis was managed; consider also the teamwork aspects and the way in which the "systems issues" helped or hindered patient care. Seek to change those aspects of the situation that impeded optimum management.

Reading about crisis management is not enough. As with pilots, military personnel, athletes, and musicians, actual practice of skills is important. The Anesthesia Crisis Resource Management (ACRM) course that we pioneered,[1] and that is now replicated around the world (and in a diverse variety of health care domains), teaches concepts about crisis management found in this book, but its centerpiece is simulation and debriefing. It is widely believed that skilled and intensive debriefing after simulations greatly augments the learning that takes place and hopefully allows the translation of these lessons to the real workplace.

However, even those who do not yet have easy access to a simulation program can practice these skills through role-playing or verbal simulation. These can be augmented by applications for smartphones and tablet computers that replicate and control virtual replicas of patient monitors. Even on our own we can prepare for crises by systematically reviewing, aloud, what we would do in a variety of problem situations. Many pilots and astronauts have described doing this at home, even to the extent of touching the controls on a paper mockup as they would use the controls in the cockpit, in order to prepare themselves for the simulator exercises and the actual flights that truly put them to the test. Our responsibility to our patients demands the same commitment.

Chapters 1 and 2 begin with a comprehensive look at a theory of decision making and crisis management in anesthesia. Chapter 1 provides a theoretical background on the psychology of the anesthesia professional during routine patient care and during crisis management. Chapter 2 provides concrete advice on how to forestall crises and how to manage the situations should they arise. Chapter 3 discusses options on how to learn or to teach the principles of ACRM, with or without simulation. Chapter 4 gives an overview of debriefing that can accompany either real case experiences or simulation sessions. Together these chapters provide the fundamental basis for lifelong learning about the management of tough situations and for becoming the very best anesthesia professional that you can be.

REFERENCE

1. Howard SK, Gaba DM, Fish KJ, et al. Anesthesia crisis resource management training: teaching anesthesiologists to handle critical incidents. Aviat Space Environ Med 1992;63:763.

Chapter 1
Fundamentals of Dynamic Decision Making in Anesthesia

This book is about decision making and crisis management in anesthesia. What is a *crisis*? It is "a time of great danger or trouble whose outcome decides whether possible bad consequences will follow."[1] For our purposes, the time of great danger is typically a brief, intense event or sequence of events that offers a clear and present danger to the patient. Almost by definition, a crisis requires an active response to prevent injury to the patient; it is unlikely to resolve on its own. Of course, the best way to deal with a crisis is to prevent it from occurring in the first place. An old saying is that "it is easier to stay out of trouble than to get out of trouble."

Skilled crisis management in anesthesia is no mystery. It demands that the anesthesia professional, while under stress and time pressure, *optimally* implements standard techniques of diagnosis and treatment for the patient. Medical knowledge and skills are essential components of the decisions and actions performed during crises, but they are not enough. To actually make things happen quickly and safely for patient management, the anesthesia professional must manage the entire *situation*, including the environment, the equipment, and the patient care team. These management skills include aspects of cognitive and social psychology and even sociology and anthropology. In this chapter we delineate the underlying conceptual foundations of patient safety, and in the next chapter we provide specific practical principles about crisis management. Chapter 3 reviews how to train clinicians to enact these principles, and Chapter 4 covers the art and science of debriefing about crisis management after real patient care events or after simulation scenarios. The remainder of this book (Catalog of Critical Events in Anesthesiology) offers specific recommendations for the recognition and management of a large variety of crisis situations.

ANESTHESIOLOGY, BY ITS NATURE, INVOLVES CRISES

Why is a book on medical crisis management addressed to anesthesia professionals (this term encompasses anesthesiologists, nurse anesthetists, and anesthesia assistants)? What makes anesthesiology and a few other medical domains (such as intensive care medicine, emergency medicine, obstetrics, neonatology, and surgery, to name a few) different from most other medical fields? The answer, to a large extent, is that the clinical environment of anesthesiology is dynamic, and this dynamism interacts very strongly with the complexity of the environment.[2] The combination of complexity and dynamism makes crises much more likely to occur and more difficult to deal with. Thus the expert anesthesia professional must be skilled and therefore trained in crisis management. Following the work of Woods[3,4] and of Orasanu and Connolly,[5] we address some of the aspects of anesthesia that make it a "complex, dynamic world," namely, that it is event-driven and dynamic, complex and tightly coupled, uncertain, and risky (for the patient).

Event-Driven and Dynamic

The anesthetized patient's state changes continuously. Unpredictable and dynamic events are frequent. The initiation of many events is beyond the anesthesia professional's control, such as when the surgeon inadvertently transects a major vessel or when a patient with a previously unknown allergy suffers anaphylaxis.

Complex and Tightly Coupled

In technologic systems, complexity stems from a large number of interconnected components. The patient is the main "system" of interest to the anesthesia professional. Patients are intrinsically very complex, and they contain many components, the underlying functions of which are imperfectly understood. Unlike industrial or aviation systems, patients are not designed, built, or tested by humans, nor do they come with an operator's manual.

Some physiologic systems are buffered from changes in others, whereas certain core components, such as oxygen (O_2) delivery and blood flow, are tightly coupled and interact strongly.[6,7] Anesthesia ablates some protective and compensatory physiologic mechanisms and will force the patient's systems to become more connected. The patient's physiology may also become tightly joined to external systems such as ventilators or infusions of hemodynamically active drugs.

Although the medical equipment connected to the patient is not as complex as that found in aircraft or spacecraft, it often consists of a proliferation of independent devices with multiple, nonstandardized interconnections. Devices are typically designed in isolation by engineers so that interactions between devices, or among the equipment, the patient, and the human operator, may not be adequately addressed in the design phase. These factors increase the complexity of the domain.

Uncertain

The patient as a system contains inherent uncertainties. The medical world knows very little about the underlying causes of specific physiologic events, although the general physiologic principles involved can be described. The true state of the patient cannot usually be measured directly but must be inferred from ambiguous patterns of clinical observations and data from electronic monitors. These data are imperfect because, unlike industrial systems (which are designed and built with sensors in key areas to measure the most important variables), separate, predominantly noninvasive methods are used to measure the variables that are easiest to monitor. Most physiologic functions are observed indirectly through weak signals available at the body surface and thus are prone to various sorts of electrical and mechanical interference. Even the invasive measurements are vulnerable to artifacts and uncertainties of interpretation.

Even if the anesthesia professional could know the exact patient state, the response of the patient to interventions is extremely variable. Even in "normal" patients, genetic or acquired differences in reflex sensitivity, pharmacokinetics, or pharmacodynamics can yield a wide range of responses to a given dose of a drug or to a routine action (e.g., laryngoscopy). In diseased or traumatized patients, or in the presence of acute abnormalities, these responses may be markedly abnormal, and patients may "overreact" or "underreact" to otherwise appropriate actions.

Risky

The decisions and actions taken by anesthesia professionals can determine the outcome for the patient. Even for elective surgery involving healthy patients, the risk of catastrophe is ever-present. Death, brain damage, or other permanent injury may be the end-result of many pathways that can begin with fairly innocuous triggering events. Each intervention, even if appropriate, is associated with side effects, some of which are themselves catastrophic. Furthermore, many risks cannot be anticipated or avoided. Unlike a commercial flight, which can be delayed or aborted if a problem occurs, immediate surgery may be necessary to treat a medical problem that is itself life-threatening. Balancing the risks of the anesthesia and surgery against the risk of the patient's underlying diseases is often extremely difficult.

HOW DO CRISES ARISE?

A crisis is often perceived as sudden in onset and rapid in development, but, at least in retrospect, one can usually identify an evolution of the crisis from underlying triggering events. Figure 1-1 illustrates this process. In this model, underlying factors lead to specific triggering events, which initiate a problem. A problem is defined as an abnormal situation that requires the attention of the anesthesia professional but is unlikely, by itself, to harm the patient. Problems can then evolve and, if not detected and corrected by the anesthesia professional, they may lead to an adverse outcome for the patient. We consider this process in detail.

Problems Often Result from Latent Underlying Conditions

The events that trigger problems do not occur at random. They emerge from three sets of underlying conditions: (1) *latent errors*, (2) *predisposing factors*, and (3) *psychological precursors*.

Latent Errors

Latent errors, as described by Reason,[8] are "...errors whose adverse consequences may lie dormant within the system for a long time, only becoming evident when they combine with other factors to breach the system's defenses. [They are] most likely to be spawned by those

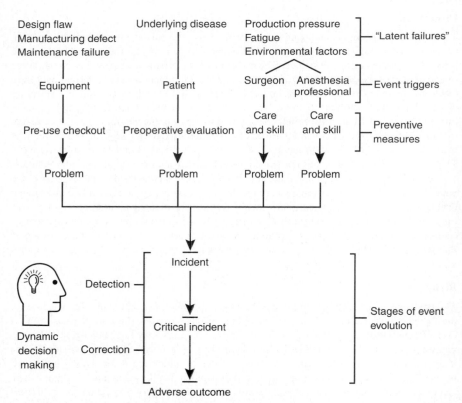

FIGURE 1-1 The process by which problems are triggered and then evolve during anesthesia. Interrupting this process can be accomplished by preventive measures or by dynamic detection and correction of the evolving event.

whose activities are removed in both time and space from the direct control interface: designers, high-level decision makers, construction workers, managers, and maintenance personnel."

Such latent errors exist in all complex systems. Reason describes them as "resident pathogens," which, like microorganisms in the body, remain under control until sets of local circumstances "combine with these resident pathogens in subtle and often unlikely ways to thwart the system's defenses and bring about its catastrophic breakdown"[8] (Fig. 1-2).

In anesthesia, latent errors can result from administrative decisions regarding scheduling of cases, assignment of personnel to staff them, and the priorities given to such things as rapid turnover between cases. They can also result from the design of anesthesia equipment and its user interfaces or how drug vials and ampules are designed and labeled or supplied to the anesthesiologist. Manufacturing defects and failures of routine maintenance are also latent errors.

Organizational Culture Factors

Safety in other industries of high intrinsic hazard is known to be a property primarily of systems rather than individuals. Organizations that perform successfully under very challenging conditions, with very low levels of failure, are termed "high reliability organizations" (HROs).[9-12] The first HRO to be studied was the flight deck of aircraft carriers. Others include certain military organizations, commercial aviation, electric power grids, and firms handling large-scale electronic financial transactions. Based on direct observation of HROs, investigators have determined that a key element of high reliability is a "culture of safety" or a "safety climate" permeating the organization.[13-17] Several features of safety culture or climate are as follows:

• A commitment to safety is articulated at the highest levels of the organization and translated into shared values, beliefs, and behavioral norms throughout all organizational levels.

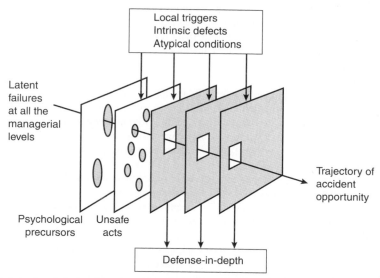

FIGURE 1-2 Reason's model of accident causation. Accidents (adverse outcomes) require a combination of latent failures, psychological precursors, event triggers, and failures in several layers of the system's "defense-in-depth." This model is functionally equivalent to that shown in Figure 1-1. *(From Reason J. Human error. Cambridge: Cambridge University Press; 1990.)*

- The organization provides the necessary resources, incentives, and rewards to allow this to occur.
- Following standard operating procedures and safety rules is a part of the behavioral norms.
- Safety is valued as the primary priority, even at the expense of "production" or "efficiency." Personnel are rewarded for erring on the side of safety, even if they turn out to be wrong.
- The organization proactively manages safety and carefully monitors ongoing safety processes and operating procedures.
- Communication among workers and across organizational levels is frequent and candid.
- Unsafe acts are rare, despite high levels of production.
- There is openness about errors and problems; they are reported when they occur.
- Organizational learning is valued; the response to a problem is focused on improving system performance.

Think for a moment how your organization compares to these safety ideals and where it could improve its performance. To the extent that a health care organization or work unit maintains a culture of safety, it can reduce the occurrence of latent errors and bolster flexible defenses against the accident sequences that do get started. However, there are many challenges to a culture of safety, particularly the erosion of safety in the search for throughput and revenue. Such forces can lead to "production pressure"[6,18]—internal or external pressure on the anesthesia professional to keep the OR schedule moving along speedily, with few cancellations and minimal time between cases. When anesthesia professionals succumb to these pressures, they may fail to perform adequate preoperative evaluation and planning or neglect to conduct pre-use checks of equipment. Even when preoperative evaluation does take place, overt or covert pressure from surgeons (or others) to proceed with elective cases despite the existence of serious or uncontrolled medical problems can cause anesthesia professionals to do things that are unsafe.

In 1994 we conducted a survey of California anesthesiologists concerning their experience with production pressures.[18] We found that 49% of respondents had witnessed an event in which patient safety was compromised owing to pressure on the anesthesiologist. Moreover, 32% reported strong to intense pressure from surgeons to proceed with a case they wished to cancel; 36% reported strong to intense internal pressure to "get along with surgeons"; and 45% reported strong pressures to avoid delaying cases. Significantly, 20% agreed with the statement, "If I cancel a case, I might jeopardize working with that surgeon at a later date." The economic pressures are obvious.

Production pressure also leads to *haste* by the anesthesia professional, which is another psychological precursor to the commission of unsafe acts. In the survey, 20% of respondents answered "sometimes" to the statement, "I have altered my normal practices in order to speed the start of surgery," while 4% answered "often" to this statement, and 20% of respondents rated pressure by surgeons to *hasten* anesthetic preparation or induction as strong or intense.

Comparable results were found in a survey of residents in anesthesiology.[19] In a similar survey conducted by Johnson in 2001,[20] such pressures and experiences were again found for anesthesiologists. Although the study has not been repeated in nearly 20 years, we think that production pressures have only increased in the interim.

We also have conducted surveys across all hospital employees in multiple institutions in studies involving tens of thousands of personnel, and have documented that production pressures exist throughout the hospital and are not unique to anesthesiology.[16,21,22] Moreover, we found a threefold greater rate of responses indicative of a lack of safety culture for health care personnel (18%) than for naval aviators (6%) given matched questions concerning safety culture.[15,17] Thus health care institutions do not yet have as strong a culture of safety as they should.

Local Predisposing Factors and Psychological Precursors

The final set of underlying features consists of latent psychological precursors, which predispose the anesthesia professional or surgeon to commit an unsafe act that triggers a problem. The primary psychological precursors are traditionally referred to as *performance-shaping factors*, and include such elements as fatigue, boredom, illness, drugs (both prescription and recreational), and environmental factors such as noise and illumination. Factors of work culture in general, and safety culture in particular, are also important to consider. Different combinations of psychological factors are discussed in detail in a number of review articles[23-26] and general strategies to deal with performance-shaping factors and safety culture are discussed in Chapter 2.

Triggering Events

Each problem is initiated through one or more triggering events. Historically, anesthesia professionals have been most concerned about events that they create themselves, such as esophageal intubation or drug swaps, but these are relatively rare compared with events that are triggered in other ways. Triggering events can come from (1) the patient, (2) the surgery, (3) the anesthesia, or (4) the equipment.

The Patient

Many problems occur *de novo* owing to the underlying medical pathology of the patient. For example, studies of myocardial ischemia in the perioperative period[27-29] demonstrate that ischemia often occurs without any significant change in hemodynamic status or any known causal effects of anesthesia.

The Surgery

Surgical stimulus alone is a profound trigger of many physiologic responses, including hypertension, tachycardia, laryngospasm, and bronchospasm. Problems linked to the patient's medical pathology may be precipitated by routine actions of the surgeon. Also, unplanned events, such as surgical compression of organs or transection of vital structures, can rapidly evolve into serious problems.

The Anesthesia

Induction and maintenance of anesthesia can precipitate problems in patients even in the absence of significant underlying medical disease. Actions or errors on the part of the anesthesia professional can directly jeopardize the patient, as when central venous cannulation causes a pneumothorax. An operation may require standard but complex maneuvers that may trigger problems, such as turning the patient to the prone position. Especially in patients under general anesthesia and with neuromuscular blockade, the body's own protective mechanisms are blunted or obliterated, making the patient more vulnerable to the anesthesia professional's actions.

The Equipment

General anesthesia is maintained and the patient's vital functions are monitored by using electromechanical equipment. Should this equipment fail, the patient can suffer irrevocable harm. However, it is very rare for an equipment malfunction, *by itself*, to harm the patient immediately. Examples of this might include electrocution, fires, and airway overpressure events. More typically, an equipment failure stops a life support or monitoring function, which can in theory be performed in another way if the failure is identified and the necessary backup systems are available and functional. Equipment problems often *contribute* to difficulties in handling other problems, either because they usurp the attention of the anesthesia professional or because the treatment of the main problem requires the use of equipment that itself has failed.

Prevention of Problems

Reducing or eliminating the latent factors that predispose patients to problems would be the most effective strategy to improve safety.[8] This might include changes in organizational structure, work procedures, safety culture, or staffing, However, most of these factors are the result of a complex evolution of medical practice and economics in combination with historical and political factors; identifying and changing them is a difficult, slow, and frustrating process. Moreover, there are external circumstances that cannot be controlled even in principle (e.g., trauma, disasters, terrorism). Therefore the individual anesthesiologist must adopt effective strategies for preventing problems targeted at individual cases, making specific checks for triggering factors, and taking corrective action as necessary. Such pre-case checks include (1) the patient, (2) the surgeon and anesthesia professional, and (3) the equipment.

The Patient

The anesthesia professional begins by using traditional forms of medical decision making in preoperative evaluation of the patient and in planning the anesthetic. During this evaluation, the anesthesia professional considers the patient's medical status, the urgency of the surgery, and whether any further treatment can make the patient a better risk. This is a crucial opportunity for the anesthesia professional to prevent adverse outcomes for the patient. If surgery can proceed, there may still be additional preventive measures that should be implemented to deal with specific medical conditions (e.g., rapid sequence induction [RSI] in patients with a bowel obstruction) or to prepare for specific surgical procedures (e.g., use of a double lumen endotracheal tube for thoracic surgery). In Chapter 2, we will emphasize the necessity of developing a sound anesthetic plan for the patient that takes each of these measures into account. In many cases, however, there are competing goals, which will prevent a perfect plan from being developed. The optimal plan in such cases must be a compromise among the various risks, benefits, and costs.

The Surgeon and Anesthesia Professional

Surgeons and anesthesia professionals have a duty to perform their jobs with appropriate care and skill. They must honestly determine whether their own ability, fitness, and preparation match those demanded by the planned procedure. Chapter 2 covers in detail how anesthesia professionals can deal with possible deteriorations in their performance so as to prevent harm to the patient.

The Equipment

A thorough pre-use check of critical life-support equipment is considered mandatory before the induction of anesthesia. The anesthesia machine encompasses O_2 delivery, ventilation, and gaseous anesthesia delivery systems. Monitors incorporate many alarms that need to be set correctly and turned on. When intravenous (IV) infusions are a primary component of the anesthetic or hemodynamic management, these are not coupled to the anesthesia machine, and they need to be checked thoroughly as well. In addition, the anesthesia professional should ensure that appropriate backup equipment is available for all life-critical functions (e.g., a self-inflating bag for ventilation).

Problems Will Inevitably Occur Despite Attempts to Prevent Them

Despite attempts to prevent the occurrence of problems during anesthesia, experience shows that problems of varying severity occur in a large percentage of cases. The exact frequency of problems is not known. Existing studies probably have underestimated the occurrence of problems because they depended on written reports of the case by the anesthesia professionals rather than real-time, objective recording of the events. Despite their limitations, two studies offer some data concerning the frequency of problem events.

In the Multicenter Study of General Anesthesia,[30] 17,201 patients received general anesthesia under specific protocols with random stratification to receive one of four anesthetic techniques (each of the three common volatile anesthetic agents or narcotics plus nitrous oxide). The anesthesia professionals observed the patients for the occurrence of any of a large variety of carefully defined perioperative "outcomes," that is, adverse events ranging from minor, such as sore throat or hypotension (i.e., systolic blood pressure reduced by more than 20% from baseline), to serious, such as myocardial infarction (MI) or death. Based on our definition of a "problem," most of the outcomes measured in this study would constitute a perioperative condition that could evolve into one that might harm the patient. The researchers observed 34,926 defined outcomes in the 17,201 patients. Clearly, some patients experienced more than one outcome while others had none, but 86% of patients faced at least one undesirable outcome. Although most events were minor and caused no injury to the patient, over 5% of patients had one or more *severe* events requiring "significant therapy, with or without full recovery." This incidence is probably a lower limit for severe events because the entry criteria of the study excluded critically ill patients and emergency cases in which evolving problems of a severe nature more likely might occur.

In another study, Cooper and associates[31] found that "impact events," which were "undesirable, unexpected, and could cause at least moderate morbidity," occurred in 18% of patients either in the OR or in the postanesthesia care unit (PACU) and 3% of all cases involved a "serious" event. These, too, are probably lower limits, because, for technical reasons, the study excluded patients electively destined for an intensive care unit (ICU). Extrapolating from both of these studies, it seems that at least 20% of cases involve a problem event requiring intervention by the anesthesiologist, and approximately 5% of cases involve a potentially catastrophic event. The actual frequency of problems may be higher in practice settings with greater than average case complexity.

The exact mortality rate of patients related to anesthesia care is uncertain.[32] Deaths resulting from administration of anesthesia in relatively healthy patients undergoing routine surgery are rare, but even for this restricted category the rate is approximately 1 per 250,000 (0.4 per 100,000 cases). Overall, perioperative deaths related to anesthesia may be as high as 1 per 1400 cases.[33] This makes the frequency of a fatal accident in surgery attributable solely to anesthesia 45 times higher than that of any fatal airline accident in the United States. There are about 25,000 to 30,000 airline flights per day in the United States and there are very few serious incidents or accidents, although the exact number is unknown. The *total* accident rate from *all causes* (not including terrorist acts) for scheduled airline flights from 2002 through 2011 was 0.29 per 100,000 departures. Air carrier accidents with one or more fatalities occurred at a rate of 0.009 per 100,000 departures. In fact, according to the National Transportation Safety Board, in the years 2007 to 2011 there was only a single fatal airline accident! (http://www.ntsb.gov/data/table6_2012.html). Relative to aviation, anesthesia has a long way to go to optimize patient safety.

How Do Problems Evolve into Adverse Outcomes?

Once a problem occurs, there are various possibilities for its future evolution. The problem may be self-limited or may continue to exist without any threat to the patient. It can increase in severity. It can trigger new problems (cross-triggering) within the patient or within the anesthesia/surgery system; the new problems may be more threatening than the original problem. Multiple small problems in several different subsystems can together create a more serious situation than any one of them alone (combination). A problem triggered by one factor may interfere with the management of problems triggered by others (triggered failure of recovery), or it may distract the anesthesia professional's attention from other more serious problems.

Although there are no universally accepted criteria for categorizing the states of evolution of a perioperative problem, we term the next state an *incident*—a problem that will not resolve on its own and is likely to continue evolving. A *critical incident* is an incident that can *directly* cause an adverse patient outcome. Further information on the nature of critical incidents comes from studies by Cooper and colleagues[34-36] at Massachusetts General Hospital in Boston. These studies pioneered the investigation of incident pathways and collected data both retrospectively and prospectively on critical incidents, which they defined as

... a human error or equipment failure that could have led (if not discovered or corrected in time) or did lead to an undesirable outcome ranging from length of hospital stay[37] to death.

Each event was categorized by its primary cause: human error, equipment failure, disconnection (a special type of equipment failure), or other. For human errors, a distinction was made between *technical errors* in performing appropriate actions and *judgment errors* in which the actions occurred as planned but were inappropriate. In addition to these categorizations, the authors collected information on a variety of "circumstances that conceivably could have contributed to the occurrence of an error or to a failure to promptly detect an error;" these were termed *associated factors*.

Table 1-1 shows the distribution of the 25 most frequent critical incidents reported in these studies. Note that the true incidence of such events is unknown because the denominator of total cases from which these events were taken is unknown. Although the distribution of events may have changed somewhat since the original studies in the late 1970s and mid-1980s,

TABLE 1-1 MOST FREQUENT CRITICAL INCIDENTS	
Incident Description	**Number of Incidents**
Breathing circuit disconnection during mechanical ventilation	57
Syringe swap	50
Gas flow control technical error	41
Loss of gas supply	32
Intravenous line disconnection	24
Vaporizer off unintentionally	22
Drug ampule swap	21
Drug overdose (syringe, judgment)	20
Drug overdose (vaporizer, technical)	20
Breathing circuit leak	19
Unintentional extubation	18
Misplaced endotracheal tube	18
Breathing circuit misconnection	18
Inadequate fluid replacement	15

TABLE 1-1 MOST FREQUENT CRITICAL INCIDENTS—Cont'd	
Incident Description	**Number of Incidents**
Premature extubation	15
Ventilator malfunction	15
Misuse of blood pressure monitor	15
Breathing circuit control technical error	15
Wrong choice of airway management technique	13
Laryngoscope malfunction	12
Wrong intravenous line used	12
Hypoventilation (human error only)	11
Drug overdose (vaporizer, judgment)	9
Drug overdose (syringe, technical)	8
Wrong choice of drug	7
Total	507

Data from Cooper J, Newbower R, Kitz R. An analysis of major errors and equipment failures in anesthesia management: considerations for prevention and detection. Anesthesiology 1984;60:34-42.

TABLE 1-2 ASSOCIATED FACTORS IN CRITICAL INCIDENTS	
Associated Factor	**Number of Incidents**
Failure to check	223
First experience with situation	208
Inadequate total experience	201
Inattention or carelessness	166
Haste encouraged by situation	131
Unfamiliarity with equipment or device	126
Visual restriction	83
Inadequate familiarity with anesthetic technique	79
Other distractive simultaneous anesthesia activities	71
Teaching in progress	60
Excessive dependency on other personnel	60
Unfamiliarity with surgical procedure	59
Lack of sleep/fatigue	55
Supervisor not present enough	52
Failure to follow personal routine	41
Inadequate supervision	34
Conflicting equipment designs	34
Unfamiliarity with drug	32
Failure to follow institutional practice	31

Data from Cooper J, Newbower R, Kitz R. An analysis of major errors and equipment failures in anesthesia management: considerations for prevention and detection. Anesthesiology 1984;60:34-42.

critical incident studies have been repeated in many settings and countries during the ensuing 3 decades, with similar results.[38-40]

Table 1-2 presents the kinds of associated factors that were found for these critical incidents. These are familiar themes, which provide concrete examples of the latent factors, and the frequency of "failure to check" as an associated factor reinforces this chapter's previous discussion of measures to avoid equipment failures.

The Anesthesia Professional Is Responsible for Detecting and Correcting Problems Early in Their Evolution

The primary weapon of crisis management is the *detection* and *correction* of evolving problems, incidents, critical incidents, and adverse outcomes. Reason[8] described the multiple points of interruption of evolving incidents as "defense-in-depth." As shown in Figure 1-3, adverse outcomes only occur when an incident is triggered as described earlier, it evolves into a critical incident, *and* the defense-in-depth fails. Ideally the defenses succeed before an adverse outcome occurs, but even if patient injury occurs, the anesthesia professional must still be involved in mitigating the severity of the injury.

A MODEL OF DYNAMIC DECISION MAKING IN ANESTHESIOLOGY

We have created a functional model of the details of the dynamic decision-making processes used by anesthesia professionals to detect and correct problems. This model (Fig. 1-4) posits several different cognitive levels operating simultaneously: a sensorimotor level acquires and feeds information first to a procedural level of rapid assessment and decision making, supported by a more complex level of abstract reasoning as necessary.

This three-level process is then overseen by a layer of supervisory control that executes a repeated loop of "Observation, Decision, Action, and Reevaluation." The entire process is overlaid by another level of knowledge about when and how to use certain strategies for learning or problem solving or, as in this case, for concentrating on dynamic decision making and resource management. This is also known as "metacognition" (the awareness and understanding of one's own thought processes [See "Metacognition, Supervisory Control, and Resource Management."])[41] Various forms of metacognition—modulating one's own thinking processes—occur in everyday life as well. For example, when about to merge onto a busy highway, a good driver may decide to minimize distractions (e.g., asks passengers to stop talking), shift attention to high-value data streams (e.g., the driver's door rear-view mirror), and call up preplanned strategies for inserting the car into a stream of traffic. Skilled drivers often perform this with little conscious effort, but these acts of altering their own thinking are part of what sets good drivers apart from merely adequate ones. This kind of dynamic alteration in one's thinking is necessary for anesthesia professionals managing challenging situations. The rest of this section reviews the details of our model of the different levels at which thinking occurs.

Decision making in anesthesiology simultaneously involves both the typical decisions of routine care and the non-routine decisions made during the management of problems or crises. For any given case, the anesthesia professional executes a variety of tasks, including checking equipment, establishing appropriate vascular access, inducing and maintaining anesthesia, securing the airway, positioning the patient, administering drugs as needed, terminating the anesthetic, and either awakening the patient or transporting the patient to the ICU or PACU while still anesthetized. In addition, the anesthesia professional must perform tasks for the surgeon, maintain a clean work space, and interact with the OR personnel.

How is it possible to do so many things simultaneously in a complex and dynamic environment? The secret involves aspects of information processing that are now well known to cognitive scientists and computer scientists. They are

Parallel processing
    Working at different levels of mental activity
    Performing more than one task simultaneously
Multitasking or multiplexing
    Performing one task at a time, but switching rapidly from one set to another
Iteration
    Performing a sequence of actions repetitively

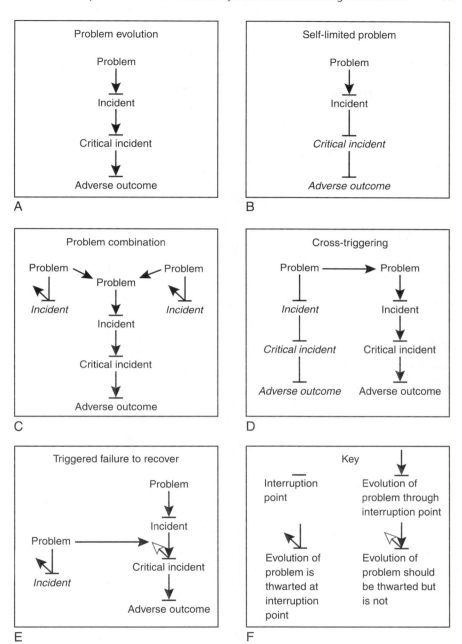

FIGURE 1-3   Schematic depiction of five examples of possible pathways for problem evolution and interaction. **A,** Problem evolution: a single problem evolves into an adverse outcome. **B,** Self-limited problem: a problem evolves into an incident but fails to evolve into a critical incident in the absence of any intervention. **C,** Problem combination: two typically minor problems combine to trigger a more serious problem. **D,** Cross-triggering: a problem fails to evolve but triggers a new problem, which evolves into an adverse outcome. **E,** Triggered failure to recover: one usually minor problem makes it impossible to interrupt the evolution of another problem. **F,** Key to symbols.

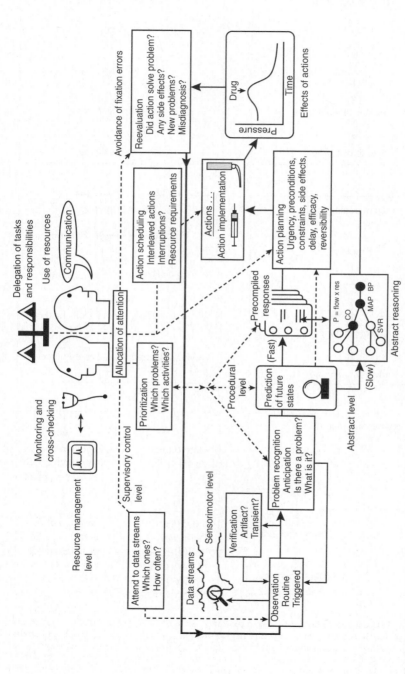

FIGURE 1-4 Our model of the anesthesia professional's complex process of intraoperative decision making. As described fully in the text, there are five levels of mental activity. There is a primary loop (*heavy black arrows*) of observation, decision, action, and reevaluation. This loop is controlled by higher levels of supervisory control (allocation of attention) and resource management. *BP*, Blood pressure; *CO*, cardiac output; *MAP*, mean arterial pressure; *P*, pressure; *res*, resistance; *SVR*, systemic vascular resistance.

Expert performance in anesthesia involves these features in a repeated "loop" of observation, decision, action, and reevaluation. An important feature of this loop is that there is little or no distinction between diagnostic and therapeutic activities. In fact, the anesthesia professional's attention is such a scarce resource that its allocation is extremely important in nearly every aspect of dynamic decision making.

Observation of incoming data is the first step in decision making. Without data that are transformed by interpretation into "information" and then into "meaning," no other processing is possible. Data streams typically involve direct visual, auditory, or tactile contact with the patient, routine electronic monitoring, special (sometimes invasive) monitoring systems (e.g., transesophageal echocardiography), and communications from other personnel. The plethora of simultaneous data streams in even the most routine case is a challenge for anesthesia professionals to interpret consistently.

Vigilance is defined as the capacity to *sustain* attention. It plays a crucial role in the observation and detection of problems and is a necessary prerequisite for meaningful care of the patient (it is the motto of the American Society of Anesthesiologists). Vigilance can be degraded by the performance-shaping factors mentioned previously, and it can be overwhelmed by the sheer amount of information and the rapidity with which it is changing. Although vigilance is essential, it alone is not enough to preserve patient safety. It is a *necessary, but not sufficient, component* of decision making and crisis management. The vigilant observer may err in making observations or in the many steps beyond observation that are required to make decisions and manage crises successfully.

VERIFICATION

In the OR environment the available data are not always reliable. Most monitoring is noninvasive and indirect and is therefore prone to *artifacts* (false data). Brief *transients* (true data of short duration), which will quickly correct themselves, can occur. Neither artifacts nor transients should be interpreted as indicating a problem requiring precipitous action. To prevent them from skewing the decision-making process, many critical observations must be verified before one can act on them. This requires the use of all available data and information and cross-checking different related data streams rather than depending solely on any single datum without sensible interpretation.

Having recognized a problem, how does the expert anesthesia professional respond? The classical paradigm of decision making involves a careful comparison of the evidence with various causal hypotheses that could explain the problem. This is followed by a careful analysis of all possible actions and solutions.[42] This approach, although powerful, is relatively slow and does not work well with ambiguous or scanty evidence. Many perioperative problems faced by anesthesia professionals require quick action to prevent a rapid cascade to a catastrophic adverse outcome, and solution of these problems through formal deductive reasoning from first principles is just too slow. Like all dynamic decision makers, anesthesia professionals use approximation strategies to handle these ambiguous situations. Psychologists describe these strategies as heuristics. One heuristic involves categorizing the event as one of several generic problems, each of which encompasses many different underlying conditions. Another is to gamble on a single diagnosis (frequency gambling[31]), initially choosing the single most frequent candidate event. In preparing for a case, the anesthesia professional may adjust a mental index of suspicion for recognizing certain specific problems that are anticipated for a particular patient or surgical procedure. The anesthesia professional must also decide whether the data can be explained by a single underlying diagnosis or multiple causes.[32] This decision is important because excessive attempts to refine the diagnosis can be very costly in terms of allocation of attention.

Use of heuristics is typical of expert anesthesia professionals and often results in considerable time saving in problem solving. Like all heuristics, these approaches are two-edged swords. As we will see in the section on "Reevaluation" of data, both frequency gambling and inappropriate allocation of attention solely to expected problems can seriously derail problem solving when these gambles do not pay off.

PREDICTION OF FUTURE STATES

Problems must be assessed in terms of their significance for the future state of the patient. Predicting future states[33] based on the occurrence of seemingly trivial problems is a major part of the anticipatory behaviors that characterize expert crisis managers. Those problems that are already critical or that can be predicted to evolve into critical incidents receive the highest priority. Prediction of future states also influences action planning by defining the time frame available for required actions.

PRECOMPILED RESPONSES

The initial responses of experts to most perioperative events arise from precompiled rules or response plans for dealing with the specific type of event.[43,44] One model refers to this process as "recognition-primed decision making."[45-47] In the hands of an experienced practitioner, precompiled responses to common problems are retrieved and executed rapidly. Traditionally, these responses were acquired through personal experience alone, although a few that involve major catastrophes (e.g., advanced cardiac life support [ACLS]) were explicitly codified and taught systematically. The use of optimum response procedures is extremely variable, even among experts. For this reason, we developed the Catalog of Critical Events in Anesthesiology (Section II) to allow anesthesia professionals to study and practice optimized routines for handling a large variety of events. On the other hand, even optimized responses are destined to fail when the problem is not caused by the suspected etiology or when it does not respond to the usual actions. For this reason (among others), performing anesthesia using only precompiled response procedures is impossible. Even when quick action must be taken, careful reasoning about the problem using fundamental medical knowledge should take place in parallel. This may involve a search for high-level analogies (e.g., "this case is similar to that one last week, except that...") or true deductive reasoning from the deep knowledge base and careful analysis of all possible solutions.

METACOGNITION, SUPERVISORY CONTROL, AND RESOURCE MANAGEMENT

Based on the research in simulation, on studies of mental workload, and work processes during real anesthesia care, we believe that anesthesia professionals' abilities to modulate their own thinking through supervisory control and resource management are the key components of crisis management.

Supervisory control includes managing observation of data streams, prioritizing diagnostic and therapeutic alternatives, and actively managing workload. Rather than being totally at the mercy of periods of rising workload, the anesthesia professional takes active steps to prepare for them. There are a variety of strategies for workload management, but each has caveats:

Distributing workload over time—this requires remembering later to do tasks that were postponed. This involves "prospective memory,"[48] remembering to do something in the future, a process that is particularly prone to disruption.

Anticipation and planning is a key principle of Anesthesia Crisis Resource Management (see Chapter 2). In some cases, there are quiet times that can be used to prepare for the next phases of a case (e.g., drawing up reversal agents, completing charts, etc.).

Distributing workload across other personnel—this requires communication with other personnel and continuous coordination of their efforts.

Simplifying tasks to match the resources available—this requires that the most critical tasks and goals are identified correctly, and also runs the risk that simplification could leave some needed tasks undone.

The "supervisory controller" in the mind allocates the scarce resource of *attention* during multitasking. For the anesthesia professional, this supervisory controller must determine how frequently different data streams are observed, what priorities are given to routine tasks versus potential or actual problems, and how to schedule actions so that the necessary attention and motor resources will be available to execute them. Such intensive demands on the anesthesia professional's attention could easily swamp the available mental resources. Therefore the ideal anesthesia professional strikes a balance between acting quickly on every small perturbation (which requires concentration and may distract attention from a larger, more pressing problem) versus adopting a more conservative "wait and see" attitude. This balance, which can be described as "aggressively underreacting," must be constantly shifted as the situation changes. Although it is important to avoid immediate action on small, distracting problems, it is critical that true crisis situations be identified and addressed promptly. When serious problems are detected, it is vital to switch from "business as usual" to "emergency mode" as erring too far in the direction of "wait and see" can be particularly catastrophic. We have observed this failure in simulation scenarios.

Supervisory control and resource management also involve the optimum planning of *actions* and the scheduling of their efficient execution. Often there are multiple actions that are appropriate, yet they cannot all be done at once. Each action must be interwoven with myriad other activities that are ongoing. The expert anesthesia professional considers many factors in planning and adapting optimum action sequences, including

Preconditions necessary for carrying out the actions (e.g., it is impossible to assess regional myocardial wall-motion abnormality if an echocardiography machine is not present)

Constraints on the proposed actions (e.g., it is impossible to check the pupils when the head is fully draped in the surgical field)

Side effects of the proposed actions

Rapidity and ease of implementing the actions

Certainty of success of the actions

Reversibility of the actions and the cost of being wrong

Cost of the actions in terms of attention and resources

ACTION IMPLEMENTATION

A particular hallmark of anesthesiology is that the decision maker does not just decide what action is required but is involved directly in the implementation of actions. Executing these actions requires substantial attention and may in fact impair the anesthesia professional's mental and physical ability to perform other activities (e.g., when an action requires a sterile procedure). In performing actions, a variety of errors of execution, termed *slips*, may occur. These are actions that do not occur as planned, such as turning the wrong switch or making a syringe swap. Norman[49] has categorized errors of this type as

Capture error: A common action taking over from the one intended (e.g., a "force of habit")
Description error: Performing the correct action on the wrong target (e.g., flipping the wrong switch)
Memory error: Forgetting an item in a sequence
Sequence error: Performing an action out of sequence from other actions
Mode error: Actions appropriate for one mode of operation but incorrect in another mode (for example, if the BAG/VENTILATOR selector valve on the anesthesia machine is left on the BAG "mode" but no one is squeezing the bag—thinking that the ventilator is working—the patient's lungs will not be ventilated)

Some of the risks caused by slips in anesthesia have been addressed through the use of *engineered safety devices*, which physically prevent incorrect actions. For example, anesthesia machines have interlocks that physically prevent the simultaneous administration of more than one volatile anesthetic agent. Other interlocks physically prevent the selection of a hypoxic mixture of O_2 and nitrous oxide. As anesthesia machines have become more heavily automated, new kinds of engineered safety have become possible—the software can sense abnormal states, can activate backup systems, or advise the anesthesia professional of the appropriate action. However, this has come at a price, not only in terms of money but also in terms of complexity and the introduction of new failure mechanisms. Machines prevalent 30 years ago had no need for electrical power. They were rugged mechanically and worked well most of the time. New machines require AC power and battery backups, and, because they are run by embedded computers, they can sometimes fail and need to be rebooted, a process that can take several minutes. Just as in aviation—which made a transition from mechanical dials and controls to computerized "glass cockpits" and "fly by wire"—such automation remains a two-edged sword.

REEVALUATION

Successful dynamic problem solving under uncertainty requires the supervisory control level to initiate frequent reevaluation of the situation. The initial diagnosis and situation assessment can be incorrect, especially when the available cues do not precisely identify a problem. Even actions that are appropriate to the problem are not always successful and sometimes cause serious side effects. Furthermore, the anesthesia professional often must handle more than one problem at a time. Only by frequently reassessing the situation can the anesthesia professional adapt to dynamically changing circumstances. The reevaluation process returns the anesthesia professional to the "observation" step but with specific assessments in mind:

• Did the actions have any effect (e.g., did the drug reach the patient)?
• Is the problem getting better, or is it getting worse?
• Are there any side effects resulting from previous actions?
• Are there any other problems or new problems that were missed before?
• Was the initial situation assessment or diagnosis correct?

The process of continually updating the situation assessment and of monitoring the efficacy of chosen actions is termed *situation awareness*, a concept that has been used extensively in aviation and more recently in health care[50,51]

RESOURCE MANAGEMENT

The general cognitive processes of observation, decision, action, and reevaluation, with oversight and modulation through supervisory control, are a natural part of the work of professionals in any dynamic domain. These processes are typically acquired through apprenticeship and mimicking role models. Overlaying these processes is another layer of metacognition and control known as resource management. Enhancing this component of flight crew decision making was found to be very important in improving aviation safety and we have found it equally important in the work of anesthesia professionals. Hence, we have devoted the entirety of Chapter 2 to describing in detail the components of "Anesthesia Crisis Resource Management."

REFERENCES

1. Webster's New Twentieth Century Dictionary. New York, Simon and Schuster; 1979.
2. Gaba D, Evans D, Patel V. Dynamic decision-making in anesthesiology: cognitive models and training approaches. In: Advanced models of cognition for medical training and practice. Berlin: Springer-Verlag; 1992. p. 122.
3. DeKeyser V, Woods D, Masson M, Van Daele A. Fixation errors in dynamic and complex systems: descriptive forms, psychological mechanisms, potential countermeasures, Technical report for NATO Division of Scientific Affairs; 1988.
4. Woods D, Johannesen L, Cook R, Sarter N. Behind human error: cognitive system, computers, and hindsight. In: Wright Patterson Air Force Base. Crew Systems Ergonomics Information Analysis Center; 1994.
5. Orasanu J, Connolly T, Klein G, et al. The reinvention of decision making, decision making in action: models and methods. Norwood, NJ: Ablex Publishing Corp.; 1993. p. 3.
6. Perrow C. Normal accidents. New York: Basic Books; 1984.
7. Gaba DM, Maxwell M, DeAnda A. Anesthetic mishaps: breaking the chain of accident evolution. Anesthesiology 1987;66:670-6.
8. Reason J. Human error. Cambridge, Mass: Cambridge University Press; 1990.
9. Rochlin G, La Porte T, Roberts K. The self-designing high reliability organization: aircraft carrier flight operations at sea. Naval War College Rev 1987;42(Autumn):76.
10. Roberts K, Rousseau D, La Porte T. The culture of high reliability: quantitative and qualitative assessment aboard nuclear powered aircraft carriers. J High Technol Manage Res 1994;5:141.
11. Sagan S. The limits of safety. Princeton, NJ: Princeton University Press; 1993.
12. Gaba D. Structural and organizational issues in patient safety: a comparison of health care to other high-hazard industries. Calif Manag Rev 2000;43:83-102.
13. Weick K. Organizational culture as a source of high reliability. Calif Manag Rev 1987;29(2):112-27.
14. Roberts K. Some aspects of organizational cultures and strategies to manage them in reliability enhancing organizations. J Manage Issues 1993;5:165-81.
15. Gaba D, Singer S, Sinaiko A, Bowen J, Ciavarelli A. Differences in safety climate between hospital personnel and naval aviators. Hum Factors 2003;45:173.
16. Singer SJ, Gaba DM, Geppert JJ, et al. The culture of safety: results of an organization-wide survey in 15 California hospitals. Qual Saf Health Care 2003;12:112.
17. Singer SJ, Rosen A, Zhao S, Ciavarelli AP, Gaba DM. Comparing safety climate in naval aviation and hospitals: implications for improving patient safety. Health Care Manage Rev 2010;35:134-46.
18. Gaba D, Howard S, Jump B. Production pressure in the work environment: California anesthesiologists' attitudes and experiences. Anesthesiology 1994;81:488.
19. Healzer JM, Howard SK, Gaba DM. Attitudes toward production pressure and patient safety: a survey of anesthesia residents. J Clin Monit Comput 1998;14:145.
20. Johnson K. Anesthesiologists and organizational behavior: the operating room culture: emerging informal practices (abstract). Anesthesiology 2001;95:A1100.
21. Singer SJ, Gaba DM, Falwell A, et al. Patient safety climate in 92 US hospitals: differences by work area and discipline. Med Care 2009;47:23-31.
22. Singer SJ, Hartmann CW, Hanchate A, et al. Comparing safety climate between two populations of hospitals in the United States. Health Serv Res 2009;44:1563-83.
23. Howard SK, Gaba DM, Rosekind MR, Zarcone VP. The risks and implications of excessive daytime sleepiness in resident physicians. Acad Med 2002;77:1019.
24. Gaba DM, Howard SK. Patient safety: fatigue among clinicians and the safety of patients. N Engl J Med 2002;347:1249.

25. Howard SK, Rosekind MR, Katz JD, Berry AJ. Fatigue in anesthesia: implications and strategies for patient and provider safety. Anesthesiology 2002;97:1281-94.
26. Weinger MB, Ancoli-Israel S. Sleep deprivation and clinical performance. JAMA 2002;287:955.
27. Slogoff S, Keats A. Does perioperative myocardial ischemia lead to postoperative myocardial infarction? Anesthesiology 1985;62:107.
28. Slogoff S, Keats A. Further observations on perioperative myocardial ischemia. Anesthesiology 1986;65:539.
29. Knight A, Hollenberg M, London M, et al. Perioperative myocardial ischemia: importance of preoperative ischemic pattern. Anesthesiology 1988;68:681.
30. Forrest J, Cahalan M, Rehder K. Multicenter study of general anesthesia. II. Results. Anesthesiology 1990;72:262.
31. Cooper JB, Cullen DJ, Nemeskal R, et al. Effects of information feedback and pulse oximetry on the incidence of anesthesia complications. Anesthesiology 1987;67:686-94.
32. Cooper J, Gaba D. No myth: anesthesia is a model for addressing patient safety (editorial). Anesthesiology 2002;97:1335.
33. Buck N, Devlin H, Lunn J. The report of a confidential enquiry into perioperative deaths. London: Nuffield Provincial Hospitals Trust; 1987.
34. Cooper JB, Newbower RS, Long CD, McPeek B. Preventable anesthesia mishaps: a study of human factors. Anesthesiology 1978;49:399-406.
35. Cooper JB, Long CD, Newbower RS, Philip JH. Critical incidents associated with intraoperative exchanges of anesthesia personnel. Anesthesiology 1982;56:456-61.
36. Cooper J, Newbower R, Kitz R. An analysis of major errors and equipment failures in anesthesia management: considerations for prevention and detection. Anesthesiology 1984;60:34-42.
37. Cullen DJ, Nemeskal AR, Cooper JB. Zaslavsky A, Dwyer MJ. Effect of pulse oximetry, age, and ASA physical status on the frequency of patients admitted unexpectedly to a postoperative intensive care unit and the severity of their anesthesia-related complications. Anesth Analg 1992;74:181-8.
38. Utting J, Gray T, Shelley F. Human misadventure in anaesthesia. Can Anaesthetists Soc J 1979;26:472-8.
39. Craig J, Wilson M. A survey of anaesthetic misadventures. Anaesthesia 1981;36:933-6.
40. Chopra V, Bovill JG, Spierdijk J. Accidents, near accidents and complications during anaesthesia. A retrospective analysis of a 10-year period in a teaching hospital. Anaesthesia 1990;45:3-6.
41. OED Online. Oxford University Press, http://www.oed.com.laneproxy.stanford.edu/view/Entry/245252?redirected From=metacognition; March 2013 [accessed April 19, 2013].
42. Kahneman D. Thinking, fast and slow. New York: Farrar, Straus and Giroux; 2011.
43. Rasmussen J. Skills, rules, and knowledge; signals, signs, and symbols, and other distinctions in human performance models. IEEE Trans Syst Man Cybernet 1983;13:257-66.
44. Reason J, Rasmussen J, Duncan K, Leplat J. Generic error-modeling system (GEMS): a cognitive framework for locating common human error forms. In: Rasmussen J, Gunter SK, Leplat J, editors. New technology and human error. Chichester: Wiley; 1987. p. 63-83.
45. Klein G. Recognition-primed decisions. In: Rouse WB, editor. Advances in man–machine systems research, vol. 5. Greenwich, Conn: JAI Press; 1989. p. 47-92.
46. Klein G, Orasanu J, Calderwood R, Zsambok C. A recognition-primed decision (RPD) model of rapid decision making. In: Klein G, Orasanu J, Calderwood R, editors. Decision making in action: models and methods. Norwood, NJ: Ablex Publishing Corp.; 1993. p. 138-47.
47. Klein G. Sources of power: how people make decisions. Cambridge, Mass: The MIT Press; 1998.
48. Stone M, Dismukes K, Remington R. Prospective memory in dynamic environments: effects of load, delay, and phonological rehearsal. Memory 2001;9:165-76.
49. Norman D. Categorization of action slips. Psychol Rev 1981;88:1-15.
50. Sarter N, Woods D. Situation awareness: a critical but ill-defined phenomenon. Int J Aviation Psychol 1991;1:45-57.
51. Gaba DM, Howard SK, Small SD. Situation awareness in anesthesiology. Hum Factors 1995;37:20-31.

Chapter 2
Principles of Anesthesia Crisis Resource Management

RESOURCE MANAGEMENT IS A CRUCIAL SKILL FOR ANESTHESIA PROFESSIONALS

The concept of resource management is borrowed directly from the domain of aviation. It should be no surprise that we turned to other complex, dynamic systems such as aviation and nuclear power for useful parallels. These industries have directly addressed issues of optimal crisis management performance by the humans "in the loop." In the case of military aviation, the need to optimize human performance systematically has been evident since before World War II and still exists. These efforts have been spurred by the need to recruit and train large numbers of pilots and by the pilots' very cogent desire to stay alive in the air. Commercial aviation learned much from military aviation, and the last 30 years have seen intensified efforts to improve human performance issues among aircrews and air traffic controllers. For the nuclear power industry, it was largely the accident at Three Mile Island (and later the Chernobyl catastrophe) that demonstrated the importance of human factors in the safe performance of these reactors. For many years these industries have recognized that maximizing safety and productivity requires an understanding of individual and group cognitive psychology aimed at changing organizational structure, equipment design, operational protocols, and crew training.

For example, in 1979 a thorough analysis[1] of 60 airline accidents, including data from cockpit voice and flight data recorders, disclosed lethal decision-making errors by individual crew members or inadequate teamwork by crews. These findings were confirmed in detailed simulator studies of flight crews.[2] As a result of these investigations of crew performance, the aviation industry embraced a training philosophy originally called "cockpit resource management" (CRM)—later "crew resource management." In the CRM approach, crews are instructed not only in the technical "nuts and bolts" of managing crises such as engine fires, but also in how to manage their individual and collective resources to work together optimally as a team.

There have been six generations of CRM in aviation, and CRM has now been adapted not only to health care (as described more fully in this chapter) but also to other diverse domains including maritime operations, spaceflight, and firefighting. Many issues concerning resource management in these various dynamic domains are not yet completely understood. More than 25 years of experience and study of the CRM approach in aviation, health care, and elsewhere has demonstrated that effective resource management is an important component of managing challenging situations. Successful conduct of an anesthetic depends on more than just having the requisite medical knowledge and technical skills. These must be translated into effective *management of the situation*. In this chapter we provide core concepts and a set of practical principles to guide you in improving or refreshing your case management skills. These principles should be useful for any anesthesia case, but they are particularly important in difficult or complex cases and in crisis situations.

Between 1989 and 1990 we first adapted aviation's crew resource management to anesthesiology, naming our approach and course Anesthesia Crisis Resource Management (ACRM). We changed the term *crew* to *crisis* because the term crew is not as familiar to most health care personnel as the concept of crisis. The term *crisis resource management* (hereafter considered roughly synonymous with aviation's *crew resource management* and using the

TABLE 2-1 KEY POINTS OF ANESTHESIA CRISIS RESOURCE MANAGEMENT	
Cognitive Components of Dynamic Decision Making	**Team Management Components**
Know the environment	Call for help early enough to make a difference
Anticipate and plan	Designate leadership
Use all available information and cross check it	Establish role clarity
Allocate attention wisely	Distribute the workload
Mobilize resources	Communicate effectively
Use cognitive aids	

same generic acronym of CRM) has been widely adopted within the health care community. This choice of terminology has unintentionally led to several misconceptions. One is that ACRM says nothing about how to prevent crises. Another misconception is that the ACRM principles apply only to patients who are already in a serious state and thus do not pertain to management in mildly abnormal or anomalous situations that have not deteriorated catastrophically. As will be seen shortly, anticipation and planning is a key element of ACRM that includes recognizing risks, preventing anomalies, optimizing safety in ordinary patient care, and handling early states of deterioration to prevent the development of a full-blown crisis.

Whether at an early stage or at the height of a crisis, ACRM encompasses the ability of the anesthesia professional to command and control *all* the resources at hand to execute the anesthesia as planned and respond to problems that arise. This is, in essence, the ability to translate the *knowledge* of what needs to be done into effective team activity in the complex and ill-structured *real world* of perioperative settings. In ACRM, the fundamental principles fall into two categories: decision-making components and team management components. In this chapter we will describe these principles in detail and offer practical advice about how to implement them in the real world (Table 2-1).

KNOWING THE ENVIRONMENT AND AVAILABLE RESOURCES

Your different work environments (e.g., OR, PACU, ICU, emergency department) contain many individuals, systems, and physical objects that you must coordinate to manage the patient optimally. Some resources are obvious, such as the anesthesia machine; others are not very obvious, such as use of the scrub nurse to perform manual ventilation during a major catastrophe. You or the rest of the team are very unlikely to identify all the relevant resources in the heat of the moment unless you have given them some serious thought beforehand. Resources can be categorized as self, OR personnel, equipment, cognitive aids, plans, systems, and other external resources. We discuss each of these in detail as follows.

Self

Your professional knowledge and skills are your most important resource because they enable you to take direct action to protect the patient or to supervise the use of the other resources at your disposal. However, like all resources the self resource is neither omnipotent nor inexhaustible. Many factors will limit your ability to care for the patient optimally. As discussed in the previous chapter your *attention* is a scarce resource, and you must learn to use it wisely. A significant part of these principles of crisis management will address ways in which you can best divide your attention between the various tasks at hand and the various problems you face.

Remember, too, that as a human being your performance is not constant. It will vary both over the course of a day and from day to day, and it is affected by many performance-shaping factors such as fatigue, stress, illness, and medication. Fortunately, good anesthesia practice does not typically demand continuous peak human performance, but *any* case could call on more personal reserves than you have available.

Your personality and style of interaction with others is important in achieving the optimum use of yourself as a resource. As will be discussed more fully in this chapter ideal interactions blend respectful assertiveness and decisiveness with calm rational leadership and decision making. Your underlying temperament may be more or less easily adapted to this style.

The responsibility for providing good patient care is yours. You should be sensitive to any degradation of yourself as a resource, whether you detect it yourself or are told about it by others. You must respond appropriately to changes in your performance status; a patient should never suffer for your decision to "tough it out." No one will thank you for going ahead with a case if you cannot do your job properly and a catastrophe then ensues.

What can you do if you find that your performance is lagging? Under some circumstances, if you are ill, sleep-deprived, or preoccupied with a personal matter, you may need to postpone the case or insist that someone replace you. The organizational structure of your practice should provide for such situations. If you are currently in training, think about this when you evaluate the practice opportunities available to you after graduation.

If your ability is less severely degraded, you may still need to mobilize additional resources to maintain adequate performance levels. You could, for example, ask a colleague to assist you with particularly difficult parts of a case, or you could alert the circulating nurse to be ready to help you more than usual. You might also set the alarm limits on your monitors more stringently than you otherwise would and raise their audio volume so that you can be alerted early to potential problems. For impairments linked to your overall level of arousal (such as fatigue or illness) there are specific countermeasures that you can take to raise your arousal level. These have been summarized in the literature[3-5] and include things such as standing rather than sitting throughout the case, conversing with OR personnel, strategically using caffeine (before or during periods where high alertness is needed but not too close to an upcoming sleep period), or trying to obtain a short nap before beginning a case (which may be feasible unless the situation is truly emergent).

Hazardous Attitudes and Production Pressure

Your *attitudes* are an important component of your abilities. They can affect your performance just as strongly as physiologic performance-shaping factors. In addition, psychologists studying judgment in aviators have identified five attitude types as being particularly hazardous, and they have developed specific antidote thoughts for each hazardous attitude[6] (Table 2-2). Aviation psychologists instruct pilots to actually verbalize the antidote thought whenever they find themselves thinking in a hazardous way.

The invulnerability and macho attitudes are particularly hazardous for anesthesia professionals. The belief that a catastrophe "cannot happen to me," and that your expert performance allows you to do anything, can make you cavalier about planning and executing patient care. It can alter your thresholds for believing abnormal data or for recognizing problems, thereby leading to the fixation error of "everything's OK."

Hazardous attitudes are compounded by production pressures (see Chapter 1) and by the lack of a culture of safety in the work unit or institution. The economic and social realities of practice can cause these pressures to become *internalized* by anesthesia professionals, who then develop hazardous attitudes they might otherwise have resisted. For example, the surgeon will no longer need to overtly push you to go ahead with a case that should be canceled if you

TABLE 2-2 EXAMPLES OF HAZARDOUS ATTITUDES AND THEIR ANTIDOTES	
Hazardous Attitude	**Antidote**
Antiauthority: "Don't tell me what to do. The policies are for someone else."	"Follow the rules. They are usually right."
Impulsivity: "Do something quickly—anything!"	"Not so fast. Think first."
Invulnerability: "It won't happen to me. It's just a routine case."	"It could happen to me. Even 'routine cases' develop serious problems."
Macho: "I'll show you I can do it. I can intubate anybody."	"Taking chances is foolish. Plan for failure."
Resignation: "What's the use? It's out of my hands. It's up to the surgeon."	"I'm not helpless. I can make a difference. There is always something else to try that might help."

Modified from Aeronautical decision making. Advisory circular number 60-22. Washington, DC: Federal Aviation Administration; 1991.

have already altered your own approach to conform to the surgeon's wishes. Of course, there may be valid reasons to proceed with a questionable case when medical urgency demands it. Under these conditions the usual protocols for elective case management must be adapted to seek the best outcome for the patient.

In the final analysis, *you* must ensure that the patient's benefit is the primary criterion in such decisions, and you should establish a bottom line of safe planning, pre-use equipment checks, and patient preparation beyond which you will not be pushed. Even if surgeons, nurses, or administrators have pressured you to do things that you do not think are safe, *they* will *not* thank you if the patient suffers, nor will they come to your defense should litigation arise.

To simplify these decisions, many institutions have developed multidisciplinary written consensus guidelines on the preoperative preparation of patients that address the appropriate workup for patients with various medical conditions in different surgical urgency categories. This approach is analogous to preestablished "flight mission rules" used in spaceflight operations. "Flight mission rules are agreements among NASA management, flight crew personnel, flight operations personnel, and others on courses of action to take in non-nominal (abnormal) in-flight situations."[7] These are intended to encapsulate detailed objective analyses and to isolate decisions from the pressures of the "heat of the moment." Centers that utilize preoperative evaluation clinics that apply such guidelines have reduced the number of day-of-surgery cancellations for medical causes while maintaining appropriate standards of patient safety.[8]

Operating Room Personnel

The other members of the OR team are also important resources. The surgeon and anesthesia professional (and other team members) will all feel responsibility for the patient, but it is the surgery that actually provides definitive benefits to the patient. Anesthesia itself has no therapeutic benefit. From the viewpoint of the anesthesia professional, surgeons have other important roles. The surgeon may know the patient well and may be able to give you important information about underlying medical or surgical conditions that could not be obtained from the patient or from the chart. Most surgeons are also more capable than you are to perform certain important technical procedures that might be needed to manage a crisis.

Nursing and technical staff each has a duty to safeguard the patient by using their specialized knowledge and skills within their defined scope of practice. Effectively using them as resources, while not exceeding their limits, is essential to achieving good outcomes. As we shall see, *every* person in the OR can help you manage a complex situation.

The OR is a relatively unique team environment. Each discipline—anesthesia, nursing, surgery, etc.—may have multiple individuals in its "crew" (e.g., a primary surgeon plus one or more assistants, an attending anesthesiologist plus a nurse anesthetist or resident). The crews then come together to work as a "team." There are rarely fixed crews or teams of personnel that always work together, but rather pools of individuals forming the crews and teams. Moreover, on different days even the same team may be working on vastly different sorts of cases. Depending on the size of the work unit, you may occasionally or regularly work with the same set of people. In other settings, such as working in a "locum tenens" position, or on a cardiac arrest response team ("code team") you may have never met the other members of the team. Until the last decade health care has not placed much emphasis on attitudes of team orientation and cohesion, relying instead primarily on the ethos of individual clinical responsibility. The variability in team makeup places a premium on the ability of individuals to form a coherent team when the going gets tough, and it places a burden on you as a team leader to manage the team's resources appropriately (see later section on Leadership and "Followership").

Your institution can also adopt mechanisms to help promote team orientation. As one example of such an approach, over the last 2 years the code team at one of our hospitals (VA Palo Alto Health Care System) has adopted twice-daily (8 AM and 10 PM) 5-minute code team briefings where all members gather in a convenient spot to introduce themselves, to review key aspects of code management, and to provide a heads-up on unstable patients whose condition could deteriorate to a cardiac arrest. Merely knowing who the other team members are that day has proven to be extremely valuable to improve team cohesion.

Equipment

Although clinical observation and direct manipulation of the patient are important skills for anesthesia professionals, they are not enough for optimal practice. Anesthesia care in the industrial world requires considerable equipment, including gas delivery systems, ventilators, monitors, infusion pumps, and OR tables. Although errors in equipment use can directly cause harm to the patient, or can trigger accident sequences, the use of every piece of equipment to its best advantage will maximize your ability to obtain a good clinical outcome. In order to achieve this goal you must

- ensure that the relevant routine equipment is present and is working properly
- ensure that critical backup equipment is immediately available (e.g., a self-inflating bag for emergency ventilation), and
- know how to operate each piece of equipment you use, including knowledge of its operating characteristics in both normal and abnormal circumstances

In commercial aviation, pilots are "type-rated" and can only fly aircraft of the type for which they are certified. For example, a captain type rated only for a Boeing 737 cannot act as pilot in command on a Boeing 747 regardless of the number of hours of total flying experience. Furthermore, aircrews receive extensive training in the operation of the aircraft's systems. Our own experience as clinicians and teachers in real and simulated anesthetic cases suggests that many anesthesia professionals are not sufficiently knowledgeable in the operation of their equipment. These devices are the tools of the trade and knowing how to use them is just as important as, if not more important than, knowing about physiology and pharmacology. It is *our responsibility* as anesthesia professionals to acquire this knowledge and skill. The operation of many devices is not intuitive, and there are often hidden pitfalls in their operation that can lead to a failure to function properly. Although the human-factors engineering and anesthesia professions are attempting to address these difficulties, they will never be solved completely, which makes it important for you to be well versed in the individual operational features of your equipment.

Cognitive Aids

The human factors literature demonstrates conclusively that cognitive functions such as memory and arithmetic calculation are fallible, even more so during periods of stress. A particular vulnerability exists for "prospective memory"—remembering in advance to do something that has been postponed.[9-11] Pilots and professionals in all domains of intrinsic hazard make extensive use of a variety of written, electronic, or mechanical "cognitive aids"[4] to help support thinking and execution of complex tasks. These aids relieve decision makers of having to memorize every piece of information that might be needed for all possible cases. Although a few written checklists and protocols have been widely used in health care for many years (e.g., the Malignant Hyperthermia Association of the United States protocol for treating malignant hyperthermia [MH]), cognitive aids until recently have not been prominent in anesthesia. Even the language frequently used in health care to describe such aids shows how little they are valued—they are sometimes called "cheat sheets" or "crutches," and people apologize for "having to look it up."

We have been long-time pioneering advocates of a completely different philosophy that encourages the use of cognitive aids as a sign of strength. The attitude toward cognitive aids may be changing. For example, working with this book's authors in 2003, the National Center for Patient Safety of the Veterans Health Administration produced a set of cognitive aids on the recognition and management of 16 serious perioperative events printed on laminated sheets. A study of the use of the cognitive aids suggested that they were beneficial to VA anesthesia professionals.[12] Other research by several authors of this book has demonstrated that (1) medical and technical performance is better during a simulated crisis (e.g., MH) when a cognitive aid is used,[13] and (2) it can be very helpful to the anesthesia professional leading the team if there is a "reader" whose job is to read the relevant aid to the team and keep track of whether the relevant tasks have been performed.[14] A group from Boston has published results from simulation testing of 12 "crisis checklists" demonstrating a substantial reduction in failure of adherence to critical steps in management when the checklists were used.[15,16] In 2014 multiple papers and editorials in a single issue of *Anesthesia and Analgesia* discussed a number of important issues about cognitive aids and their implementation.[17-21]

The Catalog of Critical Events in Anesthesiology (Section II of this book) can be used as a cognitive aid during case management, but it has not been optimized for use as an emergency aid in the heat of the moment. The Stanford Anesthesia Cognitive Aid Group (SACAG), which includes two of this book's authors as members, has conducted many years of simulation testing of cognitive aids meant for intraoperative use. These have evolved with increasing levels of optimization through enhanced graphic design and attention to usability. SACAG has now produced an Emergency Manual for Anesthesia, comprising 23 cognitive aids for perioperative events (Figs. 2-1 and 2-2) (an earlier version of the cognitive aids was published as an Appendix in the textbook Manual of Clinical Anesthesiology[22]). These cognitive aids have been placed in all anesthetizing locations in the Stanford family of teaching hospitals. The manual is now available for free throughout the world as a downloadable portable document format file under a Creative Commons license (allowing free use of the document as is, without unauthorized modifications, and with attribution of the author). To download the manual go to http://emergencymanual.stanford.edu. Users can print out the manual locally, and instructions are given on best choices of printing paper, binding, and placement in perioperative patient care settings. The impetus to use cognitive aids has also been fostered by the widespread adoption of the World Health Organization (WHO) Safe Surgery (preoperative) Checklist (see http://www.who.int/patientsafety/safesurgery/en/) promulgated in part by noted patient safety advocate Atul Gawande, MD.[23] The use of the WHO

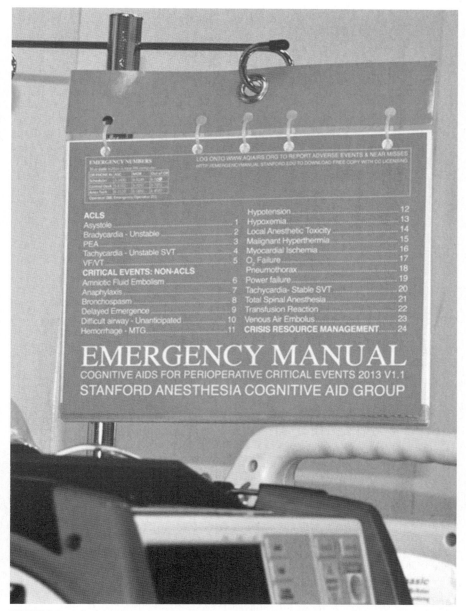

FIGURE 2-1 Anesthesia Emergency Manual by the Stanford Anesthesia Cognitive Aid Group (SACAG) shown hanging on a crash cart. A full-size physical manual such as this has distinct advantages (and some disadvantages) compared to pocket-size or smartphone types of manuals. SACAG core contributors, in random order: Howard S, Chu L, Goldhaber-Fiebert SN, Gaba DM, Harrison TK. *(From Stanford Anesthesia Cognitive Aid Group: Emergency Manual: cognitive aids for perioperative critical events. Creative Commons BY-NC-ND, 2013; photo courtesy David M. Gaba.)*

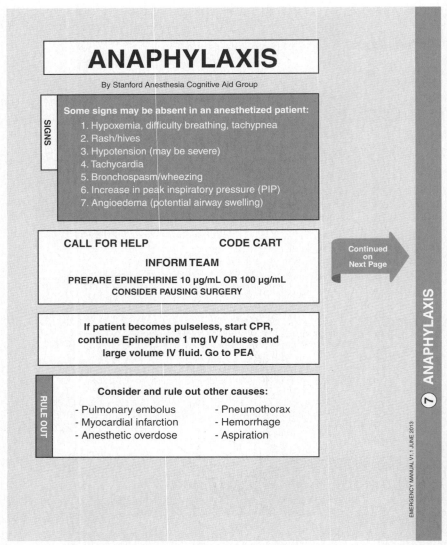

FIGURE 2-2   First page of the anaphylaxis event in the SACAG Emergency Manual. This illustrates some of the elements of graphic design (by SACAG member Larry Chu, MD) that enhance the readability and usability of this manual.

checklist, incorporating a preoperative timeout, has now become ubiquitous in the immediate preanesthesia process.

Mnemonics are another form of cognitive aid; they are learning techniques to assist in information retention and retrieval. They are often auditory in nature, such as an acronym or memorable phrase. For example, a phrase to remember the names of the carpal bones is "some lovers try positions that they can't handle." A frequently used mnemonic for preoperative anesthesia workspace preparation is MS MAID (monitors, suction, machine check, airway equipment, IV equipment, drugs). Another example is the mnemonic checklist THRIVE for preparation for weaning from cardiopulmonary bypass (CPB), developed by one of this book's authors after he witnessed and heard about "near-miss" cases in which key items (such as ventilation) were omitted:

*T*emperature is acceptable.
*H*emodynamics and cardiac function are acceptable.
*R*hythm is acceptable.
*I*nfusions are selected as desired and are infusing properly.
*V*entilation is taking place at the rate and volume desired.
*E*lectrolytes are acceptable.

Although other personnel (including the surgeon) can provide important cognitive support, their memory is also fallible. It is probably better to use a written aid or call the hospital pharmacist to determine how to mix and dose a drug that is rarely used rather than rely solely on your memory or the memory of someone else who is not completely familiar with the medication.

Reference works and handbooks contain a wealth of useful information on the medical and anesthetic management of virtually every type of condition. Many anesthesia professionals also use written tables and lists that contain information on the preparation of drug infusions and their appropriate dose ranges. By law, each drug approved by the U.S. Food and Drug Administration (FDA) comes with a package insert containing extensive information on the drug's characteristics. These are compiled in widely available references and are also available on the internet. The internet has become an increasingly useful cognitive aid and may be available on computer terminals, tablets, and smartphones in hospital settings. The medical literature can be queried directly via PubMed (www.pubmed.gov) and there are a variety of open or proprietary sites with well-researched evidence-based summaries of best practice. Accessing internet-based resources in the middle of a case is a two-edged sword. Useful information may be acquired but at the cost of significant distraction and increase in mental workload. If extensive interaction with a computer is needed it is probably best to have someone else assist you.

Bedside use of aids embedded on tablet computers and smartphones is also becoming more common. In addition, these devices bring mathematical calculators immediately to hand for anesthesia professionals. Under stress the ability to perform calculations—even simple addition or multiplication—degrades quickly. We encourage you to use a calculator to compute drug doses (especially for unfamiliar drugs or patient weights) rather than to rely only on memory or on-the-spot mental arithmetic. Of course people make errors with calculators too, so the results of any calculation also need to be checked for sensibility by the anesthesia professional.

The patient's medical record is a key source of information that contains the current and past medical history as well as the results of laboratory and radiologic tests. The advent of electronic medical records has made it possible to access data for patients in your system more expeditiously. Your anesthetic record is another important source of information, especially if you have not been present for the entire case. Always double-check your recollection of important data with the written source. Additional case information may also be obtained from the data stored as trends within the monitoring equipment in use.

We encourage you to seek out cognitive aids of all types and to use them whenever possible. Obviously there are some limits to this—you cannot be an effective anesthesia professional if you have to look up everything. But our experience, in real patient care and in simulated cases, shows that even when the aids are available their value is underestimated.

Where cognitive aids have not been published formally, we encourage you to develop and produce them for yourself, in concert with others in your practice, or through professional societies.

Systems and Other External Resources

In most sites in which surgery is performed (hospitals and stand-alone outpatient surgery centers) the OR is a subsystem linked to other systems. Thus there may be *many* external resources available to assist you in preventing or managing adverse events. For example, such system resources include preoperative assessment clinics, postoperative care units, laboratory services, blood bank, radiology, consulting physicians (most commonly cardiologists and neurologists used for crisis management), engineers, risk managers, and administrators. Experience shows that the best use of systems resources is difficult, and in fact the interface between systems can itself be a source of errors. You must consider in advance how you will mobilize and utilize these resources and communicate with them. Knowing where the key sites (such as the blood bank) are physically located as well as their phone numbers will help; this is information that lends itself to cognitive aids posted in clinical work areas. If you work in more isolated locations, such as a surgeon's private office, you are responsible for knowing what resources are available and what plans exist should a problem develop, making it necessary to obtain help or transfer a patient to a higher level of care.

Regional and national resources also exist. A good example is the MH hotline in the United States (1 800 MH HYPER), which can provide expert advice in the management of patients with suspected MH susceptibility or with full-blown MH. Keep in mind, however, that contacting the hotline should not interfere with carrying out critical tasks of patient management. If extra personnel are available, one person can be delegated to contact the hotline.

There is also telephone or online technical support offered by poison control centers and by many manufacturers of drugs and medical devices. Such contact information should be available on the internet. For example, such technical support has been especially helpful in the management of patients with cardiac pacemakers or implanted defibrillators.[24]

Plans and the Work Environment

Resources can be mobilized and used "on the fly," but the best use of resources requires advance planning. The plans themselves become key resources because they enable you to manipulate the situation more quickly. Appropriate plans come in three forms: *A work environment plan* for resource mobilization in a specific work setting; an *anesthetic plan* for dealing with the particular problems of a specific patient; and *emergency procedures* for the management of critical incidents. A good program of quality management or quality improvement is of enormous value to all forms of planning. It is the mechanism by which knowledge of past adverse events can be translated into changes in practice that minimize their recurrence.

Work environment plans should incorporate a detailed knowledge of each environment in which you care for patients, whether it is an OR, a PACU, or a remote setting such as a magnetic resonance imaging (MRI) suite. The equipment and external resources available in each setting may differ, and you will *not* be able to use them effectively unless you plan in advance. It sounds obvious, but our experience shows that clinicians often fail to know what they have available, where it is, and how to use it. Know the contents of your anesthesia carts, including emergency use items such as flashlights, resuscitation drugs, and pressure infusion sets. Know the location and operating characteristics of emergency equipment. Learn to operate the available defibrillators and to troubleshoot minor problems. Know what other equipment exists and where it is located, such as spare O_2 cylinders and regulators (and become familiar with changing cylinders and regulators), MH carts, difficult airway equipment, fire extinguishers, and battery-powered monitors. Think about the location of critical external resources such as satellite laboratories or pharmacy stations so that you can instruct runners how to get back and forth. Know how to call for help and how to call a "code" in the event of a cardiac arrest or other major emergency. Every facility has its own procedures and code alert language (e.g., "code blue" for a cardiac arrest, "code red" for a fire, "code silver" for an active shooter). Find out who will respond to a code both day and night. If you are not sure who to contact, call the facility's telephone operator (usually dial 0). If you are not in a hospital or other all-hours facility, you may need to call outside the institution for help, for example dialing 911 (in the United States) to reach the dispatcher for paramedic, police, and fire departments.

Construction of the Anesthetic Plan

Preoperative evaluation of the patient and construction of a suitable anesthetic plan is an important task that you perform to prevent the occurrence of events that can evolve into adverse outcomes. The plan delineates how you will conduct the anesthetic, how you will deal with the problems you are likely to face, and what other resources you must mobilize to meet the anesthetic goals for the case. A sound plan matches the anesthetic technique to the patient's disease state, the technical requirements of surgery (e.g., position of the patient), the anesthesia equipment available, and the skills of the anesthesia professional. It also includes specific backup procedures and contingency plans to be used if the original plan fails or needs to be changed. Often, faulty plans occur when underlying disease states are missed or ignored because of inadequate data gathering during preoperative evaluation. Poor planning may also result from the invulnerability type of hazardous attitude. **A faulty anesthetic plan will expose the patient to risk even if it is carried out perfectly**.

Generalized Emergency Procedures

Systematically prepared emergency procedures are used in virtually all complex dynamic work environments, not because the operators are ignorant or stupid, but because experience has shown that even well-trained, intelligent people need decision-making support during rapidly changing problem situations. Every licensed pilot (including the purely recreational pilot) is taught specific emergency procedures for a variety of contingencies. In the case of large commercial aircraft the emergency procedure manuals are quite extensive. Pilots are expected to memorize certain critical portions of each procedure and then to rely on the manual (and *not* on their memory) for the rest of the procedure. Airline pilots practice these procedures regularly during simulator-based recurrent training programs.

The situation in medicine in general (including anesthesiology) has been considerably different. Responses were described in a formal fashion for only a few extremely severe events (e.g., CPR, MH). For the most part, anesthesia professionals were expected to learn responses to adverse events solely by experiencing them. Each teaching anesthesia professional may have a favorite "clinical pearl" concerning emergency responses to hand down to trainees, but few pass these on consistently. For most practitioners serious adverse events are uncommon, and even those responses that were once second nature are soon forgotten for lack of use. It is for this reason that we created the Catalog of Critical Events in Anesthesiology for this volume and the Anesthesia Emergency Manual (see earlier section on Cognitive Aids).

Briefings

For planning to be most effective it should ensure the coordination of all members of the patient care team. This begins with greeting the patient (the most important member of the team) just prior to surgery. In addition to identifying the patient and surgical site properly, this meeting allows further clarification of the plan.

It is important to ensure that all members of the anesthesia crew and the rest of the OR team (surgeons, nurses, technicians) agree with and understand the plan. Aspects of the surgical procedure, such as the desired patient position and the extent of planned dissection, may alter the plan; if these are not clearly defined on the surgical schedule, the surgeons must be consulted. If predictable problems might necessitate changing plans or aborting the procedure, this should be specifically discussed in advance with the surgical team.

Over the last 10 years there has been a major movement to formalize such briefings. The WHO began a "Safe Surgery Saves Lives" campaign, creating a preoperative checklist to be used in a mandatory preoperative briefing involving surgeons, anesthesia professionals, nurses, and others. In these briefings an important element is to define likely critical events and patient specific considerations. This is an opportunity to delineate contingency plans and who will determine when to switch from the initial plan to a backup one.

Handoffs from one anesthesia professional to another,[25] or from the anesthesia professional to the PACU staff, are also important times for a different kind of formal briefing. There is considerable research ongoing about handoffs of many kinds in health care. Although many different protocols have been suggested, none has proven to be ideal. This puts the burden on you to determine the best mechanism to conduct such briefings. The less formal and very rapid kind of briefing that is needed when a helper arrives in a crisis is discussed more fully later in this chapter.

CASE MANAGEMENT BEHAVIORS

The discussion of resources should help you *prepare* to provide good anesthesia care at any time. We now turn to the question of how to act optimally *during* intraoperative patient management. Every strategy that you might choose is a two-edged sword, ideal for some situations but inadequate for others. Optimal care therefore requires constantly balancing and adapting your behavior to the changing situation.

Anticipation

We have stressed the need to anticipate the requirements of a case in advance. One aspect of this is to have a high index of suspicion for the medical problems that you might expect to encounter because of a patient's underlying diseases. You should look for these and make preparations to treat them. However, the risk of this strategy is that other problems that mimic the one you expect may in fact occur. It is important to keep an open mind and to make sure that you consider other possibilities (see discussion of reevaluation in the section titled Repeatedly Assess and Reevaluate the Situation).

Throughout the case you need to maintain awareness of every change that occurs in your environment. As mentioned in Chapter 1 pilots call this "situation awareness." The goal is to "stay ahead of the game." You can easily fall behind if the situation changes radically or quickly or if you fail to devote sufficient resources to meet the changes. When you find yourself getting seriously behind the events of a case, regardless of the reason, you *must* either slow down the progress of the case (e.g., ask the surgeon to hold off from significant actions while you catch up) or mobilize additional resources (see Call for Help—Early Enough to Make a Difference) so that you can catch up and get ahead. Staying behind for any prolonged period exposes the patient to risk.

Vigilance and Allocation of Attention

Vigilant observation of the patient is the necessary (although insufficient) starting point for expert case management. In discussing the self-resource, we mentioned several performance-shaping factors and hazardous attitudes that can globally degrade your vigilance. There are two other factors that can specifically degrade your vigilance whenever they exist in a case: one is *distractions*, the other is a *high task load*.

Distractions of various kinds occur during every case. They include activities that are important to other OR personnel, such as surgeons taking photographs, nurses counting surgical instruments or entering data in the computer, or phone calls from the ICU asking for the surgeon's instructions on a patient's care. Your attention to the patient can suffer if you assist in these activities. For example, if there is a phone at the anesthesia workstation, it should not be used routinely for phone calls that are not important to you. Nurses or clerks can transcribe laboratory results or relay messages between the surgeons and the ICU.

Routine tasks can be very distracting. The use of transesophageal echocardiography has been shown to alter the vigilance of anesthesiologists to the occurrence of secondary tasks.[26] Rotating the operating table (especially 180 degrees) or repositioning the patient on the table (e.g., prone or lateral) is also a high workload distracting activity. Increasingly, anesthesiologists interact with patient data management systems. As pilots have discovered, spending too much time "heads down" at the computer can reduce vigilance for key events in the "cockpit."

Distractions can also include music, social conversation, and jokes. Each of these activities is appropriate under the right circumstances. They can make the work environment more pleasant and promote the development of team spirit, but they can also seriously lessen your ability to detect and correct problems. You must take charge of modulating these activities so that they do not become distracting. If the music is too loud, insist that the volume be reduced or that it be turned off (a rule of thumb is that the pulse oximeter volume should always be louder than the music or conversation). When a crisis occurs, *all* distractions should be eliminated or reduced as much as possible.

Tenney and colleagues[27] have described how interruptions and distractions are prime contributors to the evolution of small problems into major catastrophes. Distractions are problematic because of a known human weakness in "prospective memory"—remembering in advance to do something. These "remembered intentions" are particularly prone to disruption by distractions and interruptions. Besides modulating potential distractions, other strategies can help to reduce the likelihood of forgetting a task because of interruptions or distractions (an error of prospective memory). Take the example of being interrupted when you have turned off the ventilator for an appropriate reason. There are various strategies to deal with this. Some anesthesia professionals leave their finger on the ventilator switch. Other strategies include putting a small sign on the ventilator to remind you that it is off, or executing a checklist periodically after turning off the ventilator to ensure it has been turned on again when appropriate (see THRIVE example previously mentioned). As a last resort in this example, properly set alarms should warn you of apnea should you forget to turn the ventilator back on.

Allocation of Attention During Varying Task Loads

Allocation of attention is a dynamic process through which you must constantly prioritize the tasks requiring your attention. You *should* handle critical items quickly and leave the less critical problems for when you have ensured the stability of the patient. On the other hand, you should deal with minor problems when the task load is low because they might otherwise evolve to something more significant. You can also use times when the workload is low to prepare for upcoming high workload periods, such as emergence from anesthesia or termination of CPB.

It is important to maintain vigilant assessment of the patient even while you continue to carry out a myriad of routine tasks and interact with students, teachers, subordinates, or supervisors. If you suspect that a problem is developing, allocate your attention primarily to problem recognition and patient evaluation until you prove to yourself that all is well. Whatever tasks occupy the OR team, at least one individual should be watching the patient's condition at all times. The task load can quickly become excessive, making you so busy that it will be *impossible* to maintain vigilant situational awareness. If you find yourself in this situation, you must mobilize additional resources to help you carry out the needed tasks and watch the patient. A frightening example from aviation that has proved compelling in the training of anesthesia professionals is that of the airliner (Eastern 401) that crashed because all of the cockpit crew were preoccupied with a faulty indicator light for nose gear deployment. The crew failed to notice that the autopilot had become disengaged—in other words, no one was flying the plane (a web search will show multiple sources for information about the details of this flight).

Use All Available Information

No single piece of information tells the whole story. Considerable controversy has been generated since the early 1970s concerning the relative merits of direct clinical observation versus the use of electronic and mechanical monitoring devices. This is a false dichotomy; *neither* clinical observation nor any single monitor currently in use gives the entire picture. The goal is to utilize *all* the information at hand to help you care for the patient. The challenge is to learn how to integrate data from every possible source, giving each datum its appropriate weight toward a decision.

Similarly, it is important to pay attention to the patient care activities of surgeons and nurses. Be very aware of the medications drawn up on the surgical field. A number of catastrophes have resulted from errors in dilution or administration of such drugs. If something unusual appears to be happening with the surgery, insist on finding out what is going on. Comments and concerns of other team members may not be addressed to you but may give early warning of an impending problem or provide critical information on how the problem can or cannot be solved.

The Burden of Proof Is on YOU to Ensure That the Patient Is Safe

Every type of observation has possible artifacts. Alarms from electronic monitors often occur repeatedly but falsely. A "cry wolf" syndrome can develop in which the anesthesia professional *assumes* that an alarm is false, even when it is really true. Alarm sounds are typically distracting, and they seem to trigger a "make it stop" response in anesthesia professionals, whose first (and sometimes only) move is to turn off the alarm.[9] This assumption can lead to catastrophe for the patient. When a monitor alarm sounds or when a question of patient safety is raised by your own observations or those of others, the burden of proof is on you to *first* determine that the patient is safe, and *then* to deal with any technical problems. Your evaluation of the patient can include checking alternate electronic monitors, but you should always remember to check the patient and equipment using all your senses, including your eyes (visual inspection), ears (auscultation), and touch (feeling the pulse). Some anesthesia professionals describe their overall practice style as always assuming that the patient might be in trouble, and then continuously proving to themselves that the patient is really safe.

MANAGING AN IMMEDIATE CATASTROPHE

Although crises typically evolve from smaller problems, it is not uncommon to be suddenly faced with a serious event. Regardless of the cause, when a catastrophic problem presents suddenly, highly practiced emergency procedures must be used to maintain life and brain function until a more specific plan can be implemented.

Immediate Life-Support Measures for Catastrophic Situations

- Call for help.
- Ensure that the patient has a pulse and that the BP is acceptable.
- If there is no pulse or absent (or very low) BP.
- Begin CPR and ACLS protocols: Good CPR is critical and takes precedence over everything else. End-tidal carbon dioxide (ET CO_2) CO_2 <10 mm Hg or diastolic pressure <20 mm Hg suggests poor CPR or vascular tone requiring improvement.
- Maintain ventilation and oxygenation. If in doubt about the ventilation system or O_2 supply, use a backup system or O_2 source.
- Turn off all anesthetics in use and increase the fraction of inspired oxygen (FiO_2) to 100% with high fresh gas flows. As you proceed, also verify that the measured inspired O_2 concentration approaches 100%.
- Support the circulation with fluids and vasopressors as necessary (or per ACLS). Double-check vasoactive or anesthetic infusions for proper setting and flow rate.

Team Management Components

Teamwork is a complex topic. Table 2-3 gives an overview of some of the broader issues involved in teamwork. However, in this chapter we present some of the practical aspects of the key points of ACRM concerning team management.

TABLE 2-3   TEAMWORK COMPETENCIES FOR KNOWLEDGE, SKILLS, AND ATTITUDES

Knowledge Competencies	Skills Competencies	Attitude Competencies
• The team's mission, objectives, norms, and resources • What coordination strategies are appropriate in what situations • Accurate understanding of typical tasks and problems shared by the team • How tasks must be sequenced • How teams communicate and arrive at decisions • How characteristics of individual teammates affect the team • How to manage interaction with other teams or individuals	• Adaptability and flexibility of decision making and action • Task coordination, including distribution of workload • Shared situation awareness • Monitoring teammates' performance and backing them up when necessary • Decision making • Communication • Team leadership • Interpersonal relations, including conflict resolution	• A shared vision of team goals • Belief in importance of teamwork and team efficacy (belief that the team is superior to any individual) • Team cohesion (attraction and loyalty to team) • Mutual trust between team members

Modified from Salas E, Burke C, Cannon-Bowers J, Kraiger K. What we know about designing and delivering team training: tips & guidelines. In: Kraiger K, editor. Crating, implementing, and managing effective training and development: state-of-the-art lessons for practice. San Francisco: Jossey-Bass; 2002.

Leadership and "Followership"

We believe that in many OR crises the senior anesthesia professional involved in the case will be best equipped to manage the situation and should take the leadership role. In some cases another team member will be more experienced with the particular situation, and he or she may assume leadership even if junior in rank to the rest of the team. In any event, it is important that the team understands who is in charge.

What does it mean to be a leader? In practical terms leadership is primarily a matter of deciding what needs to be done, prioritizing the necessary tasks, assigning them to specific individuals, and ensuring that they get done. To fulfill these leadership functions the anesthesia professional must have good technical knowledge and skills and must remain calm and organized. The leader's command authority is vital to maintaining control of the situation, but control should be accomplished with full participation of the team. The team should share information and suggestions from all its team members. When junior members of the team have vital information or are in a better position to manage the crisis, they need to convey that fact assertively to the team leader(s). The American Airlines Crew Resource Management course incorporates a saying that covers these situations: "Authority with participation, assertiveness with respect" (personal communication, Rand McNally, MD, CRM instructor, American Airlines, 1991).

The instructors at the Center for Medical Simulation in Boston express the leadership issues as establishing "role clarity" for the leader and the followers. They point out that the leader will need to establish his or her position then step back briefly to assess the situation. An important part of the leader's role is to articulate a *plan* that the whole team can follow rather than just delegating specific tasks and responsibilities.

There are several different options that will make it possible for leaders and followers to work together. The best option will depend on the situation, the individuals involved, their level of experience, and their personalities. For example, suppose you—an anesthesia professional—arrive to help in a crisis. Depending on the situation, you might do the following:

- Give advice or carry out tasks only as requested (unless you are very inexperienced, restricting your contribution only to this restricted role is probably a waste of your talent)
- Provide advice or suggest tasks to be done without being asked specifically to do so
- Work as co-equal leader with the original anesthesia professional (this can be very effective, but it requires strong cooperative work and communication)
- Take over the primary leadership role if the original anesthesia professional requests it or is grossly ineffective at managing the situation (although this would be an uncommon event, it may be necessary on occasion)

Declare an Emergency Early Rather than Late

Clinicians sometimes delay making the switch from "business as usual" to crisis management, even as a situation worsens. Often this represents denial that a catastrophe is really occurring (the fixation error of "everything's OK"), and it may also reflect fears of upsetting the surgeons, altering the OR routine, or appearing weak and incompetent. Declaring an emergency mobilizes needed resources and quickly communicates to the team that a crisis is at hand. There is a risk in declaring an emergency prematurely or too frequently—too many false alarms will make the team less likely to believe you in the future (the "cry wolf" syndrome). But the risk of *not* responding quickly to an emergency usually far exceeds the risk of doing so. The leader can vary the level of urgency as necessary and the declaration can always be cancelled if the problem resolves.

A Spectrum of Options in Declaring an Emergency

Sometimes anesthesia professionals act as though they have only two options in dealing with surgeons—keep quiet or demand immediate cessation of surgery. Actually there are many options and the most appropriate will depend on the severity of the situation and the specific nature of the problem. If the chances of real difficulty are low you may only need to increase your own level of awareness, double-check information, and make appropriate preparations and interventions. But as the actual or potential situation increases in severity or likelihood, you may need to express these concerns to the rest of the team (see later section, Good Communication Makes a Good Team). Choosing an option requires an informed and explicit discussion between the anesthesia professional and surgeon, possibly involving others. When the patient is experiencing medical or anesthetic problems, surgical activities that are not absolutely necessary pose the risk of triggering additional complications or worsening the underlying diseases, problems that will only add to the complexity of the situation. Remember that you share the patient with the surgeon. Don't just assume that you both are "on the same page." Some of the options you have for coordinating with the surgeon (in increasing order of severity) are as follows:

- Inform surgeon of the problem but allow surgery to continue with heightened awareness of the issues.
- Advise continuation of surgery but with some modest limitations or alterations in the surgical plan.
- Suspend surgery temporarily with final resolution to be determined. This provides time to assess the situation and to monitor the effects of interventions without necessarily changing the surgical plan.
- Advise the surgeon to continue, but with major changes in surgical plan, and in such a way that it can be completed more quickly than usual.
- Demand that surgery be aborted as soon as possible. Have incisions closed or if necessary have the wound packed and covered quickly. However, remember that merely moving the patient to another site, such as the ICU, does not treat the problem and may only shift the burden to other clinicians. Be certain that aborting surgery and moving the patient is really the best option for the patient.

Good Communication Makes a Good Team

Communication between team members is crucial in a crisis. It is the glue that molds separate individuals into a powerful team. The leader must communicate the appropriate sense of urgency for a situation without inducing panic. You should notify the surgeons and nurses of ongoing problems and concisely convey to them the nature of the problem, what you need them to do (or not do), and your immediate plans. Order them to suspend or abort the surgery if necessary. Conversely, you should be prepared to help the surgeons or nurses in any reasonable way when they encounter problems, as long as you can also maintain safe assessment of the patient and control of the anesthetic course.

Good team communication is a complex skill. We have observed many instances of poor communication between team members in both real and simulated OR settings. The following are some principles of good communication that you should practice to become a more effective team leader:

- **Do not raise your voice** unless absolutely necessary. However, as the leader you may need to ask for silence forcefully so that you can be heard.
- **State your commands or requests as clearly and as precisely as possible.** This is very difficult in a crisis, and it takes practice.

- **Avoid making statements into thin air** (e.g., "We need a nitro drip" or "Could somebody do..."). Whenever possible, address statements or questions to specific people and be sure that they know you are speaking to them.
- **Close the communication loop.** Provide and request acknowledgments of critical communications. Pilots are required by law to "read back" clearances such as "cleared for takeoff." OR personnel can and should do the same. Verify ambiguous messages; if you are not sure what someone said, clarify it with that person.
- **Foster an atmosphere of open exchange among all OR personnel.** Listen to what other people have to say regardless of their job description or status. They may know something important about the patient or the situation that you do not. If you are in charge, you must decide whether their information needs to be acted on, but you cannot make that decision if you are not aware of it. Others may detect errors that you or other team members have made, thus saving you from significant mistakes and helping you to recover from errors.
- **Should conflict arise, concentrate on *what* is right for the patient rather than on *who* is right** (a slogan learned from an American Airlines CRM course). You can sort out the interpersonal issues at another time. The patient is depending on the team to work together.

COMMUNICATION TECHNIQUES

Many anesthesia professionals are able to implement these principles, and good communication is a part of their daily practice. However, experience shows that it is sometimes hard to translate the principles into effective communication. A generic approach has been taught in CRM courses:

(1) Open the communication channel (e.g., "Hey, Bill . . .")
(2) Express an "owned" emotion (e.g., "I am concerned")
(3) Express the content of the emotion (e.g., ". . . concerned that the BP is very low")
(4) Express a possible solution (e.g., "Do you think you can retract less on his vena cava?")
(5) Close the loop (e.g., "What do you think about that?")

It is very useful to package all this together into a coherent whole. Rapidly indicating what is going on and what your plan is will often mollify surgeons' worries and coordinate the needed urgent care of the patient. Thus, when a problem "X" is apparent and you either need to let the surgeon know about it or to respond to some comment by the surgeon, a useful formula is as follows:

(1) "X is happening" or "I'm aware of X."
(2) Here is (or I am aware of) the significance of X and what it means.
(3) Here is what I have done/am doing/or planning to do about X.
(4) Here's what I expect to happen about X over time.
(5) Here is my plan for dealing with X.
(6) Here is what I can do to help you or what you can do to help me with X.

Here are two examples of this formula in action. Suppose the surgeon says, "The BP's too high—get it down!" You might say, "I'm aware the BP just shot up. I'm working on it with <name drug A>. It should come down soon, and if not I'm going to give more <drug A> or start some <drug B>. In the meantime, is it OK if I put the head of the table up to see if that helps?"

Or, for example, suppose you discover signs of possible MH, but you are not certain what is happening, you might say, "Hey <surgeon's name>—I'm concerned that this patient may have a serious metabolic problem. The ET CO_2 is rising despite my increasing the minute ventilation, and the heart rate is up despite deep anesthesia. It's even possible the patient has MH, a lethal problem triggered by anesthetics. I'm going to draw a blood gas and change my anesthetic technique just in case it is MH. Maybe you can stop operating for a few minutes to lessen the surgical stimulus until we get this sorted out. Then we'll see what we have to do."

Distribute the Workload

When a crisis occurs, the leader must distribute the workload across all the resources at hand. A common scene in an OR crisis is to have a handful of people seriously overworked while others stand around with nothing useful to do. Anesthesia professionals must exercise leadership by assigning specific tasks and responsibilities to individuals according to their skills. In general, experienced individuals should perform the most critical tasks. A major crisis is not a good time for students, interns, or inexperienced residents to practice invasive procedures, although there may be key tasks that they will be suited to perform. Simulation now provides opportunities for inexperienced personnel to learn to manage even time-critical lethal crises.

When skilled help is available it may be useful to delegate *responsibility for specific issues* to a colleague, not just *isolated tasks*. This will allow the individual to make plans, mobilize resources, and distribute the workload. Of course you will need to keep each other apprised of the progress on the various issues.

Ideally, the leader should remain free enough of manual tasks to observe the evolving situation and to direct the team. The team leader should only become involved in manual tasks if specific expertise is *necessary* to ensure their correct and timely completion. This is especially true if the manual task requires intense concentration or imposes limitations on the leader's ability to think and act. If this is the case, the leader must then delegate the responsibility to another team member until that critical task is done. This should be an explicit handover of responsibility.

You should look for overloads and failures in your performance or that of the team. If someone is becoming overloaded, allocate more help to their task or take away some tasks previously assigned to them. If a task is not getting done by one individual, ask someone else to try, either along with or in place of the first individual. If *you* are becoming overloaded, you will have to distribute more tasks to others, if possible, or restrict your own attention only to the most critical items.

Call for Help—Early Enough to Make a Difference

Everyone agrees that it is sometimes best to call for help in managing a patient. For novice anesthesia professionals, this is frequent (in fact they are not expected to perform induction, emergence, and other critical phases of a case without supervision and help). It is less frequent, but still critically important, for experienced anesthesia professionals. Many situations that would spin out of control if help was delayed can be readily resolved with appropriate and timely assistance.

Although the experienced anesthesia professional can handle more alone than the novice can, here are some general criteria for when help is needed that apply to everyone. Help is needed when:

The patient's condition is
- already catastrophically bad (e.g., cardiac arrest; "can't intubate and can't ventilate")
- bad and getting worse (e.g., "can't intubate and getting harder to ventilate")
- not responding to the usual treatments (e.g., hypotension, ST segment depression)
- known to require help to deal with (e.g., major trauma, MH)

Or when you, the primary anesthesia professional,
- need to accomplish more tasks in less time
- are overloaded with task demands
- are not sure what's going on and need a second opinion or
- are asked by another team member if you want some help (if they ask you, chances are you probably could use the help!)

You should determine whether personnel with special skills are needed and mobilize them immediately. Different types of help may be needed or available. It is helpful to articulate what kind of help you really want. It is also important to know how best to use the different types of help that will arrive. Here are some of the kinds of help that may be needed/available:

- Muscle help (more people to lift/move patient or equipment)
- Transport help (people to take items or messages from one place to another)
- Help with a specific technical skill (e.g., someone who can place/interpret the transesophageal echocardiogram; someone who knows how to place a chest tube or perform a tracheostomy)
- General technical skill (nursing or medical)
- Thinking help (another clinician who can help decide what is wrong and what should be done)
- A senior person with more "clout" in the system who can reinforce the decisions of a more junior clinician or who sometimes can more readily overcome administrative barriers

To get the best help, you will need to know in advance who you will call, how you will contact them, and how you will use them when they arrive. In a major OR facility during regular working hours, the assistance needed may be instantly at hand. In fact, in such situations your challenge may be how to utilize the large number of helpers who may show up. However, in smaller facilities, or at night, on weekends, or on holidays there may be little help available. If necessary you may need to call for help from the emergency room or from the ICU, call a hospital-wide "code," or even call 911. If you ask for such assistance, make sure that the staff of the surgical suite know what is going on so that they can direct the help to your location rather than turning them away at the door! You may also need to contact colleagues at home, either for "telementoring" advice over the phone, or to ask them to come in to the hospital to help.

Know How to Utilize the Help Available from Every Member of the Team

Anesthesia Professionals and Surgeons

Other anesthesia professionals and surgeons have a knowledge and skill base similar to yours, so you can use them to perform or supervise critical tasks, for second opinions on difficult decisions, and as a check of your own accuracy and completeness. Most surgeons are better equipped than you to carry out critical procedures such as performing a tracheostomy or insertion of a chest tube. However, some surgeons, especially very specialized physicians such as ophthalmologists, may have less skill at these procedures than you do. You need to take these aspects of the situation into account as you plan for the next steps of an evolving crisis.

Nurses and Technicians

Skilled nonanesthesia professional personnel (nurses, anesthesia technicians) can be used for tasks within their scope of training. They also are likely to know where to find drugs and equipment. Try to avoid sending all the skilled personnel out of the room for minor tasks when you may need them to help you manage something more critical.

Nonmedical Personnel

Even personnel with no medical training, such as orderlies and housekeepers, can be used for important tasks under your direction. They can obtain supplies, remove trash, or help you move the patient. They can also be employed as runners to external resources such as the blood bank, laboratory, or pharmacy. If you use them as runners, make sure that they know where to go and that they have clear messages to convey or specific instructions on what to bring back to you.

Briefing the Helpers

How you brief the incoming helpers can be critical, especially when they are skilled clinicians. On the one hand, they need to know enough about what is going on and what has already been done to be most effective at rendering assistance. On the other hand, you can channel their thinking so much (taking them "down the garden path") that they cannot effectively act as a "fresh set of eyes." A quick synopsis of the situation should be followed by any request for a time-critical task and then an invitation to double-check and verify important data. Many health care settings have been encouraging the use of the SBAR protocol for briefings, especially in nursing.[28] SBAR stands for "situation, background, assessment, and recommendations/requests." This structure is intended to be a template for a very succinct and focused description of what is going on and what is needed. When anesthesia professionals come to the aid of their colleagues, the SBAR approach is an appropriate guide. Each element may be much abbreviated while still communicating the essence of the crisis.

Optimize Your Actions

As you begin to take action in response to a crisis, it will be important to structure your activities in an optimal fashion. If the patient's condition is deteriorating, you should quickly perform "generic" actions that buy time for more definitive ones. The initial life-support protocol is one example. In a crisis, escalate *rapidly* to therapies that have a high chance of success if the more routine therapies fail. Never assume that the next action *will* solve the problem. You must constantly be thinking of what to do next in case your current actions cannot be implemented or do not succeed. Think through the consequences of major *irreversible* actions, such as extubation or neuromuscular blockade, *before* initiating them. Once these bridges are burned, you are committed to a course of action from which it may be difficult to recover.

Repeatedly Assess and Reevaluate the Situation

It is critically important to perform a repeated reevaluation of the patient. No crisis manager can be certain of success at any stage in the event. It is crucial to keep thinking ahead (anticipate and plan). Do not *assume* that anything about the situation is certain—double-check all critical items. Anesthetic overdoses, syringe or ampule swaps, vasoactive infusions, and hypoventilation or hypoxia are frequent causes of acute events. Mentally review all the actions that you have taken in the preceding few minutes. Force yourself to look at the vaporizers and any infusions even if you believe that they were not in use.

After initiating critical life-support measures and stabilizing the patient's condition, you can stand back and think more abstractly. Think about the causal chain leading to the problem; try to understand the underlying causes and see that they have been or are being addressed. Remember that any single data source may be erroneous; cross-check redundant data streams to verify important data. Make sure that *all* available data are used, including the surgeon's observations, laboratory data, radiographs, and historical information from the patient's current and old charts.

Fixation Errors

Faulty reevaluation, inadequate plan adaptation, and loss of situation awareness each can result in a type of human error termed *fixation error*.[29] This type of error is extremely common in dynamic situations. Fixation errors are prominent among the performance failures observed by our laboratory's studies of anesthesiologists' responses to simulated critical incidents and occurred among both novice residents and experienced practitioners.

Incorrect initial diagnoses are to be expected given the complexity and uncertainty of the data available to the anesthesia professional. What makes this a fixation error is the *persistent* failure to revise a diagnosis or plan in the face of readily available evidence that suggests a revision is necessary. There are three main types of fixation error that should be understood, namely:

This and only this

This is the persistent failure to revise a diagnosis or plan despite plentiful evidence to the contrary. The available evidence is interpreted to fit the initial diagnosis or attention is allocated to a minor aspect of a major problem.

Everything but this

This is the persistent failure to *commit* to the definitive treatment of a major problem. An extended search for information is made without ever addressing potentially catastrophic conditions.

Everything's OK

This is the persistent belief that no problem is occurring in spite of plentiful evidence that it is. Abnormalities may be attributed to artifacts or transients. A failure to declare an emergency or to accept help when facing a major crisis may stem from denial that a serious situation is actually occurring.

Ways to Break Fixation Errors

The defining aspect of fixation errors is that they persist over time. Therefore continuous reevaluation should be able to prevent them or break them.

For "This and only this"

The very act of repeated reevaluation using all available data is the best antidote for this fixation. Cross-checking of data sources and constant questioning of one's mental model will usually disclose the invalidating evidence.

For "Everything but this"

The question of commitment is a difficult one. At what point do you quit collecting information and "go for it" on the most serious likely occurrence? There is no magic answer, but you should err on the side of providing definitive treatment for any suspected problem that requires it, especially if the risks of treatment are low in comparison with those of the problem. During simulations we have seen this fixation error in the context of MH, in which there is reluctance to admit that such a major event is occurring, and the life-saving treatment is delayed too long.

For "Everything's OK"

Remember that the burden of proof is on you. For every abnormality you must assume that the patient is *not* OK until you satisfy yourself otherwise. Similarly, you must assume that any abnormality represents the worst possible diagnosis until you can determine what is actually going on.

DOCUMENTATION OF CRISES

Your primary task is always to *attend to the patient first*. Never let record keeping prevent you from taking care of the patient; yet, good documentation of a crisis is important to its overall management. It will help you determine what happened and how to avoid further complications throughout the remainder of the case. Your documentation will be critical for meaningful quality assurance review and in defending against possible litigation.

The use of automated record keeping and OR data management systems is becoming more common as part of the overall conversion to electronic health records. The data stored in such systems is often far more granular than the data points on the visible anesthesia record. Even when an automated record system is not in use, most modern patient monitoring systems automatically store considerable trend data to help you later make an accurate reconstruction of the record, or to help you and your colleagues understand what happened after the crisis is over. Other useful data sources include hard-copy printouts made during the case as well as records kept by nurses. Therefore it is extremely helpful to ensure the activation as needed of electronic and human recorders at the first sign of a crisis. At the end of the case, do not allow anyone to turn off or reset any monitors or record keeping equipment until you have verified that data have been permanently stored, or you have made a hard-copy printout of all trend plots and data logs. Depending on the device, there is a risk that the data could become erased. If you are not sure how to make or verify permanent recordings or hard copies, put a sign on the equipment instructing OR staff to leave the electronic equipment alone and find someone else to assist you who is more familiar with the equipment. If enough skilled staff are available during an event, assign one of them the task of being timekeeper and recorder. Make sure that they receive all relevant details about drugs administered and laboratory data (including the time each specimen is sent to the lab).

When multiple data sources are used, it is wise after the event to reconcile the time on all clocks (including the clocks within the monitors). In the absence of a master clock, the various electronic devices, wall clocks, and wristwatches will frequently be out of synchronization by minutes. It is relatively simple for a few people to note the time showing on all clocks approximately simultaneously.

Because taking care of the patient is the most important activity, you must suspend manual recording of vital signs whenever necessary if your full attention must be devoted to the patient. Retrospective reconstruction of the timeline of data is appropriate when it could not be credibly recorded in real time. NEVER ALTER THE RECORD, whether recorded automatically or by hand by you or others. If the anesthesia record or other document contains an error that could influence some aspect of the patient's future care, you can note the corrections in a subsequent entry. If it is absolutely necessary for clarity and ongoing patient management, in the paper record draw a light line through the erroneous entry (to maintain its legibility). Record date and time for every entry you make in the chart. It is especially important to sign or initial any changes you have made. Many automated record keeping systems have audit trails that capture all changes or annotations made to the record.

Debriefing After a Crisis

After a case in which a crisis has occurred it is wise to conduct a debriefing of the team to review what transpired, how the team performed, and what individual, team, and systems lessons can be learned from the event (see Chapter 4 for more details about debriefing techniques). If the event involved, or could result in, serious harm to the patient, this debriefing may need to involve quality/risk management and be constituted as a formal quality management activity. Ideally the debriefing would be conducted for the entire team, including anesthesia personnel, nurses, surgeons, and any other relevant parties, but it may still be valuable even if only the anesthesia personnel debrief themselves. Debriefing should be a constructive self and group critique, not a blame session. Experience with debriefing after simulation sessions has taught us that nearly every challenging situation will have positive and negative aspects of performance to consider. There are few absolutely right or wrong answers, even for medical and technical issues. Rather, usually there are pros and cons to each action, or to each strategy, and the relative merits of the various alternatives can be discussed. When definite errors are identified, personnel should understand that the error was made and should attempt to determine how it happened and how it might be prevented in the future. It does no one any good to deny or overlook distinct errors in care. The focus of debriefing, besides individual growth, should be on systems improvement.

FOLLOW-UP AFTER A MAJOR CRISIS

Stay Involved in the Patient's Care

After a serious perioperative event your responsibility to your patient does not end when the patient is transferred to a ward or to an ICU. In such situations it is even more important than usual for you to stay involved in the case. Make sure that appropriate consultations are obtained as needed to diagnose or manage the patient, to establish a prognosis, or to begin rehabilitation. Be aware that the opinions and statements of surgeons or consultants may not always be correct. Communicate with them and review their notes. Ensure that they are appropriately informed and do not allow any misinformation, speculation, or erroneous conclusions written by consultants to go unchallenged in the record.

Use Your Institution's Follow-up Protocol

Many institutions have a formal protocol for dealing with serious anesthesia-related events. A protocol for this purpose was first developed and published in 1993 by the Risk Management Committee of the Harvard Medical School's Department of Anaesthesia.[30] It is available on the website of the Anesthesia Patient Safety Foundation (http://www.apsf.org/resources_safety_protocol.php). Your institution may have adopted its own protocol—if so, you should follow it. As we have already described, the first item of this protocol is to attend to the patient. The next step is to contact the head of the department or the clinical practice. Someone from the anesthesia practice needs to take charge of the follow-up activities.

A second important feature of any protocol is the necessity of impounding any equipment or supplies that could be at fault. This is done not only to preserve the physical record of what transpired for possible quality management or root cause analysis, but also to ensure that any faults are corrected so that other patients are not injured. It is tragic enough to have a failure contribute to the injury of one patient, but sequential injuries to multiple patients have been known to occur. Make sure that the next patient does not also suffer as a result of an uncorrected failure.

Even if it is unlikely that equipment failures played any role in the event, the Harvard protocol recommends a routine inspection before the equipment is returned to service. If there is any suspicion of a drug problem, ampule swap, or syringe swap, you should impound all syringes, ampules, vials, sharps containers, and trash. It may be necessary to examine the vials, ampules, or syringes used or even to have assays of their contents conducted. If there is any question of equipment failure, the equipment should be stored in a secure location and labeled "Do Not Touch," and it should not be altered or manipulated in any way. Especially if equipment is a likely suspect in the event, resist the impulse to experiment with the equipment to determine whether a fault occurred; you might impede discovery of the real cause.

You may also have a responsibility to report the failure to the manufacturer and (in the United States) to the FDA under the Safe Medical Devices Reporting Act. Similarly, if problems or contamination of a drug is found, you may need to inform the FDA. The risk management, biomedical engineering service, and pharmacy departments of your institution should be able to help you determine whether and how to make such reports.

The Medical Record

You should ensure that the medical record is complete, including an appropriate summary of the event. Make sure that the record truthfully reflects what happened; to the best of your ability reconstruct it objectively. Record the *facts* of the case as you know them, not speculation or interpretation. When you contact your insurance carrier, your attorney may ask you to write a separate summary of the event. Such a document may be shielded from discovery under attorney-client privilege. Be careful not to speculate about the events with other personnel except as necessary to provide proper care to the patient or as part of duly constituted quality assurance. These conversations could be discoverable in litigation, and any ill-considered speculations about what might have happened may later create unnecessary difficulties in defending your actions.

There is some controversy about what to do with hard-copy printouts and strip charts from monitors; should they be placed in the patient's chart, attached to the quality assurance report, kept elsewhere, or discarded? If printouts are placed in some charts and not others, serious questions could be raised about how the decision to place the printouts was made. If the printouts are attached to the quality assurance report, they may not be admissible in court to support your case without releasing the entire quality assurance file on the case. Discarding the printouts will impede the quality assurance process in determining what happened and what, if any, changes are needed to avoid similar events in the future. You should consult with risk managers and attorneys before adopting an institutional or departmental policy.

Speak with the Patient's Family

Whenever a serious crisis has occurred in the OR, it will be necessary to inform the patient and/ or the family or guardian. There is a growing movement to expand what patients and families are told about adverse events and about any errors in care that may have occurred. Policies and standards on this issue have been adopted by The Joint Commission (www.jointcommission.org), the National Patient Safety Foundation (www.npsf.org), and the Veterans Health Administration, among others.[31] There is now general agreement that disclosure of errors affecting care or outcome is necessary, although there remains controversy on the topic. A review article in 2012 by Souter and colleagues[31] gives a good overview of the issues. Several other articles provide guidance on how to deliver bad news to patients or families.[32-36] Although you may never have to disclose a death or serious injury related to anesthesia care, the principles in these sources apply not only to major catastrophes, but to all sorts of unexpected news. Nearly all anesthesia professionals will need to discuss with patients or families less serious but still unwelcome outcomes (such as unexpected hospitalization after ambulatory surgery, or unexpected admission to the ICU).

Several models of disclosure have been articulated and different ones are in use at different institutions. These models include (a) having a single person from the institution—usually a risk manager—responsible for all disclosures in concert with the relevant clinician; (b) having a team of disclosure experts to help clinicians; (c) training many clinicians to be disclosure experts themselves; (d) just-in-time disclosure coaching, in which the relevant clinician(s) conducts the disclosure session following a predisclosure coaching session with an expert.[37] If your institution has these resources, they should be used whenever possible. However, in our experience it may not always be possible to mobilize risk managers or coaches in time for the initial contact between the anesthesiologist and the patient or family after an event has occurred. Regardless of the disclosure model, it is very important that whenever possible you and the surgeon should speak to the patient or family together. Practically speaking, this is sometimes difficult when the patient is alive but critically ill, because you are likely to be involved in stabilizing or transporting the patient long after at least one of the senior surgeons is free. If the surgeon can wait until you are available, this is ideal. In the event that the surgeon or someone else has already discussed the situation with the patient or family, you should still speak with them as soon as you can. This will give you a chance to explain anesthesia-related issues more accurately and thoroughly than what has been conveyed by others, and allows you to (re)establish a relationship with the patient or family for the ongoing discussions of the patient's status and the determinations of what happened.

When discussing the case with the family, outline the steps currently being taken to care for the patient. Once again, tell the family the *facts* of the case as you know them, not speculation as to what might have happened. As Bryan Liang, MD, PhD, JD, puts it:

The theme of disclosure and all resultant discussions with the patient and/or the family should be objectivity. A descriptive method is important substantively because a full systems assessment generally has not been completed by the health care entity. Any conclusions regarding the error are therefore premature at best and misleading at worst, and, again, they may have negative legal consequences as an admission of fault.[37]

If a definitive explanation of the event is already known unequivocally, you can communicate it (e.g., for a case of one of the authors, during a redo sternotomy for cardiac surgery, the reciprocating chest saw transected the aorta, and despite resuscitative efforts the patient died—what happened was really not in question). More commonly, even though you may suspect a cause, its likelihood is still uncertain. In such cases, after stating the facts regarding what happened, let the patient and/or family know that the situation is being analyzed carefully, generally how such an analysis is conducted, and that there will be continued communication with them regarding the review.[37] You can correct any misconceptions that the family may have by your explanation of the facts, but try not to make your explanations too complex.

There is some debate about how any expressions of empathy or sorrow (e.g., "We are so sorry that this event has occurred to you.") should be made because of the legal complexities about such statements in different jurisdictions. General expressions of empathy and sorrow are probably all right, whereas expressions of specific personal regret or sorrow could be problematic. As of 2011, 36 jurisdictions had adopted laws that prevent statements of sorrow (e.g., sympathy or benevolence), on their own, to be admissible in court and used against clinicians. Statements of fault may still be admissible. A few states have similarly shielded the statement of an apology, in and of itself, from being used against the clinician during litigation (see, e.g., http://www.ncsl.org/issues-research/banking/medical-liability-medical-malpractice-laws. aspx). You may wish to determine the laws on these matters where you practice.

Regardless of the circumstances of the initial contact with the patient or family after an event, you will need to inform a variety of parties, including your practice, your institution (presumably risk management), and your insurer. If you are in an academic setting, a large multidisciplinary group practice, an independent group, or a solo practice, your legal situation may be quite different for each venue. If you are an independent practitioner not employed by the same institution as the hospital or surgicenter, you will still have certain responsibilities to the institution as a member of the professional staff. You should fully understand the legal relationships among you, your practice, and the institution.

Quality Management Reporting Systems

Because there are usually systems causes for an event, the same thing is likely to happen again to somebody else. Only changes in the way the system does business are likely to have a widespread and lasting beneficial effect. Analyzing events and planning systems changes is beyond the scope and ability of individual anesthesia professionals or the crew involved in a particular case. Event reporting and analysis systems applicable to the case will vary. Anesthesia departments are required to have internal quality assurance and quality improvement programs. They also typically have a confidential morbidity and mortality (M&M) conference where difficult cases are discussed.

Therefore, after any salient event, you should complete your department's standard quality assurance report and attach a copy of the anesthesia record and any summaries that you have put in the chart. This will ensure that you and your colleagues can thoroughly review the events of the case in the appropriate quality assurance forum. Make sure that all quality assurance materials are appropriately labeled "Confidential Quality Assurance Document." Do not share these confidential documents or information with family members; they exist solely for the purpose of evaluating and improving patient care.

You should submit a report to a confidential or anonymous external reporting system. Each country may have one or more systems for submitting reports. For example, for more than 4 years Germany has had the Confidential Incident Reporting System—https://www.cirs-ains.de/). In the United States, an event reporting system allowing either confidential or anonymous reporting has been operated since 2011 by the Anesthesia Quality Institute (AQI)—the Anesthesia Incident Reporting System (AIRS—https://www.aqihq.org/airs/airsIntro.aspx). Because AQI is a federally qualified Patient Safety Organization under the Patient Safety and Quality Improvement Act of 2005 (Patient Safety Act), reports to AIRS and its work products are shielded from discovery in litigation.

Stress Management for the Anesthesia Professional After a Perioperative Catastrophe

Caring for a patient who suffers a perioperative catastrophe can be extremely stressful. In some cases the stress can degrade your performance capabilities, and it can adversely affect both your mental and physical health.[38,39] Syndromes analogous to posttraumatic stress disorder can develop. Despite the fact that survey results indicate that most anesthesiologists have gone back to clinical work immediately after a catastrophic case,[38] we advise that unless emergency patient care requires it, you should *insist* that someone else complete the rest of your assigned cases. Even when emergencies require your immediate attention, you should seek relief from other members of your practice as soon as they can come in. Remember that the other patients should receive the complete attention of their anesthesia professional.

Anesthesia residents or student nurse anesthetists may need special attention after a catastrophe, whether or not they were in any way responsible. Often they are shunted aside to let more experienced personnel manage the crisis. But they may make premature judgments of what the event means for their suitability for anesthesia practice. Attending staff or supervisors should be sensitive to the impact of a catastrophe or patient death on their students. The role of prophylactic therapy using "critical incident stress management" or "psychological debriefing" (a psychotherapeutic technique distinct from clinical debriefing) is controversial. Evidence-based reviews of randomized controlled trials did not show any benefit—or indeed suggested some risk of damage—when these techniques are used for primary and secondary victims of traumatic events.[40] Whereas other reviews[41] argue that the studies and systematic reviews each have flaws that call into question the conclusion that these prophylactic techniques are inadvisable, the overall consensus at this time appears to be that immediate psychological debriefing is not required.

Short- or long-term support services for anesthesia professionals and other OR personnel who have been involved in an OR catastrophe may be available if they need it, either through the anesthesia department under the aegis of the department chief or within the institution through the medical staff office or risk manager. These offices or your own insurer or attorney may also be able to assist you in seeking professional advice or counseling should you require it.

REFERENCES

1. Billings CE, Reynard WD. Human factors in aircraft incidents: results of a 7 year study. Aviat Space Environ Med 1984;55:960-5.
2. Ruffell-Smith H. A simulator study of the interaction of pilot workload with errors, vigilance, and decisions. (Technical memo 78482) Moffett Field, Calif: NASA-Ames Research Center; 1979.
3. Howard SK, Rosekind MR, Katz JD, Berry AJ. Fatigue in anesthesia: implications and strategies for patient and provider safety. Anesthesiology 2002;97:1281-94.
4. Smith-Coggins R, Howard SK, Mac DT, et al. Improving alertness and performance in emergency department physicians and nurses: the use of planned naps. Ann Emerg Med 2006;48:596-604 604 e1-3.
5. Rall M, Gaba D, Howard S, Dieckmann P. Human performance and patient safety. In: Miller R, Eriksson L, Fleisher L, Wiener-Kronish J, Young W, editors. Miller's anesthesia. 7th ed. Philadelphia: Churchill Livingstone; 2010.
6. Aeronautical decision making. Advisory circular number 60-22. Washington, DC: Federal Aviation Administration; 1991.
7. Keyser L. Apollo experience report: The role of flight mission rules in mission preparation and conduct (NASA TN D-7822). Washington, DC; 1974.
8. van Klei WA, Moons KG, Rutten CL, et al. The effect of outpatient preoperative evaluation of hospital inpatients on cancellation of surgery and length of hospital stay. Anesth Analg 2002;94:644-9 table of contents.
9. Stone M, Dismukes K, Remington R. Prospective memory in dynamic environments: effects of load, delay, and phonological rehearsal. Memory 2001;9:165-76.
10. Dieckmann P, Reddersen S, Wehner T, Rall M. Prospective memory failures as an unexplored threat to patient safety: results from a pilot study using patient simulators to investigate the missed execution of intentions. Ergonomics 2006;49:526-43.
11. Loukopoulos L, Dismukes R, Barshi I. The multitasking myth. Farnham, England: Ashgate Publishing Limited; 2009.
12. Neily J, DeRosier JM, Mills PD, et al. Awareness and use of a cognitive aid for anesthesiology. Jt Comm J Qual Patient Saf 2007;33:502-11.
13. Harrison TK, Manser T, Howard SK, Gaba DM. Use of cognitive aids in a simulated anesthetic crisis. Anesth Analg 2006;103:551-6.
14. Burden AR, Carr ZJ, Staman GW, Littman JJ, Torjman MC. Does every code need a "reader"? Improvement of rare event management with a cognitive aid "reader" during a simulated emergency: a pilot study. Simul Healthc 2012;7:1-9.
15. Ziewacz JE, Arriaga AF, Bader AM, et al. Crisis checklists for the operating room: development and pilot testing. J Am Coll Surg 2011;213:212-7 e10.
16. Arriaga AF, Bader AM, Wong JM, et al. Simulation-based trial of surgical-crisis checklists. N Engl J Med 2013;368:246-53.
17. Gaba DM. Perioperative cognitive aids in anesthesia: what, who, how, and why bother? Anesth Analg 2013;117:1033-6.
18. Augoustides JG, Atkins J, Kofke WA. Much ado about checklists: who says I need them and who moved my cheese? Anesth Analg 2013;117:1037-8.
19. Goldhaber-Fiebert SN, Howard SK. Implementing emergency manuals: can cognitive aids help translate best practices for patient care during acute events? Anesth Analg 2013;117:1149-61.
20. Tobin JM, Grabinsky A, McCunn M, et al. A checklist for trauma and emergency anesthesia. Anesth Analg 2013;117:1178-84.

21. Marshall S. The use of cognitive aids during emergencies in anesthesia: a review of the literature. Anesth Analg 2013;116:1162–71.

22. Chu L, Fuller A. Manual of clinical anesthesiology. Philadelphia: Lippincott Williams & Wilkins; 2011.

23. Gawande A. The checklist manifesto: how to get things right. New York: Metropolitan Books; 2009.

24. Atlee JL, Bernstein AD. Cardiac rhythm management devices (part II): perioperative management. Anesthesiology 2001;95:1492-506.

25. Cooper JB, Long CD, Newbower RS, Philip JH. Critical incidents associated with intraoperative exchanges of anesthesia personnel. Anesthesiology 1982;56:456-61.

26. Weinger MB, Herndon OW, Gaba DM. The effect of electronic record keeping and transesophageal echocardiography on task distribution, workload, and vigilance during cardiac anesthesia. [see comments] Anesthesiology 1997;87:144-55 discussion 29A-30A.

27. Tenney Y, Adams M, Pew R, Huggins A, Rogers W. A principled approach to the measurement of situation awareness in commercial aviation. (NASA contractor report 4451) Washington, DC: National Aeronautics and Space Administration; 1992.

28. Haig KM, Sutton S, Whittington J. SBAR: a shared mental model for improving communication between clinicians. Jt Comm J Qual Patient Saf 2006;32:167-75.

29. De Keyser V, Woods D. Fixation errors: failures to revise situation assessment in dynamic and risky systems. In: Colombo A, Saiz de Bustamonte A, editors. Systems reliability assessment. Dordrecht, The Netherlands: Kluwer Academic Publishers; 1990. p. 231-51.

30. Cooper J, Cullen D, Eichhorn J, Philip J, Holzman R. Administrative guidelines for response to an adverse anesthesia event. J Clin Anesth 1993;5:79-84.

31. Souter KJ, Gallagher TH. The disclosure of unanticipated outcomes of care and medical errors: what does this mean for anesthesiologists? Anesth Analg 2012;114:615-21.

32. Buckman R. How to break bad news: a guide for health care professionals. Baltimore: The Johns Hopkins University Press; 1992.

33. Iverson K. Grave words: notifying survivors about sudden, unexpected deaths. Tucson: Galen Press; 1999.

34. Bacon A. Death on the table. Anaesthesia 1989;44:245-8.

35. Bacon A. Major anaesthetic mishaps – handling the aftermath. Curr Anaesth Crit Care 1990;1:253-7.

36. Full Disclosure Working Group. When things go wrong: responding to adverse events. Boston: Massachusetts Coalition for the Prevention of Medical Errors; 2006.

37. Liang BA. A system of medical error disclosure. Qual Saf Health Care 2002;11:64-8.

38. Gazoni FM, Amato PE, Malik ZM, Durieux ME. The impact of perioperative catastrophes on anesthesiologists: results of a national survey. Anesth Analg 2012;114:596-603.

39. Martin TW, Roy RC. Cause for pause after a perioperative catastrophe: one, two, or three victims? Anesth Analg 2012;114:485-7.

40. Rose S, Bisson J, Churchill R, Wesley S. Psychological debriefing for preventing post traumatic stress disorder (PTSD). Art. No.: CD000560 Cochrane Database Syst Rev 2002;2002:1-45.

41. Hawker D, Durkin J, Hawker D. To debrief or not to debrief our heroes: that is the question. Clin Psychol Psychother 2011;18:453-63.

Chapter 3

Teaching Anesthesia Crisis Resource Management

This book attempts to lay out the principles of learning and teaching anesthesia crisis resource management (ACRM) in anesthesia practice. Although the principles can be summarized in a book, and even represented on a single reminder graphic, mastering and honing these skills requires various sorts of hands-on practice. Some practice can occur during real patient care. Principles of teamwork and decision making are exercised in almost every case during the delivery of patient care even when everything runs smoothly. In fact, for everyday clinical work, perhaps the issue is not lack of practice but rather that routine work can make people complacent. Perhaps with the exception of those administering anesthesia near the battlefield, in busy trauma centers, or with high volumes of unusually ill patients, the challenges of everyday cases are small compared with those seen when things go wrong. Thus many aspects of crisis management are likely to become rusty unless special mechanisms are put in place to counter this natural trend.

How, then, should people organize to teach ACRM skills? First, there are a variety of ways to become highly conversant with the principles of ACRM, and these are described in detail in Chapters 1 and 2. Being conversant with the principles means more than just knowing about them or being able to answer multiple choice questions about them. It means being able to explain them and then to recognize them when discussing cases or videos of cases (real or simulated). Finally, it means to be able to enact the principles when called upon to do so. Simulation—using various modalities—is an important technique for teaching, learning, and practicing ACRM, although it is neither the only way to do so nor the only way to get started.

METHODS TO LEARN THE PRINCIPLES OF ACRM

Articulating Key Points

One technique that we have used successfully to help people become more conversant in the principles of ACRM involves using a list of ACRM key points without describing the meaning or subelements for each point. With a group, we may hand each member an 8.5×11-inch laminated sheet, each with a different key point printed on it. We then ask each individual to describe for the group the meaning of that key point—as if explaining it to a novice. The instructor and the group then probe the individual for more clarification, and the group as a whole discusses the point and its relationship to other key points and to the issues raised in the discussion. This continues for all members of the group and/or for as many key points as time allows.

Identifying and Discussing Key Points of ACRM in "Trigger Videos"

The term "trigger video" refers to a video that is used to trigger discussion about specific issues, often those with significant affective components. Trigger videos can be created locally for specific purposes. In our experience, effective trigger videos can be made by an experienced simulation team using existing audiovisual resources and without extensive script development or acting talent. Some completed trigger videos may be available for download from online health care education resources such as the MedEd Portal operated by the Association of American Medical Colleges (AAMC—https://www.mededportal.org/). Use of this portal is free to the public, requiring only registration. One of our group's trigger videos depicting a simulation of an intraoperative cardiac arrest is available at the MedEd Portal (https://www.mededportal.org/publication/7826).

It is also possible to use commercial films or videos created for entertainment as trigger videos. For example, for more than 24 years we have used a segment from an episode of the Public Broadcasting System's NOVA television program ("Why Planes Crash") depicting a reenactment of what transpired in the cockpit during a classic airliner crash (Eastern 401).

Our European simulation colleagues, Peter Dieckmann, PhD, and Marcus Rall, MD, have highlighted the use of portions of Hollywood movies as trigger videos. Based on their advice, we frequently use the opening decision-making sequence of the film *Master and Commander: The Far Side of the World* (2003, Twentieth Century Fox, Miramax Films, Universal Studios) to trigger discussion of crisis resource management (CRM) issues, or as the basis for an exemplar role-play of a debriefing.

Using such generic videos as a vehicle for learners to recognize elements of CRM and to apply them to health care has some advantages. In general, no one in the learner group— possibly composed of individuals from various fields of health care—is an expert in the domain of the nonmedical film, thus putting everyone on an even footing. This methodology also reinforces that the key points of ACRM are really about fundamental issues of human performance and thus apply to everybody.

Regardless of the source or type of trigger videos, exactly how they are used is important. As the name *trigger video* suggests, merely showing the video is typically not sufficient; the instructor must use the film as a trigger for recognition and discussion of the key aspects of performance related to the learning objectives of the exercise. The same techniques and processes used in facilitating a simulation debriefing apply to facilitating the discussion of a trigger video.

One important way trigger videos can be used is to dramatically illustrate issues of hindsight bias. This ubiquitous human bias means that one's perceptions or analysis of a situation are strongly affected by already knowing its outcome; this is sometimes referred to as the "I knew it all along" phenomenon. Hindsight bias can be very difficult to prevent or ignore, even when people try to avoid it; thus it is ideal to present situations without the eventual outcome being known. By pausing a video before viewers learn the outcome, the viewers can discuss decisions and actions made by the protagonists in terms of what was known at the time. Similarly, if the same video is viewed without pause, the potential for hindsight bias can be made clear. Issues of hindsight bias in debriefing of simulation scenarios are discussed more fully in Chapter 4.

Analyzing Real or Simulated Cases Using the Three-Column Technique

Another technique we often use with groups is the analysis of interesting cases divided into three categories: (a) the *medical/technical* issues of care; (b) the examples of the use or nonuse of the *key points of ACRM*; and (c) the various *systems issues* underlying why things transpired the way they did, or system-oriented mechanisms to prevent errors or failures. Typically, we list each of these categories as a heading of a column on a whiteboard. At various pauses in the case narrative, we facilitate a discussion of the relevant elements for each column that were observed or triggered by the preceding case segment. The key thrust of this approach is to help learners see the interrelationships between medical/technical decisions and the actions that resulted from those decisions, and between the CRM issues and the organizations and systems they affect. These interrelationships often explain why people behave the way they do or reveal the interventions that might be most effective in preventing such adverse events from recurring.

This technique is equally applicable to analyzing simulation scenarios or to real cases, as in morbidity and mortality conferences or when swapping clinical "war stories." The three-column technique can be used whether or not there is a video of the case.

THE ROLE OF SIMULATION IN TEACHING ACRM

The previous sections of this chapter illustrate that simulation is not absolutely necessary to teach people about ACRM. When simulation is not feasible, facilitated discussions are a useful way to engage individuals in learning about these principles. Nonetheless, more than 24 years ago, we adapted the aviation paradigm of CRM for health care specifically in the context of developing a simulation-oriented approach to teaching.[1-3] As a core technique used to optimize learning and practice of ACRM, we believe that simulation has enormous advantages,[4] including that it:

- Forces learners to walk the walk, not just talk the talk
- Allows practice in a controlled, psychologically safe environment
- Allows situations that challenge behavioral aspects such as communication or leadership and followership as well as the medical/technical aspects
- Allows self-reflection with feedback from peers and experts
- Allows team members to discuss care outside of caring for real patients
- Allows discussion of hierarchy

In discussing simulation more fully, it is important to remember that it is a "technique, not a technology."[5] Simulation applicable to ACRM can be conducted in many different and complementary ways, some of which require no technology at all. Thus there are various "modalities" of simulation to consider, each with its own pros and cons. Simulations that challenge the anesthesia professional's decision making can be conducted with little or no physical realism or technology. Verbal simulation—asking "What would you do if…"—is one technique. Such verbal simulation and questioning has formed an important component of examination for specialty board certification for decades. An enhancement to verbal simulation is to use apps available for smartphones or tablets that can display and modify waveforms and numerics as if on a physiologic monitor. One downside of verbal simulation is that there are many people can "say it, "but they can't" do it." Other people can recognize a situation when the information is fed to them but when they have many different things to attend to, they do not do as well picking up cues and responding to them sensibly.

Another low-technology technique that concentrates on the behavioral skills of ACRM is role-playing. Participants interact with each other while playing the role of themselves or another team member or instructor. The goal of the interaction is to probe and challenge participants to actually *say* the things they would say in a particular situation rather than to simply describe what they *think* should be said. For example, it is one thing to suggest how best to word a conversation with a surgeon; it is another thing to actually "play it out" with someone acting in the role of surgeon. As described earlier in this book, choice of words, manner of speaking, and tone of voice are all critical to optimal interaction with other team members. Role-playing can be useful for practicing the interactions between professionals, including team members, outside consultants, patients, or family members.

A number of simulators that go by the rubric "on-screen simulator" or "microsimulator" are available. These are similar to computer games or programs—like the venerable Microsoft Flight Simulator—that present all aspects of a simulated world on the computer screen, with interaction via devices such as a mouse, joystick, or specialty inputs. These simulators are quite good at presenting some aspects of reality, including monitor waveforms, photos, animations, or videos of the patient, but are less useful, for example, at providing direct interaction between team members, although an on-screen simulation could potentially be used by a group, and could be combined with a role-playing exercise.

A nascent modality of simulation is the online, multiplayer, virtual world. Here, each individual can have an "avatar," co-located in a single virtual environment presented on the computer screen. Avatars can act in the virtual world and they can interact with other avatars (sometimes only by text messages, but often by voice). Such virtual worlds can, in principle, marry the on-screen simulator with team interaction. Advantages include lower cost and no need for team members to be located in the same physical space (in fact, in principle they can each be in opposite "corners of the globe"). As of early 2014, there are a few virtual worlds in health care, but many are still rudimentary and it is uncertain whether they can provide the clinical challenge and interactivity needed for ACRM training. However, they may improve in the future and could become important adjuncts to other modalities of simulation.

The ultimate in simulation would be full-blown virtual reality, a technique that would create experiences that are indistinguishable from the real world. The current modalities of virtual reality encompass either systems with devices like head-mounted displays and datagloves (which can provide powerful "immersion" but limited interactivity) or computer augmented virtual environments, that have multiple, large, high-resolution displays, typically occupying several walls of a room. The latter approach can provide virtual immersion while allowing for multiple players in both the virtual and physical space. Combining participants in the physical space (possibly with a mannequin and clinical equipment) with participants, "scenery," or tools in the virtual space is known as mixed reality simulation. Perhaps in the future, such virtual experiences may allow certain kinds of ACRM simulation that are hard to accomplish with any other modality.

Physical Simulation Using Mannequin-Based Simulation and Clinical Equipment

Mannequin-based simulation is the modality of simulation that is most commonly used to teach, practice, and hone ACRM skills. A computerized mannequin that can provide a number of physical cues (e.g., breath sounds, heart sounds, palpable pulses, etc.) and that allows various physical interventions (e.g., endotracheal intubation; IV drug administration) is combined with real clinical equipment (e.g., anesthesia machine) and with all the relevant personnel to present scenarios. The scenarios for ACRM training are usually chosen to incorporate challenges about decision making and actions regarding the medical and technical situation (often serious but uncommon events, such as anaphylaxis, MH, and myocardial ischemia) along with challenges in terms of interpersonal interaction and team management. Such simulations attempt to marry the physical elements inherent in real clinical care with the challenges of dynamic decision making and behavioral skills that are at the core of ACRM. This all comes at a price in terms of logistics, cost, efficiency, and realism. Plastic mannequins are poor substitutes for human beings. Not all interventions can be carried out as they would be in real patients. Getting a real OR team together in one room can be logistically difficult. Even conducting simulations with role-players who are the confederate of the instructor is expensive and difficult in practice. Some mannequin-based simulations can be conducted in situ in real patient care areas (the OR suite, for example), but others may be best accomplished in a stand-alone simulation center, which itself is an expensive proposition. Nonetheless, a large number of sites have been conducting ACRM-like simulations for anesthesia professionals. Thus it is appropriate to describe this kind of training, at least as we conduct it, and to discuss various aspects of using simulation for this purpose.

CHOICES, CHOICES, CHOICES

The field of simulation is quite diverse. Even narrowing it down to the use of mannequin-based simulation as a mechanism to focus on the key points of ACRM (rather than only focusing on the medical/technical aspects of cases), the instructor has many choices to make.[4]

Single Discipline or Combined Team?

One key choice is whether to target participants from a single discipline—such as anesthesia professionals—or to bring together teams from multiple disciplines and domains, teams of people who work together or might work together. There are pros and cons to each approach (Table 3-1). Because these approaches complement each other, the ideal situation would be to conduct single-discipline training for all members of the team and supplement it with periodic combined-team sessions.

Where to Conduct Simulation? In a Dedicated Center or In Situ?

Simulation is not necessarily conducted in a fancy simulation center. It can be done in situ, that is, in the actual work environment. For ACRM, such sites could include a clinic room, an OR, a PACU bay, or a room in an ICU. In any of these cases, the only dedicated simulation space needed is to store the mannequin when not in use. Even for those with the luxury of having a dedicated simulation center, a decision must be made whether to conduct a simulation activity in the center or in situ, because there are advantages and disadvantages to each technique, as shown in Table 3-2.

In the ideal world, one would conduct some activities in the dedicated center to take advantage of the control, sequestration, and neutral ground, while conducting other activities in situ to reap the benefits of training in the real world and the attendant systems probing that is possible.

TABLE 3-1	PROS AND CONS OF SINGLE-DISCIPLINE VS. COMBINED-TEAM TRAINING PARADIGMS	
Approach	**Pros**	**Cons**
Single discipline	Can conduct simulations with loosely scripted role-players (confederates) in roles of nonanesthesia personnel, thus providing appropriate inter-individual, inter-crew interaction Allows focus to be on issues of greatest importance to anesthesia professionals Logistically simpler to have only anesthesia professionals Allows presentation of a spectrum of behavior by nonanesthesia personnel	Does not train real teams to work as a team Markedly less learning for nonanesthesia personnel (small spillover from single-discipline sessions)
Combined team	Trains real teams to work together as a team Possible to leverage team training to change real-world safety culture Facilitates seeing issues from nonanesthesia perspectives; may allow cross-training	Logistically complex to bring entire team together at the same time Needs of each discipline may not be met Participants experience the personality and behaviors only of the personnel present at that session

TABLE 3-2 PROS AND CONS OF SIMULATIONS IN DEDICATED CENTERS VS. IN SITU

Approach	Pros	Cons
Dedicated center	Logistics are simple Optimal control over environment, including audiovisual system; setup can be done in advance Participants sequestered from demands of clinical care "Neutral ground"—not the real care environment with attendant memories and bad habits Cost of supplies can be reduced because outdated or simulated drugs, or blemished/reused supplies, can be used	Requires participants to travel—even if just on foot—to Simulation Center site (away from patient care areas) Not the real care environment—lack of systems probing of pitfalls of the real setting
In situ	The real care area, with all the familiarity and pitfalls of the actual site of work, facilitates "systems probing" Guarantees actual clinical equipment and procedures as per real work Does not require travel time of participants	Availability and logistics can be difficult and advance setup usually impossible; simulation may need to be canceled or aborted to allow real patient care Limited control over environment, including suboptimal audiovisual system Participants more vulnerable to being pulled back to clinical work Added expense of using actual clinical supplies

Is the Activity Scheduled, or Is It an Emergency "Surprise" to Participants? (Especially for In Situ Simulation)

Simulations can be conducted as prescheduled activities. In this case, everyone knows there will be a simulation exercise at a certain date and time, and that it is an exercise. Alternatively, a simulation can be a surprise for a team of clinicians. The simulation can be set up, say in an OR or pediatric acute care unit, and an emergency or code paged as if it were the real thing. When done this way, the participants do not know that it is a simulation until they hit the door of the room. Surprise mock events also can be run in the dedicated simulation center, although the location gives away the surprise. The main advantage to a surprise event, especially if conducted in situ, is that it taps the characteristics of an emergency team assembling in real time at the patient's bedside. Such surprise events are most frequently conducted for mock cardiac arrests or rapid response team calls. The surprise aspect melds well with the in situ aspect when it comes to systems probing, that is, identifying ways in which the overall organization and culture of patient care at a given site or with a given team interact with the physical environment to generate successes and failures in managing challenging clinical situations. When there is time to think ahead, problems in the system can be more easily accommodated or mitigated. When everything happens unexpectedly, hidden vulnerabilities can be revealed.

In situ simulation can also be used to probe the readiness of a new clinical facility to start real patient care and to uncover and help correct systems problems at the site and with the facility's operational procedures. At the same time, the simulations can help train personnel who will work there to be prepared for their new environment.

Should Everyone Play Their Own Role During Simulations?

With single-discipline simulations, other clinical roles may be played by actors, who in fact may be clinicians from that domain who have been hired or are volunteering to play a scripted role. When scripted individuals are acting on behalf of the instructor, they are called "confederates" and are working in association with the instructor. Sometimes a course participant is asked to be a confederate in a scenario. For example, in our ACRM simulation course, participants rotate through the role of the scrub technician. This person does not know the nature of the scenario and is tasked with assisting the confederate surgeon—typically played by an anesthesiologist instructor—who is pretending to do the surgery. The scrub technician sees things unfold from the viewpoint of a member of the surgical team, seeing and hearing bits and pieces occurring on the other side of the "ether screen." In ICU or ward settings, anesthesia professionals may be asked to play the role of the ICU nurse so that they gain the perspective of nursing staff as they assess the patient and respond to physician orders.

When playing a scripted role, we sometimes ask confederate actors to be less astute or less independently helpful than usual to put more burden on the anesthesia professional participant to react, decide, and lead. Surgeons are typically played as preoccupied with the surgery and not extensively familiar with anesthetic or medical problems. Although such scripts do not, of course, represent the best performance in these professions, they are within the spectrum of clinical response that is frequently observed, and such scripts provide more challenge to the anesthesiology participants than they would encounter if the other personnel were extremely knowledgeable and helpful.

CHARACTERISTICS OF SCENARIOS FOR USE IN ACRM TRAINING

To be useful for ACRM training rather than just for the "drill and practice" that might be relevant to learning specific clinical or psychomotor skills, simulation scenarios usually have special requirements, as follows:

- Team interaction is required. Members of the rest of the clinical team are fully interactive, whether played by real clinicians (combined-team training) or by confederates acting in the roles. Confederates often are clinicians because lay actors, no matter how skilled, usually do not have enough domain knowledge to improvise sufficiently well to respond to the various clinical queries or discussions that can arise in a challenging scenario.
- Interpersonal challenges are represented. Whether inherent in the natural team interaction, or scripted as specific learning objectives, most scenarios require handling interpersonal issues, whether among clinical team members, with patients, or with family or friends of the patient.
- The usual treatment responses are insufficient to solve the problem. Especially for house staff and experienced clinicians, scenarios typically present situations in which the usual actions are either unfeasible or will not succeed. Worst-case scenarios are common. This forces clinicians to think not only about their usual "plan A" or even "plan B," but to flexibly consider and execute plans "C, D, E," and so on.
- A single diagnosis or etiology is not obvious. A benefit of simulation is that the true cause of an event can be known (unlike real cases in which the actual cause is often unclear). However, many scenarios present confounding information that suggests several possible

TABLE 3-3	CATEGORIES OF ADDITIONAL INFORMATION IN SCENARIOS (THE "HERRINGS"*)	
Category	**Definition**	**Example**
Red herring (distractor)	Information that is completely unrelated to what is actually wrong with the patient	Patient with ruptured aortic aneurysm and a history of sinusitis
Green herring (confounder)	Information that *could be related* to what is actually wrong with the patient, but is not the actual cause	Patient with malignant hyperthermia, a fever (appendicitis), and a history of hyperthyroidism, undergoing laparoscopic surgery (CO_2 insufflation)
Blue herring (clue)	Information that is provided to the participants to aid them in solving the problem	Patient with malignant hyperthermia; surgeon says, "Hmm ... her leg seems kind of rigid"

*The term "red herring," meaning a distraction, dates back at least to the early 19th century. In the mid-1990s, our group applied the term "green herring" to mean a plausible confounder. The term "blue herring," meaning a clue, was provided to us in 2012 by a simulation colleague, Dr. Haru Okuda.

causes. Types of ancillary confounding or distracting information are categorized by a rather whimsical nomenclature stemming from the English colloquial expression "red herring." These categories are defined in Table 3-3.
• Scenarios cover a wide variety of problems. Some may be primarily about technical and environmental challenges such as power failure, O_2 failure, or faulty equipment. Some may be about ethical challenges. Others relate to specific, infrequently faced clinical conditions requiring special responses (e.g., cardiac arrest scenarios). In full-day simulation courses like ACRM, providing a mix of cases with different challenges enhances learning and spices up the day.

CREATING A CRITICAL MASS OF "REALISM"

We advise participants that no simulation can (currently) match all the elements of real life. We use a plastic mannequin to represent a patient. We take some shortcuts to be able to get through four to five cases in a day, or to not have to provide every drug in its actual form. In our experience, once a reasonable critical mass of realism is created and the clinical experience of the participants has been tapped, our instructions to suspend disbelief and the dynamic challenge of problem solving presented to them is sufficient to get them to feel like it is real and to behave that way.[6] We teach ACRM only to those with at least 2 months of anesthesia experience, which helps with creating a sense of reality.

CHARACTERISTICS OF AN ACRM COURSE

The principles of ACRM can be taught in different ways using simulation, and courses called "ACRM" or "Anesthesia Crisis Resource Management" have taken hold all over the world. In January 2013 Google searches for "Crisis Resource Management" showed 9.4 million hits, and there were 2.5 million for "Anesthesia Crisis Resource Management." We have articulated the core principles that underlie our approach to teaching ACRM via simulation[4] (http://med. stanford.edu/VAsimulator/acrm/criteria.html). We summarize our experience as follows:

- ACRM courses combine simulation scenarios and debriefings that are typically preceded by other modules. These modules include interactive discussion about the key points of ACRM, the viewing and discussion of trigger videos, analysis of a case using the three-column technique (see earlier in this chapter), and familiarization with the simulation center and simulator.
- Our ACRM courses typically last 8 to 9 hours. There are four to five participants (no fewer than three), who are scheduled so they are not "post-call" and thus can pay attention without undue fatigue. We typically use two to four expert instructors, resulting in a very high instructor-to-participant ratio. All instructors are clinical experts in anesthesiology and have special expertise and training in simulation and debriefing.
- A typical ACRM course for residents is a single-discipline course (see earlier in this chapter) of anesthesia residents, each within the same year of Clinical Anesthesia training. We usually offer ACRM for CA1s in the fall (September to December) to inculcate key principles of ACRM as early as possible. ACRM2 and ACRM3 are conducted from December through June. For CA3 residents about to graduate, preparation for the transition from being a resident to being the "final decision maker" becomes paramount. The basic structure of each ACRM course is the same, but the scenarios are more complex and involve more subspecialty anesthesia situations in the higher-level classes. Different teaching modules are grafted onto each of the levels of ACRM. Principles of ACRM are also incorporated into other simulation courses that are conducted for house staff. For experienced personnel, ACRM follows a similar path to that used with residents, with scenarios chosen and conducted to match the experience of the participants.
- ACRM simulation scenarios are conducted for approximately 20 to 40 minutes each, with each scenario followed by a debriefing session lasting 30 to 40 minutes. Participants rotate through different roles in the scenarios throughout the day. They might play the primary anesthesiologist ("in the hot seat") or the "first responder"—a participant sequestered during the scenario who responds to any call for help by the primary anesthesiologist, if and when the instructor decides that help would be available. The first responder arrives unaware of what has transpired, just as clinicians do when running into a room to help a colleague. Other roles in the rotation include the "scrub tech," who helps the instructor playing the surgeon perform the surgery and thus sees things unfold from the perspective of the surgical team, and the "observer," who watches events unfold on real-time video from the luxury of the debriefing room and can take notes on a whiteboard for later discussion. Participants are debriefed together because each has seen the same scenario, but from a different vantage point.
- Debriefings focus on triggering constructive discussion by the participants regarding key issues of ACRM and patient safety, with 60% or more emphasis on these generic principles and 40% or less on the specific medical/technical "nuts and bolts" of the particular scenario (these percentages vary depending on the scenario and the group). Video of the simulation is available and may be used, strategically, during debriefing.

Debriefing

Well-conducted simulation scenarios, especially if framed properly and linked to other teaching modalities, can offer substantial opportunities for learning on their own. This learning can be greatly enhanced, and can translate to improved real-world patient care, if the simulations are followed by a detailed debriefing session. Debriefing after ACRM simulations, and after real-world situations, is so important that we devote the entirety of the next chapter to the topic.

DOES ACRM WORK?

Does ACRM improve clinical care or change patient outcome? The very nature of the target of "crisis management" makes answering these questions very difficult, if not impossible. Although some aspects of ACRM translate well into everyday anesthesia care, the hallmark of the approach is to better prepare clinicians to handle challenging situations that arise infrequently and usually unexpectedly. To conduct prospective research on such events is nearly impossible. Moreover, these events are diverse in nature, with different etiologies, challenges, and underlying patient characteristics. Prospective data collection about the behavioral aspects of anesthesiologist performance will rarely be available. Although electronic anesthesia records are becoming more common and can document much of what is actually done, they cannot document accurately "how" these things were accomplished or by whom.

To conduct solid, randomized, controlled trials, it would be necessary to follow tens of thousands of patients cared for by thousands of anesthesiologists who were/are randomly assigned to two groups, one that receives ACRM training on a regular schedule and one that does not. As has been written elsewhere,[7] there exists no deep pocket in simulation willing to fund such lengthy and expensive studies. Unlike the pharmaceutical industry, the simulation industry does not have the capital to invest in such complex studies. Nor is there a government agency—at least in the United States—equivalent to, say, the National Cancer Institute, with the capital and the history of funding such complex studies of medical training interventions (rather than of clinical interventions such as chemotherapy protocols). Thus, although there have been studies in analogous medical situations (e.g., code team performance) and studies of similar interventions such as TeamSTEPPS, such studies have not provided level 1A (multiple, well-conducted randomized trials) evidence about these interventions,[8] nor do they directly address the questions about ACRM, including patient outcome. Commercial aviation also lacks such data, despite the fact that they already conduct yearly simulation-based and real flight–based performance assessments of flight deck personnel. Thus, although it will be useful to perform research to determine how best to conduct ACRM training and how it works, the world will continue to "vote with its feet" about whether this kind of intervention is worth supporting. We know that the status quo is insufficient. Every anesthesia professional knows that we, as individuals and teams, are never fully prepared to deal with the adverse events that rarely occur. Through ACRM, there are reasonable ways to approach these events. Such training is expensive, but not nearly as expensive as loss of life or function of a critical organ for a patient, or the financial or psychological expense to the clinician of settling or losing a lawsuit alleging suboptimal anesthesia care.

ACRM-LIKE SIMULATION TRAINING IS A REQUIRED ELEMENT OF PART IV OF THE U.S. MAINTENANCE OF CERTIFICATION IN ANESTHESIA PROGRAM OF THE AMERICAN BOARD OF ANESTHESIOLOGY

Since 2010, new diplomats of the American Board of Anesthesiology (ABA) are required to take a simulation course as a component of their Maintenance of Certification in Anesthesia (MOCA) cycle (currently every 10 years).[9] The simulation course must be held at a site endorsed by the American Society of Anesthesiologists (ASA), with a curriculum meeting minimum standards set by the ASA. While not specifying ACRM directly, the standards for the MOCA simulation that follow are clearly derived from the ACRM simulation courses that have become common around the world:

- A minimum of 6 hours of total course instruction
- Active participation in realistic (mannequin-based) simulation scenarios

- Postscenario, instructor-facilitated peer debriefing
- Management of difficult patient care scenarios (including at least scenarios involving [1] hemodynamic instability and [2] hypoxemia of any cause, including management of the difficult airway)
- An emphasis on teamwork and communication
- At least one opportunity per participant to be the primary anesthesiologist in charge (i.e., the "hot seat")
- An instructor-to-student ratio of at least one instructor per five participants

The first 2 years of experience with the MOCA Simulation Course shows that participants consistently find the experience to be realistic and relevant, and likely to result in practice change.[9] During or after the course, participants must declare the changes they intend to make to their practice. They are queried electronically by ABA 30 to 90 days after completing the course to determine whether they have made those changes and what barriers they encountered. These data are being analyzed by the ASA Simulation Editorial Board to attempt to determine the likely impact of MOCA simulation on clinical care by ABA diplomats.

SUMMARY

Anecdotes abound about the successful application of ACRM principles to challenging patient care situations. We have experienced them in our own work and have heard interesting stories from our own course participants and from other ACRM instructors. Some of these events have played out even at 30,000 feet in the management of acutely ill airline passengers. Although assembling unequivocal proof of the benefit of this training may be impossible, we strongly believe that hearts, brains, and lives have indeed been saved through ACRM training. That belief is reward enough for our efforts.

REFERENCES

1. Rosen K. The history of simulation (including personal memoirs). In: Levine A, DeMaria S, Schwartz A, Sim A, editors. The comprehensive textbook of healthcare simulation. New York: Springer; 2013.
2. Cooper JB, Taqueti VR. A brief history of the development of mannequin simulators for clinical education and training. Qual Saf Health Care 2004;13(Suppl 1):i11-8.
3. Howard S, Gaba D, Fish K, Yang G, Sarnquist F. Anesthesia crisis resource management training: teaching anesthesiologists to handle critical incidents. Aviat Space Environ Med 1992;63:763-70.
4. Gaba D, Howard S, Fish K, Smith B, Sowb Y. Simulation-based training in anesthesia crisis resource management (ACRM): a decade of experience. Simul Gaming 2001;32:175-93.
5. Gaba DM. The future vision of simulation in healthcare. Qual Saf Health Care 2004;1(Suppl 13):i2-10.
6. Dieckmann P, Gaba D, Rall M. Deepening the theoretical foundations of patient simulation as social practice. Simul Healthc 2007;2:183.
7. Gaba DM. The pharmaceutical analogy for simulation: a policy perspective. Simul Healthc 2010;5:5-7.
8. Zeltser MV, Nash DB. Approaching the evidence basis for aviation-derived teamwork training in medicine. Am J Med Qual 2010;25:13-23.
9. McIvor W, Burden A, Weinger M, Steadman R. Simulation for maintainence of certification in anesthesiology: the first two years. J Contin Educ Health Prof 2012;32:236-42.

Chapter 4
Debriefing

RUTH M. FANNING AND DAVID M. GABA

WHAT IS DEBRIEFING?

The concept of debriefing after a challenging event has become commonplace in the health care simulation world, but debriefing as we describe it in this chapter includes a systematic discussion of any immersive event, real or simulated. We explore the debriefing process and its potential to spur reflection and affect learning across a broad spectrum of clinical activities and environments. Although simulations are especially appropriate for debriefing because they are planned exercises with known challenges and learning objectives, any clinical event can provide rich material for reflective learning. The skills described in this chapter can be used to help improve patient care and safety, enhance your own clinical expertise, and uncover systems issues in any environment.

For more than 20 years, we have worked to hone our skills in debriefing, and in this chapter we hope to introduce you to some of what we have learned. Although we will mention work by many others in health care and in other industries, this chapter—like much of the rest of this book—is largely a description of how the authors view and conduct debriefing. This is not intended to be a systematic review of the literature or an exhaustive description of all debriefing techniques. We will describe what we believe to be the most important concepts and issues and will concentrate on explaining our own approaches to debriefing.

The military originated the term "debriefing" to describe a process in which individuals systematically recount events after a mission to extract information and review lessons learned,[1] whereas a "briefing" takes place as preparation before the mission. This meaning of debriefing was adopted by commercial aviation to describe postsimulation discussions. In 1990 our exploration of the aviation experience led us to adopt this postsimulation debriefing approach as the primary method of extracting the most learning out of simulations in anesthesia. This approach was then adopted widely in the rest of health care. Subsequently, the aviation industry produced training guides that delineated principles of debriefing. These sources are also of value to those working in health care. The debriefing practices we promulgated beginning in the early 1990s are consistent with subsequent aviation training guidance.[2,3]

WHAT IS THE ROLE OF DEBRIEFING IN SIMULATION-BASED LEARNING IN HEALTH CARE?

Under what circumstances, especially following a simulation activity, is a debriefing warranted? Some types of simulation and part-task training, especially those dealing with specific technical or psychomotor procedures, may incorporate sufficient guidance in the simulation device itself to make direct involvement by an instructor unnecessary. In certain circumstances, an instructor may be able to provide technical guidance and feedback without a formal debriefing. For some simulation activities, especially with early learners, other pedagogical techniques, such as having a "teacher in the room" to guide, advise, and teach during the simulation scenario, may be more appropriate than a postevent debriefing. However, for many simulation activities, especially as attendees gain clinical expertise, allowing the participants to perform their (simulated) clinical work uninterrupted is important. A detailed discussion of what transpired, after the fact, adds to the learning experience. In concert with a major expert in aviation debriefing in 2006, we wrote, "When it comes to reflecting on complex decisions and behaviors of professionals, complete with confrontation of ego, professional identity, judgment, motion, and culture, there will be no substitute for skilled human beings facilitating an in-depth conversation by their equally human peers."[4] This intuition is borne out by the empirical study by Savoldelli and colleagues,[5] which found that participants failed to improve their nontechnical performance in complex scenarios if they were not debriefed in this reflective fashion.

Of course, not all postevent debriefings are the same. *How* they are conducted, and by whom, can have a significant effect on both the learning process and the learning climate. For example, in Line-Oriented Flight Training simulation exercises, how participants felt about the overall quality of the simulation experience correlated significantly with their perception of the skills of the debriefer.[6] Participants in health care simulations share this sentiment, in which the skill of the facilitators is thought to be a key factor in the learning process and in the credibility of simulation-based learning courses. Health care simulation instructors feel even more strongly that debriefing is the most important part of realistic simulation training, that it is "crucial to the learning process," and if "performed poorly, can actually harm the trainee."[7]

DEBRIEFING DIFFERS FROM TRADITIONAL TEACHING

Not surprisingly, debriefing is considered by many instructors of crisis resource management (CRM)-oriented simulation training to be the most challenging skill to perfect.[8] Even after 24 years, the most experienced of us are still learning to debrief. The teaching environment in simulation-based learning is very different from that of the traditional classroom, and is also different from that of real clinical work. In the classroom, learning objectives are firmly set, whereas in real-life clinical situations they are dictated by clinical events. Simulations lie somewhere in between. Although learning goals exist, they may change depending on participant needs, on how the scenario progresses, or on the issues that surface during the debriefing phase itself. Especially with more experienced participants, debriefers strive to be perceived less as experts, and more as guides for participants as they work through their own self-directed and group-directed learning processes. In a debriefing discussion, the instructor often poses a few questions or comments to trigger discussion. Often the ideal question to pose may be one that "self-perplexes"—that debriefers themselves cannot answer.[9] Having started the discussion, debriefers may comment at suitable moments to redirect or refocus the conversation. Participants speak at considerable length, back and forth with each other, often without verbal input from the instructor. We encourage debriefers to use open-ended questions directed to the group as a whole rather than just to participants who have played the most active roles. The opinions of all group members are sought, and where possible, quiet individuals are drawn out. When participants direct questions at the debriefer, we encourage the instructor to reflect them back to the group rather than provide the "answer" directly.

Debriefing is different than providing "feedback." Feedback most commonly implies observations and advice by the teacher about the level of performance of the learner versus a reference level of expected performance. Although feedback can be conducted in different ways, we often see it performed as a one-way process that requires little input from the learner. Debriefing may include feedback, but debriefing implies a more nuanced interactive conversation exploring how and why a particular sequence of events occurred, and what techniques or choices could have been used to change the process and outcome. In the language of Kolb's experiential learning theory, debriefing provides the occasion for reflection as the middle component of learning, in the cycle that begins with doing, and ends with consolidation of knowledge and skill.[10]

To maximize participant-led discussions, our approach encourages debriefers to be impartial whenever possible, and to avoid making personal judgment calls on performance (e.g., "you did that really well" or "you need to improve that"), even when the participants seek a judgment. We also dissuade participants from making similar calls, always stressing the critique of the "performance" rather than the "performer."

We encourage debriefers and participants to develop a tolerance for ambiguity, to allow instructors to relinquish some control of the learning process, and to empower the participant to lead the way. Instead of talking, debriefers must learn to listen and observe, to be sensitive to nonverbal nuances and cues, and to interpret behavior so as to optimally encourage engagement and direct discussion.

On the other hand, debriefers should try not to get too distracted formulating the perfect statement or question. Fostering an engaged conversation is much more important than aiming for the most efficient or the most probing inquiries. Focusing on active listening rather than on optimal questioning is the best way to keep the conversation going. In total, all these elements can be quite a departure for many educators. Adapting their teaching style to the debriefing approach can initially be very challenging, but the increased participant engagement is rewarding in the long term.

GENERAL FEATURES OF THE DEBRIEFING PROCESS

Although there are a number of structural elements common to most debriefing sessions, the exact characteristics or value for these elements will depend on the curriculum and session.[11] The key elements of debriefing sessions typically include:

- The debriefer(s)[11] (although the learners may sometimes act as their own debriefers[12])
- The goals and objectives of the debriefing
- The participants or learners to be debriefed
- The characteristic of the event itself (usually a simulation scenario) and its impact on the participants in the session
- The participants' recollection of what transpired and the effects of hindsight bias
- The timing of the debriefing relative to the scenario, and the debriefing's phases
- The physical environment of debriefing
- Use of audio-video recordings in debriefing

The Debriefer

Who should debrief? What is the optimal number of debriefers? Do debriefers need to be subject matter experts in the area targeted by the simulation scenario? The answers to these questions start with the simulation session's learning objectives. If the main emphasis of the activity is on CRM or teamwork skills, an expert in these fields can debrief very effectively without being a clinical expert. If there is more than one debriefer, each may debrief within their skill set or area of expertise. Depending on the complexity of the scenarios and the seniority of the participant population, a clinical expert trained in debriefing may also be required to fully address clinical questions. For example, in the Maintenance of Certification (MOC) in anesthesia simulation course for board certified anesthesiologists undergoing their 10-year MOC cycle, there is a requirement that at least one instructor (presumably one who takes part in the debriefing) is a board-certified anesthesiologist.

Debriefers who debrief in pairs may complement each other, relying on implicit reading of the flow of the debriefing or on subtle signals to coordinate their efforts. Debriefing in pairs can improve the flow when one debriefer is struggling to engage the group. It also serves as a method for honing the skills of inexperienced debriefers. However, it requires skill and tact on the part of dual debriefers for it to work effectively, and logistics may dictate that the number of instructors be limited. Hence solo debriefing is common; it can be very effective, particularly if the debriefer is skilled at using a variety of debriefing techniques. Although we typically think of debriefers as coming from the faculty pool, it is possible, in certain instances, for participants who are given appropriate guidance to act as their own debriefers.[12,13] In multimodality simulations, where mannequin-based simulations also include standardized patient (SP) actors, the SPs may also contribute to the debriefing, either "in role" or as debriefers, offering a unique perspective. The debriefing process is not rigid, and it should grow and evolve within programs, depending on the availability of facilitators, their level of expertise and experience, and the needs of the participant population.

Debriefing through facilitation is more than simply "making the discussion easier." Ideally, it is a guided pathway to meaningful discourse that will encourage learning and behavior change. The exact level of facilitation and the degree to which the facilitator is involved in the debriefing process can depend on a variety of elements, such as learning objectives and overall curricular goals, the experience level of participants, and their familiarity with the simulation environment. It may also vary with the complexity of the simulation, the setting in which the debriefing occurs, and even the time available for debriefing.

The aim is to encourage the majority of the discussion and dialogue to stem from participants, in which the debriefer interjects only as necessary to keep the discussion on track to achieve particular learning objectives. Effective debriefers encourage participants by actively listening, often using nonverbal encouragement (e.g., nodding), or echoing statements made by participants.

Debriefers should be aware of the learning objectives prescribed by the curriculum, and also recognize that the stated objectives may not be those of the participants. Participant-driven learning objectives arising as part of a deep discussion may often override the pre-established learning objectives when they have special meaning to the learners and are not inconsistent with the overall goals of the curriculum. Adult participants are particularly cognizant of the relevance and applicability of what they are being taught, and may become more engaged when discussing issues that are pertinent to their needs. On the other hand, they may become frustrated or disengaged if they are not given the opportunity to discuss the issues that are most important and relevant to them.[14]

The terminology regarding levels or degrees of facilitation can be confusing. In some sources (especially Dismukes and colleagues[2,3]), a "high level" of facilitation describes debriefings that show "little input" by the instructor, favoring encouragement of conversation as described earlier. Conversely, "low level" facilitation means "much" involvement by the instructor, even to the point of lecturing. Varying levels of instructor input are appropriate for different types of simulations, different participant populations, and learning needs.

The Participants

The role of participants in the debriefing process differs considerably from that of the learner in the traditional classroom setting. Instead of being passive recipients of information, debriefing demands that participants demonstrate an ability and willingness to critically reflect on and analyze their own performance. This process involves exploring not only what happened, but why, and what lessons can be learned to improve future performance.

Participants may be homogeneous, from a single discipline, or diverse, with hierarchical elements in the case of combined-team exercises. They may have varying levels of expertise both in their clinical domains and in their prior exposure to simulation activities. All of these elements will affect the extent of instructor guidance and the styles of debriefing employed.

Sometimes participants who are longstanding coworkers can be more forthcoming when they already feel comfortable conversing with each other. Others prefer to be anonymous among participants they do not know, needing some time to get used to their co-participants before they fully open up. The debriefer needs to quickly evaluate the group dynamics and adapt the debriefing style and techniques accordingly.

The Goals and Objectives of the Debriefing

The goals and objectives may vary considerably depending on the setting, resources, participant population, and desired outcome. Debriefings of early learners may be more focused on achieving clarity of what transpired clinically and on the available management choices, with nontechnical skills having a lesser focus. As the experience of participants rises, the focus of debriefing often shifts to a greater emphasis of CRM principles and systems issues, with a secondary focus on the medical and technical specifics of the scenarios. Similarly, short debriefings following announced in situ simulations (e.g., mock codes) typically focus on discrete learning objectives, often addressing systems issues that are pertinent to the in situ environment. Debriefings following a scenario conducted for research are often intended primarily to extract more information about the decision making of participants rather than to enhance their learning.

Characteristics and Impact of the Simulation Scenario

Scenarios designed with clear debriefing aims in mind usually lead to more success in achieving learning objectives and goals. The complexity of scenarios should be tailored to the level of experience of participants and to the relevant teaching goals. Anesthesia crisis resource management (ACRM) scenarios challenge participants to make complex decisions and to formulate, adapt, and execute difficult diagnostic and treatment plans both as individuals and teams. Scenarios with such complexity allow a rich discussion of different aspects of the performance during the debriefing. The number of participants engaged simultaneously in the scenario will also affect the debriefing (e.g., a single participant, a stratified group of participants with one individual in the "hot seat," or clinical care provided "by committee" of an entire group).

Simulation demands a flexible approach to teaching and learning, forging educational opportunities from diverse, and perhaps unplanned, events or experiences. Should a scenario fail catastrophically (e.g., as a result of a serious simulator glitch), it may be appropriate to abort it, acknowledge the failure, and either forego the debriefing or conduct a discussion about the scenario case that was planned. Alternatively, when malfunctions allow the scenario to proceed in a credible clinical fashion, the instructor may decide to continue and to use the events of the scenario to achieve an evolving educational opportunity.[15] Simulation is like live theater: often "the show must go on." Having a good sense of humor about such events is usually appreciated by the participants.

Scenarios that are challenging to the "psyche" of participants or that probe ethical decision making require special attention, both in their design and the nature of the debriefing process.[16,17] These scenarios may include those in which the simulated patient dies[18] or those in which a more junior clinician is required to challenge the judgment of senior personnel.[19]

Some scenarios involve significant interaction with "family members" or nonparticipant "colleagues" who are acting as the confederate of the instructor. How these confederate roles are handled is important. If a major confederate role is played by a nonparticipant faculty member (either from the simulation team or from the real world of clinical care), it risks confusing participants. They may be unsure, either in the simulation or during the debriefing, whether the confederate is speaking in their simulation role or in their real world role. In such instances, participants should be informed of the confederate's status either ahead of the scenario (if that will not alter its impact) or prior to the debriefing. In either case, it should be clear during the debriefing from which role the individual was (during the scenario) or is (in the debriefing) speaking. The debriefing of scenarios that knowingly challenge the participants' psyche is best facilitated by instructors with the experience, training, and skill to conduct an appropriately nuanced debriefing and to recognize and handle any adverse reactions from participants. Programs should be prepared to refer participants for professional counseling should the need arise.

Recollection and Hindsight Bias

Participants' recollection of events fade and change, both during the scenario and after it concludes. Memory is imperfect and is affected by many factors. A very important factor in most debriefings is hindsight bias, introduced by already knowing the "outcome" of what transpired.[20-23] The "I knew it all along" feeling of hindsight bias is very powerful and most people are prone to it even when advised of it or trained to handle it.[24] To mitigate hindsight bias, it may be helpful to use debriefing techniques that explicitly consider all the diagnostic and treatment possibilities rather than concentrating solely on what actually transpired or what was actually wrong with the simulated patient. Using the video recording of the scenario may help clarify facts and events at various points, bypassing subjective recall. We instruct participants to "think out loud" during scenarios so that their thought processes can be captured on the recording.[25] This provides a contemporaneous record of participants' thinking and may help reduce hindsight bias during the debriefing.

Another way to counteract hindsight bias is by using scenarios that terminate before the underlying diagnosis or process becomes apparent. Participants will have genuine uncertainty as to what diagnoses or actions are best, even as they enter the debriefing. However, this may come at the cost of not letting them fully complete diagnostic and treatment steps, which itself may be frustrating. To counteract this frustration, one may consider affording participants the opportunity to practice a procedure or treatment strategy at the end of the debriefing session.

Timing and Phases of Debriefing

Debriefings often occur immediately after an exercise, but they can also be placed within a scenario, in the "pause and reflect" style of teaching.[12] Debriefings can be conducted sequentially, with a quick initial debrief followed by more in-depth debriefings of certain skills targeted to particular individuals or groups. This sequential style may be suited to "unannounced" in situ simulations such as mock codes in a hospital where participants may need to quickly leave the site of simulation to return to care for real patients. Debriefings can also be conducted remotely in time, allowing a different perspective to be explored than would prevail immediately following an event.[26]

The Introductory or Briefing Phase: To some extent, debriefing begins with the ground rules set in the introduction to a simulation course or in a briefing that immediately precedes a specific scenario. Instructors set the parameters for how simulations and debriefings are to be conducted. This includes rules of engagement, issues related to confidentiality, the recording and storage of data and its subsequent use, and the protection of participants' privacy. The process for debriefing and the expected role of participants is explained. We, like others in the simulation community, give a high priority to creating a psychologically safe environment in which open and frank discussion of performance, clinical hierarchy, and systems-based concerns can be aired. Psychological safety—the individual's feeling that the current environment is safe for interpersonal risk-taking and discussion—is an important ingredient of learning in groups.[27] In health care, it is thought that such considerations optimize learning behavior and should ultimately facilitate improvements in patient safety.[27,28]

In our programs, we usually explicitly state that we will collectively be "critiquing the *performance,* not the performer." We encourage participants to initiate and sustain the discussion during debriefing, stressing the impact of their level of engagement on their learning. We empower them to help guide the debriefing process toward learning objectives that are meaningful to them.

Defusing Phase: Immediately after the scenario concludes, even during a short walk to a debriefing room, the participants usually start a defusing or cool-down phase.[11,29] They begin to release the tension of the simulation exercise, seek and give support to team members, and often begin a debriefing discussion among themselves. Observing participants in the defusing stage can provide material for debriefing and give insights into their behaviors and actions and the team structure and dynamics. The debriefer should control the length of this phase, allowing a period of emotional release but stopping the defusing process before the participants' discussion goes too far into a haphazard analysis.

Recollection, Description, and Clarification Phase: Defusing is followed by a stage of recollection, description, and clarification of the simulation events.[30,31] The emotional impact of the experience can be explored individually or by the group as a whole.[26,30,31] As in the defusing phase, at various points in this phase, the debriefer may need to intervene explicitly to prevent participants from "jumping ahead" prematurely in their recollection and discussion of the case. This mitigates hindsight bias, and allows a more structured discussion of key points. We may say, for example, "Hold on, let's talk more fully about the current issue and we'll get to the other one in a little while." Debriefers need to learn how to exercise control to optimize the debriefing while not unduly interrupting meaningful conversation.

Generalization Phase: The third phase involves generalizing from the subjective experience of the case or scenario to a collective reflection and analysis of the issues and principles that apply to many cases. The debriefer guides the discussion, provides context as to how prior runs of the same scenario have revealed similar or different lessons, and may encourage participants to focus on approaches that can be applied to real patient care.

The Physical Environment for Debriefing

The physical environment in which debriefing takes place deserves careful consideration, especially because it can affect the degree to which participants are encouraged to engage in open discussion and reflection. For detailed or "long form" debriefings, it is usually ideal to have a dedicated debriefing room nearby, because excessive distance from the simulation exercise may lead to distraction and discourage cohesion. The layout of furniture in the room can enhance or detract from open discourse. Ideally, facilitators and participants should sit around one table (or in a circle without a table) so as to include everyone at an equal standing in the discussion. Participants who are not at the table can feel excluded from the discussion and more easily distracted. When there is more than one debriefer present, debriefers should consider where they sit relative to participants and to each other. Co-debriefers may wish to sit opposite each other so that they can better see each others' nonverbal cues.

Debriefing outside a dedicated debriefing room, such as after in situ simulations, can provide some challenges; however, regardless of the constraints of the environment, there is always a need to create a sense of respect and community among participants and instructors. Sometimes it can be helpful to have the group step away from the bedside to create a suitable environment for debriefing. When debriefing in a clinical work area, it may be especially important to ensure a safe debriefing environment and to assure participants that the goals are education, training, and systems improvement, geared toward optimizing patient safety. Safety also dictates that special care be taken to ensure that no equipment or medications that are unfit for clinical use remain in the clinical environment.

Debriefing at the site of simulation also brings some opportunities. If debriefing a systems-based issue, being at the clinical site can help the debriefer to explore the role of equipment or patient care processes on the success of clinical work. It may then allow participants to interact with the environment and to briefly recreate elements of the simulation within the debriefing session. Thus, even when a dedicated debriefing room is available, debriefers may sometimes, elect to debrief at the site of the simulation exercise, or they may do it to add variety to a day.

Use of Video in Debriefing

Following the lead of aviation CRM programs, since the very first ACRM courses in 1990, we have made it a regular practice to record both the audio and video of simulation scenarios. In the early years, we tended to replay the entire video during the debriefing, pausing it periodically to allow discussion. Ultimately we determined that this was too time consuming and redundant, and inhibited good discussion. As we have become more experienced in simulation, we still record our simulations and debriefings, but we use much less video playback for debriefing purposes and we use it more strategically. Excessive use of video playback can be distracting. Our philosophy is that the goal of the debriefing is to have the group talking about interesting and useful issues and principles, and therefore the use of video should be to enhance that process rather than to be an end in itself. As video systems in simulation centers have become more complex, there is also a growing risk of system failures, or that instructors will not be skilled in using the system. If there are problems with the video playback that cannot be resolved very quickly, it is best to avoid it entirely instead of continuing to struggle and thereby preclude or disrupt a useful discussion.

Playback segments are best selected and explicitly framed by scenario events, points of use of specific CRM principles, or diagnostic or treatment decision points. Typical examples of selections for viewing in the debriefing might be: when a clinical event is first detected or recognized, when the first responder clinician is being briefed by the primary clinician, or when critical communication is taking place between the anesthesia professional(s) and the surgical team. When video is used, the debriefers should clarify what they are illustrating or what they wish the group to observe or comment on.

Clearly, the use of video replay is not a prerequisite for a successful debriefing session.[5,32,33] In fact, a study by Savoldelli and colleagues[5] showed that, although debriefing enhanced learning, there was no additional value added by the instructors' use of video replay. It is likely that the strategic use of video can add value to debriefing, but in what context and format remains to be elucidated.

DEBRIEFING APPROACHES AND TECHNIQUES

At the Stanford Center for Immersive and Simulation-based Learning and the Veterans Affairs (VA) Palo Alto Simulation Center, we have incorporated and use many different debriefing techniques to achieve our learning objectives. In fact, participants may find any one technique used repetitively to be tiresome; thus our instructors may use a variety of styles within any given debriefing. We tailor the debriefing approach and style to the curriculum being taught and the participant population. Debriefings in many of our courses aim to strongly emphasize the concepts of CRM while addressing the medical and technical issues of the particular clinical scenario.[34-36] As part of most of our courses, particularly in the introductory phase, we teach participants the language of CRM, using several of the techniques described in Chapter 3. Familiarizing participants with these concepts allows them to participate in a constructive debriefing, using a common language with shared values. Although the full description of any particular debriefing technique is beyond the scope of this chapter, what follows are some of the commonly used ones.

The Technique of "Alternatives and Their Pros and Cons (APC)"

One of the favorite techniques of debriefers at our centers is to encourage participants to consider, for one or more key junctures of the scenario, the various *alternatives* that were available and the *pros and cons* of each. Irrespective of the situation, a clinician rarely has only a single option (even doing nothing is an alternative). Discussing the merits of alternatives is equally applicable to medical or technical decisions (e.g., What are the possible diagnoses? What information was available?) and to nontechnical issues such as communication between the anesthesia professional and the surgeon. The APC approach offers a chance to look at a situation from all angles, to "step back" from the original decisions and actions, thus depersonalizing the decision-making process. This challenges participants to think about their own thought processes and strategies involved in patient care, and it allows them the freedom to consider alternative options in the safe environment of the debriefing room.

The APC style of debriefing also fosters thinking about how the relative merits of choices may be affected by different conditions and circumstances. This can yield new insights and can also mitigate hindsight bias. It can take the focus away from what a particular participant or team did or did not do and place the focus more abstractly on ramifications of the various choices. This can be done explicitly by saying something like, "Forget about this particular case—generally speaking, what are the possible causes or treatments for the XYZ set of findings?" Participants can suggest, and then assess the options, often coming together as a group to collectively consider the best courses of action in different circumstances.

We have found the APC technique is easy for debriefers to use. They, or the participants, need only identify certain junctures where decisions, actions, or verbalizations were made. The debriefer can then ask participants to describe the different possible alternatives at that juncture and the pros and cons of each.

Debriefing with Good Judgment

A very popular and powerful technique originating at the Center for Medical Simulation in Boston is called Debriefing with Good Judgment. This approach has three main elements. The first is a conceptual model of performance that posits that actions during a simulation are driven by cognitive-emotional "frames" held by participants. The second is a commitment to assuming the best of learners; they intended to do something sensible, even when they made errors. The third component involves pairing two types of speech that are usually used in isolation from each other: *advocacy* (a statement of the instructor's point of view) with *inquiry* (a question to get at the participant's point of view). Combining these three components allows instructors to model being open about their own reasoning and judgments, and demonstrates that they are willing to subject their own thinking to the same scrutiny as do the participants in the debriefing. Because instructors cannot know what anyone was actually thinking during a simulation, the inquiry process also allows instructors to learn new things about how the participants think and feel. The goal of the Debriefing with Good Judgment technique is not only to catalyze vibrant within-debriefing conversations, but also to help faculty and participants learn to become "reflective practitioners," practitioners who can scrutinize their taken-for-granted assumptions and mental routines in a way that allows them to self-correct as well as strengthen their ability to have the difficult conversations that allow others to improve.

This technique, which utilizes research on reflective practice,[37] has been described in detail in the literature.[38,39]

Plus-Delta Technique

Another commonly used debriefing technique that has been adapted from the military is called "Plus-Delta." It asks participants to articulate what went well ("plus"), and what could be improved in the future ("delta").[8,40] We have modified the Plus-Delta nomenclature to refer instead to which elements of handling the situation went "easily" and which were "challenging." This moves the focus from "good" versus "bad" (the latter couched as "wish to change") to "easy versus hard." Our experience is that easy and hard are less-loaded terms that make it simpler for groups to discuss *why* some things were easy and others were hard. The Plus-Delta technique can be useful, especially when time for debriefing is limited, as it can get to the key points very quickly. It is also a technique that is easy for novice debriefers to use, or when participants act as their own debriefers.

Technical-Only Debriefing

Some debriefing techniques focus almost entirely on medical or technical content, and concentrate on diagnoses and treatments. These approaches often compare what transpired with what is recommended by promulgated consensus algorithms or checklists (e.g., management of a MH crisis, ACLS guidelines). Such techniques can be useful in curricula whose medical and technical learning objectives are strongly prescribed or for debriefing sessions that must be abbreviated because of time constraints. Even in a more expansive debriefing, it can be appropriate to explicitly carve out a period of time (usually a few minutes) to focus specifically on some medical or technical issues, then perhaps to return to the discussion of the broader set of CRM and systems issues.

The Three-Column Technique

As mentioned in Chapter 3, the three-column technique can be used in the debriefing of simulation scenarios. Structuring the discussion and the analysis of the case into three categories of **medical/technical**, **CRM**, and **systems-based** has been very useful. Within each category, any debriefing technique (including APC or Advocacy/Inquiry) can be useful in guiding the discussion.

Use of Silence and Nonverbal Techniques

The effective use of silence can be a powerful technique within a debriefing, but it may not be very familiar to many clinician educators. An effective silence is a pause that typically lasts at least 8 seconds. It can demonstrate the desire for discussion to come from the participants rather than the facilitator, and it can give more time for participants to formulate their comments. Such long silences can be confusing or even intimidating to participants, and we encourage debriefers to be cognizant of their body language, moving their eyes around the group, perhaps nodding, raising their eyebrows, and otherwise nonverbally encouraging participants to engage. Using verbal phatics and fillers such as "aha" and "indeed" is useful in encouraging discussion.

Debriefers often use nonverbal communication techniques. They include the physical versions of phatics and fillers, such as nodding of the head and certain hand gestures to signal understanding or to promote conversation. Other gestures may be more direct, such as putting a hand out in the "stop" sign to bring a behavior or statement to a halt. A wide variety of nonverbal cues can be effective, but it is important to remember that they may not always be interpreted in the same way by all participants.

Demonstrations or Mini-role-plays During Debriefings

Perhaps the opposite of the strategic use of silence is to sometimes ask participants to engage in practical activities triggered by questions or comments in the debriefing. For example, when a participant says something like, "Well, the team leader could have done a better job of communicating X to person A," we encourage them to do a mini-role-play on the spot in which they act out that communication, with an instructor playing the role of person A. This requires participants to practice enacting these skills rather than just talking about them. Similarly, when issues with medical equipment or supplies are raised, we encourage instructors to lead the participants in physical demonstrations or in hands-on practice with the gear during debriefing. Not only does this effectively answer the technical question, but it can also be a change of pace that keeps participants engaged and active.

TEACHING DEBRIEFING TO SIMULATION INSTRUCTORS

Debriefing and learning to debrief is challenging. Though many centers offer instructor courses that teach debriefing, and there are many workshops on the topic at the International Meeting on Simulation in Healthcare (IMSH) and other simulation conferences, these are, in essence, just introductions to the debriefing process. The key elements of debriefing instruction at the Stanford and VA Palo Alto instructor courses include: (1) a minimal amount of didactic review of the rationale for debriefing and the applicable techniques; (2) use of trigger videos of debriefings to spark discussion about effective debriefing approaches; and (3) hands-on practice of debriefing using multiple debriefing techniques, and (4) debriefing of the debriefings.

Most instructors concur with McLean[41] that although such training provides "sufficient skills to commence facilitation, it was only with experience, and in the presence of an expert role model that they became more comfortable with the process." Experienced debriefers have honed their performance over time, building on an initial set of skills, which grow with reflection, analysis, and active experimentation. Co-debriefing with more experienced instructors is a useful way to improve skills, as is reviewing videos of one's own debriefing sessions or those of exemplary debriefers.

DEBRIEFING ASSESSMENT TOOLS AND OTHER DEBRIEFING RESOURCES

As with all complex skills, there are many reasons why assessing the debriefing process might be useful. These include research on debriefing, its longitudinal improvement through self-study or expert mentorship, and quality control of debriefing performance in a group or center. To these and other ends, a few debriefing assessment tools are available. One well-known example is Debriefing Assessment for Simulation in Healthcare (DASH), which is designed to assist in evaluating and developing debriefing skills.[42] (See www.harvardmedsim.org/Research/DASH.) It incorporates six elements: establishing and maintaining an engaging learning environment, structuring a debriefing in an organized way, provoking engaging discussion, identifying performance gaps, exploring those performance gaps, and helping to improve future performance.

Another commonly used tool is Observational Structured Assessment Debriefing (OSAD).[43] (See http://www1.imperial.ac.uk/medicine/about/institutes/patientsafetyservicequality/cpssq_publications/resources_tools/osad.) This explores eight elements: approach, learning environment, learner engagement, reaction, reflection, analysis, diagnosis, and application. A five-point, behaviorally anchored rating scale is applied to each of the eight elements to assist in providing objective feedback for the debriefer.

A group from Zurich has published a hybrid self-report debriefing quality assessment scale that combines questions from DASH and OSAD.[44] They report good reliability, content validity, and reasonable convergent and discriminant validity.

The simulation community, through publications and online forums, provides support for further learning about debriefing. National and international conferences on simulation-based education offer a wide array of debriefing workshops, expert panels, roundtables, and discussions on the topic. Conference events such as Debriefing Olympics—where several debriefers independently debrief the same participants on the same (recorded) simulation session—can expose even a large audience to the debriefing techniques and styles of experienced instructors.[45] Various well-known simulation groups also offer instructor training that emphasizes debriefing skills.

RESEARCH ON DEBRIEFING

Although the simulation-based education community considers debriefing to be a vital part of the learning process, there is still much that we do not know about what kinds of debriefing are best suited to achieve various learning objectives. Tasked with addressing this question, a group at the 2011 Society of Simulation in Healthcare Research Summit on the state of the art in simulation (held as a precursor to the IMSH 2011) examined the existing research about debriefing to highlight strengths and identify areas for further study.[46] The majority of simulation studies that mentioned debriefing did so in an unsystematic fashion, with many important variables not specified. Thus at this time we do not know for sure the role that debriefing plays in achieving different outcomes of learning or of improvement in clinical practice or patient outcome. Future research is needed to answer many questions about debriefing. Among them are: What are the pros and cons of different techniques and styles for different participant populations and teaching goals? How much debriefing is enough? Only studies designed in a systematic manner with debriefing as the primary variable and attempting to control for the plethora of confounding variables could begin to answer these questions. Unfortunately, to obtain solid data such studies will likely be large, long, and complex. This will make it very difficult to obtain adequate funding, as there are no deep pockets with a vested interest in examining debriefing effectiveness.[47]

CONCLUSION

The growth over the last 20 years of simulation-based training in health care that uses post-scenario debriefing has been astounding. Like many things in health care, the community has "voted with its feet," adopting techniques and styles of debriefing that seem to work well for improving understanding and performance regarding complex issues of CRM and patient care in challenging clinical situations. Whereas the thrust of debriefing has focused on application to simulation, its utility for improving organizational learning after real case events is still to be tapped. We seem to know intuitively some of the pitfalls to avoid, but we do not yet know what will work "best" for the many different applications of debriefing in health care. It remains mostly an art based loosely on science, and it is a significant limiting factor in the ability of new instructors and new simulation centers to get the most out of their learning exercises. Although we strongly advise new debriefers to obtain credible training in the art from one of the highly experienced centers, we are also believers in Nike's "Just do it" philosophy. Much like clinical work, no matter how much training in debriefing someone acquires—even with good debriefing exercises—there is no substitute for the real thing in building and honing debriefing skills. With institutional support and a willingness to learn, it is easily possible for eager clinical educators to master the skills of debriefing and to unlock the potential of either simulation scenarios or discussions of real cases to be transformative learning experiences.

REFERENCES

1. Pearson M, Smith D. Debriefing in experience-based learning. Simul Games Learn 1986;16:155-72.
2. McDonnell L, Jobe K, Dismukes R. Facilitating LOS debriefings: a training manual. [NASA technical memorandum 112192] Moffett Field, Calif: National Aeronautics and Space Administration; 1997.
3. Dismukes K, Smith G. Facilitation and debriefing in aviation training and operations. Aldershot, UK: Ashgate; 2000.
4. Dismukes RK, Gaba DM, Howard SK. So many roads: facilitated debriefed in healthcare. Simul Healthc 2006;1:23.
5. Savoldelli GL, Naik VN, Park J, et al. Value of debriefing during simulated crisis management: oral versus video-assisted oral feedback. Anesthesiology 2006;105:279-85.
6. Wilhelm J. Crew member and instructor evaluations of line oriented flight training. In: Jensen R, editor. Sixth annual international symposium on aviation psychology; 1991. p. 326-67.
7. Rall M, Manser T, Howard S. Key elements of debriefing for simulator training. Eur J Anaesth 2000;17:516-7.
8. Fanning RM, Gaba DM. The role of debriefing in simulation-based learning. Simul Healthc 2007;2:115.
9. Dillon J. Questioning and teaching: a manual of practice. New York: Teachers College Press; 1988.
10. Kolb D. Experiential learning: experience as the source of learning and development. Englewood Cliffs, NJ: Prentice Hall; 1984.
11. Lederman L. Debriefing: toward a systematic assessment of theory and practice. Simul Gaming 1992;23:145-60.
12. Beaubien J, Baker D. Post-training feedback: the relative effectiveness of team versus instructor-led debriefs. In: 47th annual meeting of the Human Factors and Ergonomics Society. Denver; 2003.
13. Boet S, Bould MD, Bruppacher HR, et al. Looking in the mirror: self-debriefing versus instructor debriefing for simulated crises. Crit Care Med 2011;39:1377-81.
14. Knowles M, Holton III E, Swanson R. The adult learner: the definitive classic in adult education and human resource development. Burlington, Mass: Elsevier; 2005.
15. Dieckmann P, Lippert A, Glavin R, Rall M. When things do not go as expected: scenario life savers. Simul Healthc 2010;5:219-25.
16. Truog RD, Meyer EC. Deception and death in medical simulation. Simul Healthc 2013;8:1-3.
17. Gaba DM. Simulations that are challenging to the psyche of participants: how much should we worry and about what? Simul Healthc 2013;8:4-7.
18. Corvetto MA, Taekman JM. To die or not to die? A review of simulated death. Simul Healthc 2013;8:8-12.
19. Calhoun AW, Boone MC, Miller KH, Pian-Smith MC. Case and commentary: using simulation to address hierarchy issues during medical crises. Simul Healthc 2013;8:13-9.
20. Fischoff B. Hindsightforesight: the effect of outcome knowledge on judgment under uncertainty. J Exp Psych: Hum Perception Perf 1975;1:288-99.
21. Hawkins S. Hindsight: biased judgments of past events after the outcomes are known. Psychol Bull 1990;107:311.
22. Christensen-Szalanski J, Willham C. The hindsight bias: a meta-analysis. Organ Behav Hum Decis Process 1991;48:147-68.
23. Henriksen K, Kaplan H. Hindsight bias, outcome knowledge and adaptive learning. Qual Saf Health Care 2003;12(Suppl. 2):ii46-50.
24. Arkes HR, Faust D, Guilmette TJ, Hart K. Eliminating the hindsight bias. J Appl Psychol 1988;73:305-7.
25. Ericsson KA, Simon HA. Protocol analysis: verbal reports as data. Cambridge, Mass: MIT Press; 1993.
26. Petranek C. A maturation in experiential learning: principles of simulation and gaming. Simul Gaming 1994;25:513-23.
27. Edmondson A. Psychological safety and learning behavior in work teams. Adm Sci Q 1999;44:350-83.
28. Edmondson A. Speaking up in the operating room: how team leaders promote learning in interdisciplinary action teams. J Mgmt Stud 2003;40:1419-52.
29. Zigmont JJ, Kappus LJ, Sudikoff SN. The 3D model of debriefing: defusing, discovering, and deepening. Semin Perinatol 2011;35:52-8.
30. Thatcher D, Robinson M. An introduction to games and simulation in education. Hants: Solent Simulations; 1985.
31. Lederman L. Intercultural communication, simulation and the cognitive assimilation of experience: an exploration of the post-experience analytic process. In: Third annual conference of the Speech Communication Association. San Juan, Puerto Rico; 1983. p. 1-3.
32. Hamilton NA, Kieninger AN, Woodhouse J, et al. Video review using a reliable evaluation metric improves team function in high-fidelity simulated trauma resuscitation. J Surg Educ 2012;69:428-31.
33. Sawyer T, Sierocka-Castaneda A, Chan D, et al. The effectiveness of video-assisted debriefing versus oral debriefing alone at improving neonatal resuscitation performance: a randomized trial. Simul Healthc 2012;7:213-21.
34. Howard S, Gaba D, Fish K, Yang G, Sarnquist F. Anesthesia crisis resource management training: teaching anesthesiologists to handle critical incidents. Aviat Space Environ Med 1992;63:763.
35. Gaba D, Fish K, Howard S. Crisis management in anesthesiology. New York: Churchill-Livingstone; 1994.

36. Gaba D, Howard S, Fish K, Smith B, Sowb Y. Simulation-based training in anesthesia crisis resource management (ACRM): a decade of experience. Simul Gaming 2001;32:175.
37. Argyris C, Schon D. Organizational learning II: theory, method, and practice. Reading, Mass: Addison Wesley; 1996.
38. Rudolph JW, Simon R, Dufresne RL, Raemer DB. There's no such thing as "nonjudgmental" debriefing: a theory and method for debriefing with good judgment. Simul Healthc 2006;1:49-55.
39. Rudolph JW, Simon R, Rivard P, Dufresne RL, Raemer DB. Debriefing with good judgment: combining rigorous feedback with genuine inquiry. Anesthesiol Clin 2007;25:361-76.
40. Helminksi L, Koberna S. Total quality instruction: a systems approach. In: Roberts HV, editor. Academic initiatives in total quality for higher education. Milwaukee: ASQC Quality Press; 1995. p. 309-62.
41. McLean M. What can we learn from facilitator and student perceptions of facilitation skills and roles in the first year of a problem-based learning curriculum? BMC Med Educ 2003;3:9.
42. Brett-Fleegler M, Rudolph J, Eppich W, et al. Debriefing assessment for simulation in healthcare: development and psychometric properties. Simul Healthc 2012;7:288-94.
43. Arora S, Ahmed M, Paige J, et al. Objective structured assessment of debriefing: bringing science to the art of debriefing in surgery. Ann Surg 2012;256:982-8.
44. Kolbe M, Weiss M, Grote G, et al. TeamGAINS: a tool for structured debriefings for simulation-based team trainings. BMJ Qual Saf 2013;22:541-53.
45. Dieckmann P. Debriefing Olympics—a workshop concept to stimulate the adaptation of debriefings to learning contexts. Simul Healthc 2012;7:176-82.
46. Raemer D, Anderson M, Cheng A, et al. Research regarding debriefing as part of the learning process. Simul Healthc 2011;6(Suppl.):S52-7.
47. Gaba DM. The pharmaceutical analogy for simulation: a policy perspective. Simul Healthc 2010;5:5-7.

Catalog of Critical Events in Anesthesiology

Section II
Catalog of Critical Events in Anesthesiology

The following chapters contain the Catalog of Critical Events in Anesthesiology. As described in detail in the Preface and in Chapters 1 and 2, this Catalog is intended to fill a gap in the training of anesthesia professionals. Our aim is to provide a comprehensive (although not exhaustive) compilation of approaches to both common and uncommon emergency situations that can arise in the perioperative period. This is intended to make it easy to learn or review systematically how to recognize these situations and how to respond if they occur.

The first group of events are "generic"; most of them describe a *manifestation* that may be caused by a variety of potentially serious underlying events. The generic events are listed in a separate group because they initially require no further information other than the existence of that manifestation. For example, the generic event Hypotension (Event 9) presents an approach to deal with a common but potentially serious manifestation that can result from many different causes. The generic event covers the initial diagnostic and therapeutic approach to the problem and then cross-references the other events that represent specific pathophysiologic occurrences. Thus, the event Pulmonary Embolism (Event 21) is one specific cause of hypotension.

Each of the next groups relates to a single organ system (cardiovascular, pulmonary, metabolic, neurologic) because there is considerable similarity of the manifestations and responses appropriate to each system. Following the groups devoted to organ systems is a group involving equipment failures, many of which concern the anesthesia machine and the breathing circuit. Finally, there are three groups covering events of special interest in subspecialty areas of anesthesia practice (cardiac, obstetric, and pediatric anesthesia). Of course, many events in the rest of the Catalog will be of interest to specialists in these areas, but the unique occurrences faced in their environments are grouped separately.

We developed a special format for the events in the Catalog to provide a uniform, concise framework for describing them to anesthesia professionals. As this Catalog is intended to be a guidebook, not a reference text, we have not included the vast amount of explanatory and reference material that is available on each of these topics. What we do provide is the *essential material* that we believe is needed to prepare for handling specific perioperative crisis situations. The following explains the format and headings used for each event in the Catalog.

EVENT

The name of the event.

DEFINITION

The definition of the event and any common variants.

ETIOLOGY

The underlying cause(s) of the event. There is often more than one possible cause for each defined event.

TYPICAL SITUATIONS

The perioperative situations in which the event is most likely to occur. In these situations the anesthesia professional should be especially alert to the possibility of the event. If the likelihood of its occurrence is high enough, specific steps may need to be taken to prevent its occurrence or to obtain the special equipment or personnel needed to treat it if it should occur.

PREVENTION

The actions that can make the occurrence of the event less likely or that will make it easier to treat.

MANIFESTATIONS

The ways in which the event could manifest itself. These include clinical observations, monitored variables, and laboratory data. Not every manifestation will be evident for any given occurrence of the event. Some manifestations typically are seen early in the course of the event; others will only be seen late in its evolution. The manifestations are listed in their approximate order of frequency and/or importance.

SIMILAR EVENTS

This is a list of other events whose manifestations can be similar to the manifestations of this event. For some of these alternative diagnoses there are specific manifestations that clearly distinguish them from this event.

MANAGEMENT

Guidelines on what to do if this event occurs, or if there is significant suspicion that it has occurred. The suggested management is described approximately in the order of things that an experienced anesthesia professional might check or do. The items listed in bold are the initial responses that we believe to be most important.

We have chosen to produce these hierarchical textual guides rather than rigid algorithms or flowcharts because the many permutations and combinations of real situations and real patients are too complex to allow the specification of definitive independent pathways of action.

Note: Every situation is different. It may be necessary to deviate from guidelines because of the specifics of a situation.

Remember these aspects of Anesthesia Crisis Resource Management that apply to every case:

Support the circulation as necessary
Ensure adequate oxygenation at all costs
Call for help early rather than late
Tackle the most critical problems first
Reevaluate the situation frequently

COMPLICATIONS

These are the specific complications of the event, which may occur either owing to progression of the event itself or as complications of treatment.

SUGGESTED READING

This is a list of relevant literature related to the event. We have tried to give the most useful references for each event, wherever possible citing easily accessible materials. We have referenced less readily available sources whenever they are significantly better than other materials.

Note: No literature is cited as a definitive work. On occasion our opinions may differ in some respects from those stated in the references we cite. Readers are strongly encouraged to read all available material on each topic and to decide for themselves on the applicability of this work to their practice of anesthesia.

The following is a glossary of the abbreviations used in the Catalog of Critical Events.

ABBREVIATIONS

A–a	Alveolar–arterial
ABG(s)	Arterial blood gas(es)
ACC	American College of Cardiology
ACE	Angiotensin-converting enzyme
ACEI	Angiotensin-converting enzyme inhibitor
ACLS	Advanced cardiac life support
ACS	Acute coronary syndrome
ACT	Activated clotting time
ACTH	Adrenocorticotropic hormone
AD	Autonomic dysreflexia
AF	Atrial fibrillation
AFE	Amniotic fluid embolism
AHA	American Heart Association
AIDS	Acquired immune deficiency syndrome
AP	Anteroposterior
APB	Atrial premature beat
aPTT	Activated partial thromboplastin time
ARB	Angiotensin receptor blocker
ARDS	Acute respiratory distress syndrome
ASA	American Society of Anesthesiologists
ASTM	American Society for Testing and Materials
AT	Atrial tachycardia
ATLS	Advanced trauma life support
AV	Atrioventricular
AVNRT	Atrioventricular nodal reentrant tachycardia
AVRT	Atrioventricular reentrant tachycardia
β	Beta
BID	Twice daily
BiPAP	Biphasic positive airway pressure
BLS	Basic life support
BP	Blood pressure
bpm	Beats per minute
BUN	Blood urea nitrogen
Ca^{2+}	Calcium ion
C-A-B	Compressions, airway, breathing
CABG	Coronary artery bypass graft
$CaCl_2$	Calcium chloride

CAD	Coronary artery disease
cc	Cubic centimeter
CHF	Congestive heart failure
CK	Creatine kinase
Cl^-	Chloride ion
cm	Centimeter
CNS	Central nervous system
CO	Cardiac output
CO_2	Carbon dioxide
COHb	Carboxyhemoglobin
COPD	Chronic obstructive pulmonary disease
CPAP	Continuous positive airway pressure
CPB	Cardiopulmonary bypass
CPDA	Citrate-phosphate-dextrose-adenine
CPR	Cardiopulmonary resuscitation
CSE	Combined spinal-epidural
CSF	Cerebrospinal fluid
CT	Computed tomography
CVP	Central venous pressure
CXR	Chest x-ray
D5W	Dextrose 5% in water
DBP	Diastolic blood pressure
DDAVP	Desmopressin
DIC	Disseminated intravascular coagulation
DISS	Diameter Index Safety System
DKA	Diabetic ketoacidosis
dL	Deciliter
DVT	Deep vein thrombosis
EBUS	Endobronchial ultrasound
ECG	Electrocardiogram
ECMO	Extracorporeal membrane oxygenator
ECPR	Extracorporeal cardiopulmonary resuscitation
EEG	Electroencephalogram
EMLA	Topical lidocaine/prilocaine cutaneous local anesthetic
ENT	Ear, nose, and throat
$ET\ CO_2$	End tidal carbon dioxide
$ET\ N_2$	End tidal nitrogen
ETT	Endotracheal tube
FAST	Focused assessment with ultrasound in trauma
Fe^{2+}	Ferrous ion
FFP	Fresh frozen plasma
$FiCO_2$	Fraction of inspired carbon dioxide
FiO_2	Fraction of inspired oxygen
FRC	Functional residual capacity
G	Gauge
g	Gram
G6PD	Glucose-6-phosphate dehydrogenase
GERD	Gastroesophageal reflux disease
GFCI	Ground fault circuit interrupter

GI	Gastrointestinal
H^+	Hydrogen ion
H_1, H_2	Histamine receptors
H_2O	Water
HCO_3^-	Bicarbonate ion
HELLP	Hemolysis, elevated liver function tests, low platelets
Hg	Mercury
Hgb	Hemoglobin
HPV	Hypoxic pulmonary vasoconstriction
HR	Heart rate
I:E	Inspiratory:expiratory ratio
IABP	Intra-aortic balloon pump
ICP	Intracranial pressure
ICU	Intensive care unit
IgE	Immunoglobulin E
IM	Intramuscular
INR	International normalized ratio
IO	Intraosseous
ION	Ischemic optic neuropathy
IR	Interventional radiology
IV	Intravenous
IVC	Inferior vena cava
J	Joule
K^+	Potassium ion
kg	Kilogram
KOH	Potassium hydroxide
L	Liter
LAST	Local anesthetic systemic toxicity
LCR	Laryngeal closure reflex
LMA	Laryngeal mask airway
LR	Lactated Ringer's solution
LVAD	Left ventricular assist device
M	Molar (concentration)
MAC	Minimum alveolar concentration
MAO	Monoamine oxidase
MAP	Mean arterial pressure
MDI	Metered dose inhaler
mEq	Milliequivalent
metHgb	Methemoglobin
mg	Milligram
Mg^{2+}	Magnesium ion
$MgSO_4$	Magnesium sulfate
MH	Malignant hyperthermia
MI	Myocardial infarction
μg	Microgram
min	Minute
mL	Milliliter
mm	Millimeter
mmol	Millimole

MMR	Masseter muscle rigidity
MODS	Multiple organ dysfunction syndrome
mOsm/L	Milliosmols per liter
MRI	Magnetic resonance imaging
MRSA	Methicillin-resistant *Staphylococcus aureus*
MTP	Massive transfusion protocol
MVA	Motor vehicle accident
N_2	Nitrogen
N_2O	Nitrous oxide
Na^+	Sodium ion
$NaHCO_3$	Sodium bicarbonate
NaOH	Sodium hydroxide
NG	Nasogastric
ng	Nanogram
NGT	Nasogastric tube
NIBP	Noninvasive blood pressure
NIRS	Near-infrared spectroscopy
NPH	Neutral protamine Hagedorn
NPO	Nothing by mouth
NS	Normal saline
NSAID	Nonsteroidal anti-inflammatory drug
NSTEMI	Non–ST segment elevation myocardial infarction
NTG	Nitroglycerine
O_2	Oxygen
OR	Operating room
OSA	Obstructive sleep apnea
PA	Pulmonary artery
PAC	Premature atrial contraction
PACU	Postanesthesia care unit
PALS	Pediatric advanced life support
$PaCO_2$	Partial pressure of carbon dioxide in arterial blood
PaO_2	Partial pressure of oxygen in arterial blood
PCI	Percutaneous coronary intervention
PCO_2	Partial pressure of carbon dioxide
PCWP	Pulmonary capillary wedge pressure
PE	Pulmonary embolism
PEA	Pulseless electrical activity
PEEP	Positive end-expiratory pressure
PFO	Patent foramen ovale
pH	Measure of acidity or alkalinity of a solution
PIP	Peak inspiratory pressure
PISS	Pin Index Safety System
PO	Per os
PO_2	Partial pressure of oxygen
PO_4^{+++}	Phosphate
POVL	Perioperative visual loss
PR	Per rectum
PRBCs	Packed red blood cells
psig	Pounds per square inch gauge

PT	Prothrombin time
PTCA	Percutaneous transluminal coronary angioplasty
PVC	Premature ventricular contraction
q8h	Every 8 hours
RAE ETT	Ring, Adair, and Elwyn endotracheal tube
RBBB	Right bundle branch block
RBC	Red blood cell
Rh	Rhesus blood group
RR	Respiratory rate
RSI	Rapid sequence induction
RV	Right ventricle
RVAD	Right ventricular assist device
SBP	Systolic blood pressure
SC	Subcutaneous
SCAD	Spontaneous coronary artery dissection
SCI	Spinal cord injury
SGA	Supraglottic airway
SIADH	Syndrome of inappropriate antidiuretic hormone secretion
SIRS	Systemic inflammatory response syndrome
SL	Sublingual
STEMI	ST segment elevation myocardial infarction
STOP-BANG	Sleep apnea screening questionnaire
SVC	Superior vena cava
SvO_2	Venous oxygen saturation
SVR	Systemic vascular resistance
SVT	Supraventricular tachycardia
T	Temperature
T(numeral)	Thoracic (dermatomal level)
T3	Triiodothyronine
T4	Thyroxine
TAP	Transversus abdominis plane
TEE	Transesophageal echocardiography
TIA	Transient ischemic attack
TRALI	Transfusion-related acute lung injury
TSH	Thyroid-stimulating hormone
TTE	Transthoracic echocardiography
TURP	Transurethral resection of the prostate
UPS	Uninterruptible power supply
URI	Upper respiratory infection
$\dot{V}/\dot{Q}$	Ventilation/perfusion
VAP	Ventilator-associated pneumonia
VF	Ventricular fibrillation
VGE	Venous gas embolism
VT	Ventricular tachycardia
WAGD	Waste anesthetic gas disposal
WBC	White blood cell

Chapter 5
Generic Events
T. KYLE HARRISON and SARA GOLDHABER-FIEBERT

1   Acute Hemorrhage

DEFINITION

Acute hemorrhage is the acute loss of a large volume of blood and can be either overt or covert.

Overt
> Can be visualized in the surgical field, on sponges, or in the suction containers

Covert
> No outward sign of bleeding (e.g., retroperitoneal or intrapleural hemorrhage, blood loss hidden in drapes)

ETIOLOGY

Bleeding from large blood vessel (artery or vein) secondary to surgical manipulation, trauma, or disease

May be related to disorders of coagulation or therapeutic anticoagulation

TYPICAL SITUATIONS

Vascular, cardiac, thoracic, or hepatic surgery

Coagulopathy

Major trauma

Covert hemorrhage more likely when the surgical field is obscured by drapes or distant from the anesthesia professional, or during laparoscopic surgery

Delayed complication of earlier injury, surgery, or invasive procedure (e.g., surgical clip slipping off a vessel)

Occult blood loss (e.g., femoral fracture, gastrointestinal [GI] bleed)

Retroperitoneal surgery or injury

Obstetric emergencies

PREVENTION

Identify and correct coagulopathy early
> Monitor prothrombin time (PT)/partial thromboplastin time (PTT) during warfarin or heparin therapy
> Monitor activated clotting time (ACT) during intraoperative anticoagulation or after administration of protamine

Identify and institute prophylaxis for potential bleeding sites (e.g., GI tract ulcers in ICU patients)

Perform a focused assessment with sonography in trauma (FAST) examination in trauma cases to assess the presence of intraabdominal or pericardial fluid

Insert the largest possible IV catheter if you anticipate having to administer blood during
    a case

Insert arterial line if significant blood loss is anticipated

Establish an institutional massive transfusion protocol (MTP)

MANIFESTATIONS

Overt

    Blood in the surgical field

    Blood on surgical sponges, drapes, and floor

    Suction noise and accumulation of blood in suction containers

    Fall in arterial pressure and filling pressures and increased HR

    Increased pulse pressure variation during positive pressure ventilation

    Hypovolemia assessed by transesophageal echocardiogram (TEE) or transthoracic echo-
        cardiogram (TTE)

    Surgeon's comments (e.g., "Have you given any blood yet?")

Covert

    Unexplained fall in arterial and filling pressures and/or increase in HR

    Low filling pressures assessed by TEE or TTE

    Fall in mixed venous O_2 (if monitored), especially in surgery where covert blood loss is
        possible

    Increase in fluid requirements above what is expected

    Little or transient BP response to administration of an IV fluid bolus or to vasopressor

    Excessive response to vasodilator or anesthetic agents

    Unexplained fall in urine output or hematocrit (a late sign)

    Expanding abdomen or thigh, flank discoloration

    Decreased oxygenation, increased peak inspiratory pressure (PIP) if hemothorax

    Increased pulse pressure variation during positive-pressure ventilation

SIMILAR EVENTS

Hypotension (see Event 9, Hypotension)

Anesthetic or vasodilator overdose (see Event 72, Volatile Anesthetic Overdose)

Anaphylaxis (see Event 16, Anaphylactic and Anaphylactoid Reactions)

Progressively inadequate volume replacement

Occlusion of venous return by compression of the vena cava by the gravid uterus, surgical
    packing, pneumoperitoneum, or retraction

Pneumothorax (see Event 35, Pneumothorax)

Pulmonary embolism (PE) (see Event 21, Pulmonary Embolism)

Cardiac tamponade (see Event 18, Cardiac Tamponade)

Inappropriate diuretic therapy

Tachyarrhythmias

MANAGEMENT

Inform surgeons of the problem

    Keep them informed of its severity

Options for surgeon to consider:
  Convert from laparoscopic to open surgery
  Clamp bleeding vessels, hold pressure on bleeding site, or pack to temporize bleeding
  Clamp the aorta below the diaphragm (may be essential for resuscitation of the patient) (see Event 14, The Trauma Patient)
  Apply hemostatic agents
  Obtain expert surgical assistance
If the abdomen is open, cannulate a large intraabdominal vein for rapid transfusion and cannulate the aorta directly for an arterial line
Consider surgical exploration (if postoperative hemorrhage is suspected)
Increase FiO₂ to 100% with high fresh gas flow
  Replace volatile anesthetic as tolerated with opioids, midazolam
Check and verify BP and other vital signs
Treat severe hypotension with IV bolus of vasopressor
  Ephedrine IV, 5 to 50 mg
  Epinephrine, 10 to 100 μg
  Phenylephrine, 50 to 200 μg
  Repeat as necessary to maintain an acceptable BP
Activate local MTP to get emergency release of blood products
Rapidly restore circulating blood volume
  Use crystalloid, colloid, or blood to replace circulating blood volume
    For massive hemorrhage
      Transfuse a balanced ratio (1:1) of red blood cells (RBCs) to fresh frozen plasma (FFP)
      Transfuse 1 apheresis unit of platelets per 6 units of RBCs, until labs are available
If blood loss is sudden but may be controlled soon, delay giving blood and continue to give crystalloid as needed until bleeding is stopped
Depending on patient comorbidities and extent of hemorrhage, consider tolerating low-normal BP to decrease blood loss and hemodilution until bleeding is controlled
A pressurized bag of saline or colloid will run much faster than a unit of RBCs through a small peripheral IV
Dilute RBCs with saline to increase the speed with which they can be infused
Use an additional small-pore filter to avoid occluding the IV giving-set filter with debris
Warm IV fluids and use other patient warming devices to maintain body temperature (see Event 44, Hypothermia)
CALL FOR HELP if major fluid resuscitation is necessary
  If possible, the primary anesthesiologist should monitor the patient and surgical status and direct activities of OR personnel
  Additional help should
    Check and transfuse blood products, and obtain and reorder blood products when necessary
    Set up rapid transfusor device, if available
    Set up cell saver unit for autotransfusion of RBCs if blood is not contaminated

Ensure adequate IV access; consider intraosseus (IO) line

> Have a minimum of one 16-gauge or larger IV line, preferably more. In the case of severe blood loss, place at least one very large-bore IV line (such as 8.5 French catheter introducer) in a suitable peripheral or central vein. Use large-bore rapid transfusion IV tubing if available.
>
> If IV access is difficult, change a small IV cannula to a large IV cannula by using the Seldinger technique
>
> Use ultrasound guidance for more access
>
> Check IV site to make sure IV line is not infiltrated
>
> Consider IO line placement early in the resuscitation if IV access is difficult

Obtain adequate supplies of IV fluid (colloid or crystalloid)

Continue to NOTIFY BLOOD BANK of blood product needs, per local protocol

If emergency release blood products are administered (O-neg RBCs), send a new blood sample to blood bank for type and screen procedure as soon as possible and prior to transfusion of type-specific blood

Monitor hemodynamic status for adequacy of volume resuscitation

> BP and HR
>
> Central venous pressure (CVP) and/or pulmonary artery (PA) pressure
>
> TEE or TTE

Monitor labs at regular intervals: hematocrit, electrolytes, arterial blood gas (ABG), PT/PTT, fibrinogen every 30 to 60 minutes

Further transfusion of blood and blood products should be guided by lab results

Keep track of surgical events and inform surgeon periodically about resuscitation efforts

COMPLICATIONS

Coagulopathy/disseminated intravascular coagulation (DIC)

Volume overload from overshoot of fluid resuscitation

Hypothermia

Hyperkalemia

Hypocalcemia

Irreversible shock

Acute respiratory distress syndrome (ARDS)/transfusion-related acute lung injury (TRALI)

Allergic/anaphylactic reaction to blood

Transfusion-related viral infection

Myocardial ischemia, arrhythmias

Renal failure

Neurologic injury

Cardiac arrest

SUGGESTED READING

1. Young PP, Cotton BA, Goodnough LT. Massive transfusion protocols for patients with substantial hemorrhage. Transfus Med Rev 2011;25:293-303.
2. Hajjar LA, Vincent JL, Galas FR, et al. Transfusion requirements after cardiac surgery: the TRACS randomized controlled trial. JAMA 2010;304:1559-67.
3. Carson JL, Noveck H, Berlin JA, Gould SA. Mortality and morbidity in patients with very low postoperative Hb levels who decline blood transfusion. Transfusion 2002;42(7):812.
4. Niles SE, McLaughlin DF, Perkins JG, et al. Increased mortality associated with the early coagulopathy of trauma in combat casualties. J Trauma 2008;64:1459-63.
5. Burtelow M, Riley E, Druzin M, et al. How we treat: management of life threatening primary postpartum hemorrhage using a standardized massive transfusion protocol. Transfusion 2007;47:1564-72.

2   Cardiac Arrest

DEFINITION

Cardiac arrest is the absence of effective mechanical activity of the heart.

ETIOLOGY

Cardiovascular disease (e.g., myocardial infarction [MI], myocardial ischemia, cardiomyopathy, arrhythmia, valvular disease, aortic dissection)

Hypovolemia
  Surgical maneuvers or positioning that causes decreased venous return
  Hemorrhage
Hypoxemia
  Failed airway management
  Respiratory arrest
Shock (e.g., anaphylaxis, sepsis)
Bradycardia
  After neuraxial blockade or any acute vagal reflex
  After repeated doses of succinylcholine
Tension pneumothorax
Auto positive end-expiratory pressure (PEEP)
Pulmonary, venous air, or amniotic fluid embolism
Cardiac tamponade
Toxins (e.g., cocaine, methamphetamine)
Anesthetic drug-related complications (e.g., IV or anesthetic overdose, medication error, vasodilator bolus, local anesthetic systemic toxicity [LAST])
MH
Acidosis
Hypoglycemia
Electrolyte abnormalities (e.g., hyperkalemia, particularly in renal failure)
Hypothermia
Pulmonary hypertension
Transfusion reactions
Pacemaker failure

TYPICAL SITUATIONS

ACS
Arrhythmias
Major trauma
Acute hemorrhage
Shock (e.g., anaphylaxis, sepsis)
Following a respiratory arrest
Difficult intubation or ventilation
Hypoxemia (e.g., unrecognized esophageal intubation)
Hypercarbia

PE
Bradycardia during neuraxial blockade
Acute vagal reflex
Drug toxicity (e.g., contraindications to succinylcholine, local anesthetic overdose)
Tension pneumothorax
Cardiac tamponade
Direct myocardial contact with the electrocautery
Pacemaker failure
Electrolyte abnormalities (e.g., hyperkalemia, hypocalcemia)
Obstetric complications

PREVENTION

Evaluate pacemaker function prior to surgery and manage appropriately
Place a transvenous or transcutaneous pacemaker prophylactically for patients with high-grade
    atrioventricular (AV) block or significant sinus bradycardia
Treat arrhythmias with appropriate antiarrhythmic therapy and continue through surgery
Aggressively treat bradycardia/hypotension following neuraxial blockade
Treat ACS to restore myocardial blood flow
Avoid surgery and anesthesia after recent MI
Administer vagolytic drug in patients or in procedures with a high risk of increased vagal tone
    (e.g., neuraxial blockade)
Drill and practice management of unstable patients (using simulation if available)
Administer vagolytic prior to, or mixed with, anticholinesterases that cause bradycardia

MANIFESTATIONS

Unresponsive to verbal commands
Absence of pulse oximeter waveform
Loss of consciousness or seizure-like activity
No palpable carotid pulse (palpation of peripheral pulses unreliable)
        Noninvasive blood pressure (NIBP) unmeasurable
        Invasive arterial pressure without pulsations
                Mean arterial pressure (MAP) less than 20 mm Hg without CPR
Absence of heart tones on auscultation
Apnea
        Loss of, or decreased, ET CO_2
Arrhythmias (ventricular tachycardia [VT], ventricular fibrillation [VF], asystole)
Pulseless electrical activity (PEA) (rhythm in PEA may appear normal)
Cyanosis
Regurgitation and possible aspiration of gastric contents
Lack of ventricular contraction on TEE or TTE

SIMILAR EVENTS

Anaphylaxis (see Event 16, Anaphylactic and Anaphylactoid Reactions)
Pulmonary, venous air, or amniotic fluid embolism (see Event 21, Pulmonary Embolism,
    Event 24, Venous Gas Embolism, and Event 81, Amniotic Fluid Embolism)

Sepsis (see Event 13, The Septic Patient)

Acute hemorrhage (see Event 1, Acute Hemorrhage)

Medication reaction (see Event 63, Drug Administration Error)

Local anesthetic overdose (see Event 52, Local Anesthetic Systemic Toxicity)

Total spinal anesthesia (see Event 89, Total Spinal Anesthesia)

Cardiac disease (MI, ischemia [see Event 15, Acute Coronary Syndrome], cardiomyopathy, aortic dissection)

Hypotension (see Event 9, Hypotension)

Seizures (see Event 57, Seizures)

Artifacts on monitoring devices
    Electrocardiogram (ECG)
    Pulse oximeter
    Blood pressure measurement systems (NIBP or invasive)

MANAGEMENT

Treat the patient, not the monitor

Verify that there is no pulse (and that an "awake" patient has become unresponsive)
    Check pulse oximeter and ET CO_2 waveforms
    Palpate the carotid, femoral, or other pulse
        Surgeon may have better access to palpable pulses
    Check NIBP and ECG monitors and leads
    Check arterial line waveform

Immediately notify surgeons and other OR personnel of the cardiac arrest
    Call for help
    Call OR or hospital "code"
    Call for crash cart and defibrillator
    Start CPR immediately (C-A-B: compressions, airway, breathing)
    Apply defibrillation pads to chest

Turn off ALL anesthetics

Administer 100% O_2 at high flows to flush circuit of inhaled anesthetics and verify change

Begin basic life support (BLS)
    Assign someone to start chest compressions
        Compressions should be at least 100 per minute and at least 2 inches deep
        Rotate compressors every 2 minutes and monitor for fatigue of the person performing chest compressions
        Allow for complete recoil of the chest with each compression
        Minimize interruptions in compressions and keep interruptions brief (less than 10 seconds)
        Adequate compressions should generate an ET CO_2 of at least 10 mm Hg and a diastolic pressure of greater than 20 mm Hg (if an arterial line is in place). You **MUST** improve CPR quality and vascular tone if above conditions are not met.
    Airway/Ventilation
        If patient is not intubated, establish bag mask ventilation with 100% O_2 at a compression to ventilation ratio of 30:2 and prepare for definitive airway
            Place a supraglottic airway (SGA) or endotracheal tube (ETT) without stopping compressions and then ventilate at a rate of 10/minute with continuous compressions

Assign tasks to skilled responders
   Ensure adequate IV access
      If difficult IV access, place IO infusion line
   Place arterial line
   Call for TEE/TTE machine
Begin ACLS
Employ cognitive aids (ACLS algorithms) to help determine diagnosis and treatment
Diagnose and treat arrhythmias
   Determine if patient is in a shockable rhythm
      Analyze rhythm during very short breaks in CPR (e.g., during ventilation phase of
         the 30:2 compression-to-ventilation ratio or while rotating compressors)
         CPR artifact can appear as a shockable rhythm
VT/VF (shockable pathway)
   Continue high-quality CPR
   Defibrillate as soon as possible with 200 J or follow manufacturer's recommendations
   Immediately resume chest compressions after each defibrillation
      Do not check pulse or rhythm
   If a shockable rhythm persists after the initial defibrillation, continue CPR and
      administer epinephrine IV, 1 mg every 3 to 5 minutes
   Consider replacing 1 dose of epinephrine with vasopressin IV, 40 units
   DEFIBRILLATE EVERY 2 MINUTES
   Consider antiarrhythmics
      Amiodarone IV, 300 mg
      Lidocaine IV, 100 mg
   Search for treatable causes for VT/VF
      Torsades de pointes
         Administer magnesium sulfate ($MgSO_4$) IV, 2 g
      Hyperkalemia (see Event 40, Hyperkalemia)
         Administer calcium chloride ($CaCl_2$) 10% IV, 500 to 1000 mg
         Administer dextrose 50% IV, 50 g, and regular insulin IV, 10 units
      Local anesthetic toxicity (see Event 52, Local Anesthetic Systemic Toxicity)
         Administer 20% lipid emulsion (Intralipid)
      MI (see Event 15, Acute Coronary Syndrome)
If rhythm changes to non-shockable rhythm, switch to PEA/asystole pathway
PEA/asystole (non-shockable pathway)
   Continue high-quality CPR
   Administer epinephrine IV, 1 mg every 3 to 5 minutes
   Consider replacing 1 dose of epinephrine with vasopressin IV, 40 units
Search for treatable causes of PEA/asystole
   Hypovolemia (see Event 1, Acute Hemorrhage, and Event 9, Hypotension)
      Administer fluid bolus, rule out occult bleeding, administer sufficient blood
         products for massive hemorrhage or severe anemia
      Evaluate fluid status with TEE or TTE
      Inadequate preload from caval compression
         Release pneumoperitoneum
         Left uterine displacement for gravid uterus
         Return prone patient with large abdomen to supine position
         Release surgical retraction
         Disconnect breathing circuit if breath stacking (auto-PEEP) and adjust
            ventilation appropriately

Hypoxemia (see Event 10, Hypoxemia)

Ventilate and oxygenate with 100% O_2

Auscultate breath sounds

Suction ETT

Reconfirm presence of ET CO_2

Tension pneumothorax (see Event 35, Pneumothorax)

Auscultate for unilateral breath sounds

Absence of sliding pleura sign on TTE

Distended neck veins or deviated trachea

Perform emergent needle decompression at 2nd intercostal space, midclavicular line

Patient will require pleural drainage after needle decompression

Coronary thrombosis (see Event 15, Acute Coronary Syndrome)

Unexplained cardiac arrest may be secondary to MI; consider TEE or TTE to evaluate global myocardial function and regional wall motion abnormalities

Toxins (including infusions)

Confirm that IV and volatile anesthetics are off

Check all infusions

Confirm they are the correct drug and rate of administration

Discontinue if they are not indicated

If the potential for LAST exists (see Event 52, Local Anesthetic Systemic Toxicity)

Administer 20% lipid emulsion (Intralipid)

Consider Intralipid for any overdose of a lipid-soluble drug

Send toxicology screen

Cardiac tamponade

Use TEE or TTE to rule out pericardial effusion

If present, perform emergent pericardiocentesis

Electrolyte and acid/base abnormalities

Send stat labs (ABG and metabolic panel)

Evaluate for acidosis, hyperkalemia, hypokalemia, hypoglycemia, hypocalcemia

VGE (see Event 24, Venous Gas Embolism)

Acute hypotension with drop in ET CO_2

Flood surgical field with saline

Aspirate CVP catheter, if present

PE (see Event 21, Pulmonary Embolism)

Pulmonary hypertension

Use TTE or TEE to assess right ventricular (RV) function

Hyperthermia

Rule out MH (see Event 45, Malignant Hyperthermia)

Hypothermia (see Event 44, Hypothermia)

Continually reassess patient without interrupting chest compressions

Return of spontaneous circulation is indicated by

ECG and palpable pulse or BP

Pulse oximetry waveform

Increase in ET CO_2

Consider postresuscitation hypothermia for brain protection

COMPLICATIONS

Aspiration of gastric contents
Laceration of liver
Pneumothorax or hemothorax
Rib fracture
Hypoxic brain injury
Death

SUGGESTED READING

1. Neumar RW, Otto CW, Link MS, et al. 2010 American Heart Association guidelines for cardiopulmonary resuscitation and emergency cardiovascular care science. Part 8: adult advanced cardiovascular life support. Circulation 2010;122:S729-67.
2. Moitra VK, Gabrielli A, Maccioli GA, O'Connor MF. Anesthesia advanced circulatory life support. Can J Anesth 2012;59:586-603.

---

3   Difficult Tracheal Intubation

DEFINITION

Difficult tracheal intubation occurs when successful intubation of the trachea is not accomplished within the first two attempts by an experienced anesthesia professional.

ETIOLOGY

Anatomical causes of a difficult airway
    Full dentition
    Obesity/short neck
Physician factors
    Inexperience with airway management
    Failure to respond effectively to a rapidly deteriorating situation
Equipment factors
    Inexperience with equipment
    Inadequate backup or alternative airway adjuncts or intubating devices

TYPICAL SITUATIONS

Any patient with anatomy that makes direct laryngoscopy difficult
    Short "bull" neck
    Prominent maxillary incisors
    Limited range of neck or jaw movement
    Short thyromental distance
    Late stages of pregnancy
Congenital syndromes associated with difficulty in endotracheal intubation
Infections of the airway

Acquired anatomic abnormalities
> Intrinsic or extrinsic tumors of the airway
> Following radiation therapy to the head and/or neck
> Acromegaly
> Morbid obesity
> History of sleep apnea
> Tracheal stenosis
> Significant neck swelling or hematoma compressing the airway

PREVENTION

Carefully assess airway anatomy
> Samsoon and Young modification of Mallampati classification
>> Class I: Visualize soft palate, uvula, tonsillar pillars, fauces (same as Mallampati class I)
>> Class II: Visualize soft palate, uvula, fauces
>> Class III: Visualize soft palate, base of uvula only
>> Class IV: Visualize hard palate only (same as Mallampati class III)
>> Class III and IV airways are associated with increased difficulty with tracheal intubation

Assess other patient factors
> Patient's ability to cooperate with airway management plan
> Degree of difficulty with mask ventilation (e.g., facial hair, edentulous patients)
> Degree of difficulty with SGA placement (e.g., limited mouth opening)
> Degree of difficulty with surgical airway access (e.g., limited neck extension, goiter)

Create difficult airway cart with necessary supplies and equipment

Drill and practice management of difficult airway/failed intubation algorithm (using simulation if available)

MANIFESTATIONS

Expected or known difficult tracheal intubation
> Previous history of difficult airway or tracheal intubation
> Airway examination classified as Samsoon and Young's class III or IV
> Presence of other anatomic features that make the patient difficult to intubate

Unexpected difficult tracheal intubation
> Failure to intubate the trachea after two attempts by an experienced anesthesia professional
>> May be secondary to difficult laryngoscopy or difficulty passing the ETT into the trachea

SIMILAR EVENTS

Normal airway but unsuccessful intubation owing to inexperience of the laryngoscopist

MANAGEMENT

Expected Difficult Intubation

Err on the side of caution
> Review previous anesthesia records, focusing on airway management

Perform a careful airway assessment; obtain a second opinion about the airway if you are still unsure of how to proceed

Consider alternatives to general anesthesia but remember that airway management will be difficult if a major complication or inadequate anesthesia occurs

If difficult airway is known or anticipated, consider performing an awake fiberoptic intubation

This will be the safest option in most cases

Awake intubation will be harder to perform if prior attempts at direct laryngoscopy have caused bleeding, secretions, or tissue edema

Administer glycopyrrolate IV, 0.4 mg as antisialagogue

Topicalize oropharynx

Lidocaine 4% nebulized and supplement if necessary

Be aware of total local anesthetic dose administered

Consider Williams airway in oropharynx and intubate over the fiberoptic broncho-scope with a 6.0 to 8.0 ETT

Do not oversedate the patient

Awake intubation can also be performed using video-assisted laryngoscopy with topical anesthesia

Prepare contingency plans and obtain appropriate equipment (difficult airway cart)

Multiple laryngoscope blades (different sizes of Miller and Macintosh blades)

Multiple ETT sizes (at least two sizes smaller than the expected size needed)

Bougie, airway introducers

SGA (e.g., LMA)

Intubating LMA

Video-assisted laryngoscope

Fiberoptic bronchoscope

A cricothyrotomy set (will require a trained person to perform)

If cricothyrotomy would be difficult or impossible, consider CPB standby

Unexpected Difficult Intubation

Call for help (e.g., anesthesia professional, anesthesia technician and surgeon capable of establishing surgical airway)

Call for difficult airway cart

Once help arrives, have them set up additional airway equipment

Mask ventilate with 100% O$_2$; consider using cricoid pressure but release if mask ventilation is difficult

Assess adequacy of ventilation and oxygenation

Place an oral or nasopharyngeal airway

Consider two-person mask ventilation technique

If mask ventilation is possible

Optimize patient's position for intubation

Most experienced person should perform subsequent laryngoscopies

Limit intubation to three attempts

Consider intubation with video-assisted laryngoscopy

Use stylet or bougie

Use smaller ETT if difficulty in passing ETT through cords

Consider placing an SGA to be used as the primary airway device or to be used as a con-duit for fiberoptic intubation with an Aintree exchange catheter

Consider an asleep fiberoptic intubation

Consider using an intubating LMA

Consider allowing spontaneous ventilation to return if possible and awaken the patient; convert to an awake intubation or cancel the case

If mask ventilation or intubation is impossible

    Attempt to place an SGA

        If successful, consider whether to wake the patient, continue the case with the SGA, or attempt to intubate the trachea through the device with an Aintree exchange catheter as outlined earlier

    If SGA is unsuccessful, move early and aggressively to emergency cricothyrotomy or tracheostomy. DO NOT WAIT for the O_2 saturation to fall precipitously

Follow up

After an unexpected difficult intubation, ensure that the patient is informed of the complications and recommend that he or she obtain a MedicAlert bracelet (http://www.medicalert.org) to inform future anesthesia professionals about history of difficult intubation

COMPLICATIONS

Damage to airway structures

Bleeding in the airway

Airway obstruction from loss of airway reflexes or laryngospasm

Hypoxemia

Esophageal intubation

Gastric distention

Regurgitation and aspiration of gastric contents

Damage to the cervical spine during attempts at intubation

SUGGESTED READING

1. Launcelott GO, Johnson LB. Surgical airway. In: Hung O, Murphy MF, editors. Management of the difficult and failed airway. 2nd ed. New York: McGraw-Hill; 2012, chapter 13.
2. Phero JC, Patil YJ, Hurford WE. Evaluation of the patient with a difficult airway. In: Longnecker DE, Newman MF, Brown DL, Zapol WM, editors. Anesthesiology. 2nd ed. New York: McGraw-Hill; 2012, chapter 10.
3. Apfelbaum JL, Silverstein JH, Chung FF, et al. Practice guidelines for management of the difficult airway: an updated report by the American Society of Anesthesiologists Task Force on management of the difficult airway. Updated by the Committee on Standards and Practice Parameters. Anesthesiology 2013;118:251-70.

4   Emergent (Crash) Induction of Anesthesia

DEFINITION

Emergent induction of anesthesia to facilitate an immediate lifesaving intervention

ETIOLOGY

Catastrophic event that results in the immediate need for life-saving surgical intervention

TYPICAL SITUATIONS

Trauma
Stat cesarean section
Vascular catastrophes (e.g., ruptured aortic aneurysm)
Emergent surgical reexploration
    Cardiac tamponade
    Disruption of surgical anastomosis
Cath lab crash
Necrotizing fasciitis

PREVENTION

Resuscitate the patient prior to induction of anesthesia and surgical intervention
Have an OR and anesthesia workstation that is fully functional and ready for use
Have appropriate staff and equipment available
Drill and practice management of stat and urgent surgical cases (using simulation if available)

MANIFESTATIONS

Stat call to the OR, ICU, emergency department (ED), cath lab, obstetrics (OB) suite, etc., for emergent case
Patient may arrive at the OR with little notice
Stat call to patient's bedside with a decision to go emergently to the OR

MANAGEMENT

Do not transport the patient from an area where monitoring and resuscitation are occurring to the OR until it is set up and the anesthesia team and nursing staff are ready to care for the patient.

Call for additional help
    Anesthesia professionals
    Nursing staff (scrub nurse[s] and circulating nurse)
    Technical support (anesthesia and surgical support technicians)
    Surgical assistants
Prepare anesthesia equipment
    If patient is already in the OR, assign someone to monitor the patient as you set up
    Turn on anesthesia machine and monitors
    If time allows, perform **full** machine check
        At minimum, confirm that you are able to provide positive pressure ventilation with machine and circuit
        Confirm suction is functional
    Confirm presence of self-inflating bag/mask
    Confirm airway equipment, including oral airway, ETT, functional laryngoscope blades and handles
    Confirm presence of SGA (e.g., LMA) and bougie for possible difficult airway
    Confirm that video-assisted laryngoscope is present

Prepare medications

> Induction agent as indicated (ketamine, etomidate, propofol)
>
> Neuromuscular blocker (succinylcholine unless contraindicated)
>
> Emergency medications (ephedrine, phenylephrine, and/or epinephrine)

Obtain brief history and physical

> Information can come from patient, medical record, or caregivers
>> Check critical lab values
>>
>> Check whether sample has been sent to blood bank for type and cross
>
> Reassess and confirm it is a life-threatening emergency
>> Avoid crash induction if not medically necessary
>
> Assess whether the patient has allergies to any medications
>
> Assess for major cardiopulmonary disease (e.g., valvular heart disease, low ejection fraction, asthma, chronic obstructive pulmonary disease [COPD])
>
> Perform airway examination

Monitoring

> Determine what IV access and lines are functional
>> Place additional IV access as indicated
>>
>> Consider IO line if unable to quickly achieve vascular access
>
> Connect ECG, NIBP, pulse oximeter, and all invasive monitoring lines that are present
>
> Consider placement of arterial line preinduction if not already present in situ
>> Assign this task to skilled help

Induction

> Preoxygenate while setting up and placing monitors
>
> Confirm left uterine displacement for OB patient
>
> Assume full stomach
>> Consider administration of Bicitra (PO), 30 mL
>
> Modify induction dose of anesthetic based on hemodynamic parameters and patient comorbidities
>> Consider using ketamine or etomidate as an induction agent if hemodynamically unstable
>>
>> Consider IV fluid bolus while preoxygenating patient
>
> Consider video-assisted laryngoscopy as first choice for intubation
>> Turn device on
>>
>> ETT with appropriate stylet
>
> Laryngoscope, ETT, suction on and ready at head of bed
>
> Perform RSI with cricoid pressure
>> Release or manipulate cricoid pressure if unable to visualize the vocal cords or to intubate the trachea
>>
>> Ensure correct placement of ETT via ET CO_2 and auscultation
>
> If unable to intubate, move to video-assisted laryngoscope (see Event 3, Difficult Tracheal Intubation)

Postinduction

> Monitor patient
>> Expect instability and search for treatable causes
>>
>> Support as needed with vasopressors and fluid
>>
>> Consider placement of TEE to monitor myocardial filling and function
>
> Establish additional IV access as indicated
>
> Provide anesthesia as tolerated
>> Balance risk of awareness with hemodynamic stability

Obtain RBCs and other blood products as indicated
Send labs for ABG, blood glucose, and lactate as indicated
Administer appropriate antibiotics

COMPLICATIONS

Aspiration of gastric contents
Difficult intubation
Awareness under anesthesia
Cardiac arrest

SUGGESTED READING

1. Gray LD, Morris CG. The principles and conduct of anaesthesia for emergency surgery. Anaesthesia 2013;68(Suppl. 1):14-29.

5 Esophageal Intubation

DEFINITION

Esophageal intubation is the placement of the ETT in the esophagus at the time of intubation or the subsequent displacement of the ETT from the trachea into the esophagus.

ETIOLOGY

Difficulty in visualizing the larynx at the time of intubation
Difficulty in passing the ETT
Change in position of the ETT after correct placement
Dislodgement by objects placed into, or removed from, the oropharyngeal cavity

TYPICAL SITUATIONS

After a difficult or "blind" intubation
During intubation by an inexperienced laryngoscopist
After manipulation of the patient's head or neck
After placing or removing devices from the esophagus (e.g., TEE probe or nasogastric tube [NGT])
Nasotracheal intubations

PREVENTION

Use proper intubation technique for optimal visualization of the larynx
Observe the ETT passing between the vocal cords
Secure the ETT carefully before allowing movement or positioning of the patient's head
Check the position of the ETT after each change of the patient's position or manipulation of the ETT

Visualize the carina during fiberoptic intubation
Use video-assisted laryngoscopy for difficult intubations or as a confirmation of proper ETT
  placement

MANIFESTATIONS

Abnormally low or absent ET CO_2 waveform after the first few breaths
Equivocal or absent thoracic breath sounds
Breath sounds or gurgling heard over the epigastrium
Abnormal compliance during hand or mechanical ventilation
Leakage around the ETT with a normal ETT cuff volume
In the awake patient, continued vocalization after the cuff of the ETT is inflated
Visualization of the ETT in the esophagus on direct or video-assisted laryngoscopy
Inability to palpate the cuff of the ETT in the sternal notch
Regurgitation of gastric contents up the ETT
Late signs
    Decreasing O_2 saturation and cyanosis
    Hypotension
    Bradycardia, premature ventricular contractions (PVCs), tachyarrhythmias, asystole
    VT/VF

SIMILAR EVENTS

Malfunction or disconnection of capnograph
Breath sounds that are difficult to hear
Complete or partial extubation (see Event 37, Unplanned Extubation)
Endobronchial intubation (see Event 30, Endobronchial Intubation)
Severe bronchospasm (see Event 29, Bronchospasm)
Kinked ETT (see Event 7, High Peak Inspiratory Pressure)
Rupture of, or failure to inflate, the ETT cuff

MANAGEMENT

*Development of hypoxemia within 10 minutes of intubation must be assumed to be due to
esophageal intubation unless capnography demonstrates a sustained normal CO_2 waveform or video-assisted laryngoscopy clearly shows ETT passing through the vocal cords.*

Preoxygenate the patient before induction; check ET O_2
    Administer 100% O_2 until ETT placement is verified
Verify position of the ETT after intubation
    Inflate ETT cuff and check for leak
    Check for a normal ET CO_2 waveform on the capnograph
    Listen for breath sounds in both axillae and over the stomach
    Look for bilateral chest expansion
    Manually ventilate the patient; assess the compliance of the reservoir bag
    Perform direct or video-assisted laryngoscopy to visualize the position of the ETT rela-
        tive to the vocal cords

Get help if there are problems determining the position of the ETT
　Have assistant prepare fiberoptic bronchoscope to assist with ETT verification and placement
If the patient desaturates and you are unable to verify ETT placement
　Remove ETT and ventilate with 100% O_2 by mask or SGA
If esophageal intubation is confirmed
　Remove the misplaced ETT
　Ventilate with 100% O_2 by mask or SGA if O_2 saturation is <95%
　Reintubate the trachea with a clean ETT using video-assisted laryngoscope
If intubation was difficult on the first attempt or reintubation fails (see Event 3, Difficult Tracheal Intubation)
　Ventilate with 100% O_2 by mask if O_2 saturation is <95%
　Call for help and for difficult airway equipment
　Prepare to place an SGA (e.g., LMA)
　Consider waking the patient for possible awake intubation
　Prepare for possible fiberoptic intubation
　Prepare for surgical airway

After tracheal intubation, place an orogastric tube to empty the stomach

COMPLICATIONS

Hypoxemia
Hypercarbia
Cardiac arrest
Airway, pharyngeal, or dental trauma from repeated laryngoscopy
Aspiration of gastric contents
Hypertension, tachycardia
Myocardial ischemia/infarction

SUGGESTED READING

1. Salem MR. Verification of endotracheal tube position. Anesthesiol Clin North America 2001;19:813-39.

6　High Inspired CO_2

DEFINITION

A high inspired CO_2 is the presence of any CO_2 in the inspired gas.

ETIOLOGY

Decreased absorption of CO_2 in the anesthesia breathing circuit
Decreased elimination of CO_2 from the anesthesia breathing circuit (e.g., low fresh gas flow)
Increased CO_2 production by the patient (e.g., MH, fever)
Increased exogenous CO_2 in the anesthesia breathing circuit

TYPICAL SITUATIONS

CO_2 absorbent exhausted
Stuck open (incompetent) unidirectional valve in the anesthesia breathing circuit
Low fresh gas flow in nonrebreathing circuits
Sampling of CO_2 trapped under drapes in a spontaneously breathing patient (e.g., inadequate washout of exhaled gases)
Malpositioned CO_2 canister bypass valve
Artifact (e.g., water contamination of sensor, sampling rate too low)
Improper circuit assembly (e.g., Bain circuit)
Faulty position of ET CO_2 sampling port
Exogenous source of CO_2
Channeling of anesthetic gas flow through CO_2 absorbent

PREVENTION

Perform a thorough pre-use check of the anesthesia machine, including status of CO_2 absorbent
Replace CO_2 absorbent when indicated
Check function of unidirectional valves during pre-use machine check

MANIFESTATIONS

Purple (exhausted) CO_2 absorbent
　　　Color change may not be visible despite exhaustion
Capnograph waveform does not go to zero
High fraction of inspired carbon dioxide ($FiCO_2$) alarm
"Reverse flow" alarm if incompetent unidirectional valve is present
Incompetent unidirectional valve is observable

SIMILAR EVENTS

Hypercarbia (see Event 32, Hypercarbia)
Circle system valve stuck open (see Event 61, Circle System Valve Stuck Open)
Faulty gas supply (see Event 65, Faulty Oxygen Supply)
Monitor failure (e.g., zero calibration error)

MANAGEMENT

Ensure oxygenation and ventilation
Increase fresh gas flows to 10 L/min to decrease $FiCO_2$
Replace CO_2 absorbent if exhaustion detected or suspected, even if no color change is perceived
Inspect unidirectional valves for incompetence and replace valve if needed
If bypass valve (present on some older anesthesia machines) is incorrectly set, change to include CO_2 absorber assembly
Look for exogenous source of CO_2 (e.g., CO_2 cylinders)
If unable to quickly detect and correct the etiology of inspired CO_2

Ventilate with an alternate ventilating system (e.g., self-inflating bag or nonrebreathing circuit)

Maintain anesthesia with IV agents

If necessary, consider changing out the entire anesthesia workstation; this will require help

COMPLICATIONS

Hypercarbia
    Arrhythmias
    Hypertension and tachycardia
    Altered mental status
    Intracranial pressure (ICP) increase
Awareness
Complications of changing anesthesia workstation
Cardiac arrest

SUGGESTED READING

1. Pond D, Jaffe RJ, Brock-Utne JG. Failure to detect CO_2-absorbent exhaustion: seeing and believing. Anesthesiology 2000;92:1196.
2. Kodali BS. Capnography outside the operating rooms. Anesthesiology 2013;118:192-201.

7 High Peak Inspiratory Pressure

DEFINITION

A high PIP is an increase of more than 5 cm H_2O during positive pressure ventilation or a PIP greater than 40 cm H_2O.

ETIOLOGY

Breathing circuit problem
    Ventilator/bag selector switch in the wrong position
    Inspiratory, expiratory, or pop-off valve stuck in the closed position
    Intentional or unintentional addition of PEEP to the breathing circuit
    Kinked or misconnected hose in the breathing circuit or waste anesthesia gas disposal (WAGD) system
    Failure of check valves or regulators in the anesthesia machine, allowing gas under high pressure into the breathing circuit
    Use of the O_2 flush when circuit is closed
    O_2 flush control stuck in the ON position
Raised intraabdominal pressure
    Insufflation of the peritoneal cavity for laparoscopic surgery
    Obesity

Prone position
Ascites
Late-stage pregnancy
ETT problem
Kink in the ETT
Foreign body, secretions, or mucus plugging the ETT
Endobronchial, esophageal, or submucosal intubation
Herniated ETT cuff obstructing the end of the ETT
Dissection of the interior surface of the ETT, leading to narrowing
Decreased pulmonary compliance
Pulmonary aspiration of gastric contents
Bronchospasm
Atelectasis
Decreased chest wall or diaphragmatic compliance
Pulmonary edema
Pneumothorax
TRALI
Coughing or bucking on ETT
Drug-induced problem
Opioid-induced chest wall rigidity
Inadequate muscle relaxation
MH

TYPICAL SITUATIONS

During induction of anesthesia
Immediately after intubation
Light anesthesia
During laparoscopic surgery
After change in patient or head position
Following manipulation of the ETT
Patients with COPD or asthma
After adding components to the breathing circuit
During or following surgery in or near the pleural cavities

PREVENTION

Optimize medical management of patients with COPD and asthma
Check the breathing circuit and the ETT carefully before use
Place the ETT carefully and position cuff just past the vocal cords
Maintain adequate anesthetic depth and muscle relaxation
Maintain insufflation pressures at minimum consistent with surgical needs
Use care when adding components to the breathing circuit
Plan anesthetic management to minimize bronchospasm, atelectasis, or buildup of secretions
in patients at risk
Optimize mode of ventilation to minimize PIP
Minimize abdominal compression in patients in the prone position

MANIFESTATIONS

High PIP alarm

Decreased compliance of the reservoir bag during manual ventilation

Decreased minute ventilation compared to set ventilator parameters, secondary to lower tidal volumes

> Especially with pressure-controlled ventilation
>
> Little or no excursion of the chest with inspiration
>
> Reduced or altered breath sounds

Abnormal sound of the ventilator during inspiration

Decreased or abnormal ET CO_2 waveform

Fall in O_2 saturation

Profound hypotension not responsive to vasopressors or inotropes resulting from reduced venous return secondary to high PIP

Tachycardia

SIMILAR EVENTS

Faulty airway pressure gauge or airway pressure alarm

Pneumothorax (see Event 35, Pneumothorax)

MANAGEMENT

Increase the FiO$_2$ to 100% and reconfirm presence of ET CO$_2$

Verify the PIP

Switch to manual ventilation using the anesthesia breathing circuit's reservoir bag (adjust adjustable pressure limiting [APL] valve)

> Assess the pulmonary/breathing circuit compliance

If hypotensive, disconnect from circuit to rule out auto PEEP

Disconnect the Y piece from the ETT and squeeze the reservoir bag

> If the airway pressure remains high, there is an obstruction in the breathing circuit
>
> > Ventilate using a backup ventilation system (non-rebreathing circuit, self-inflating bag, or mouth-to-ETT)
> >
> > Get help to replace or repair the obstruction in the circuit
>
> If the airway pressure falls, the problem is in the ETT or lungs, not in the breathing circuit

Auscultate both sides of the patient's chest

> Listen for symmetry of breath sounds, wheezes, or crackles (rales)
>
> If breath sounds are asymmetric
>
> > Examine the ETT and rule out endobronchial intubation (see Event 30, Endobronchial Intubation)
> >
> > Check BP and HR, palpate the trachea, percuss the chest, and rule out pneumothorax (see Event 35, Pneumothorax)
>
> If breath sounds are symmetric but abnormal
>
> > Consider bronchospasm if wheezes are present (see Event 29, Bronchospasm)
> >
> > Consider pulmonary edema if crackles are present (see Event 20, Pulmonary Edema)

Exclude ETT obstruction

> Pass a suction catheter down the ETT and apply suction to clear any secretions
>
> If it passes *freely,* the ETT is unlikely to be obstructed
>
> If the ETT is markedly obstructed

Deflate the ETT cuff and check again
Consider placing fiberoptic bronchoscope to examine ETT and airway
If unable to relieve obstruction
    Consider replacing the ETT over airway-exchange catheter
    Retain ETT for later examination
    Reintubate with a new ETT
Notify the surgical team of the problem and review any possible cause
Check for other causes of decreased chest compliance
    Inadequate depth of anesthesia or muscle relaxation
    Excessive insufflation of the abdomen
    Unusual patient position or excessive surgical retraction
    Change in patient's position (e.g., slipping off prone position supports)
    Abnormal anatomy of the patient (e.g., kyphoscoliosis)
    MH (see Event 45, Malignant Hyperthermia)

COMPLICATIONS

Barotrauma
    Pneumothorax
    Pneumomediastinum
Hypotension, cardiovascular compromise
Hypoxemia
Cardiac arrest, if severe
Hypertension, tachycardia after resolution of high PIP, owing to delayed circulation time of IV
    fluid, vasopressors and inotropes

SUGGESTED READING

1. Gadsden J, Jones DL. Events. In: Gadsden J, Jones DL, editors. Anesthesiology oral board flash cards. New York: McGraw-Hill; 2011.
2. Dorsch JA, Dorsch SE. Hazards of anesthesia machines and breathing systems. In: Dorsch JA, Dorsch SE, editors. Understanding anesthesia equipment. 5th ed. Philadelphia: Lippincott Williams & Wilkins; 2008. p. 404-30.

8   Hypertension

DEFINITION

Hypertension is a rise in arterial BP of more than 20% above baseline or an absolute value of arterial BP above age-corrected limits.

ETIOLOGY

Preexisting hypertension
    Essential hypertension
    Secondary hypertension (e.g., renal or endocrine causes, preeclampsia)
Catecholamine release
    Laryngoscopy or intubation

Surgical stimulation
Emergence from anesthesia
Hypoxemia
Hypercarbia
Acute withdrawal of antihypertensive medication
Autonomic dysreflexia
Pheochromocytoma
Thyroid storm
Carcinoid syndrome
MH
Bladder distention
Cushing response to rising ICP
Administration of vasopressor medications
Anesthetic not being delivered as expected (e.g., IV, infusion pump, or volatile anesthetic administration failure)
Volume overload
Acute increase in afterload (e.g., cross-clamping of the aorta)

TYPICAL SITUATIONS

Anesthesia in patients with chronic hypertension
During intubation or on emergence from general anesthesia
Inadequate depth of anesthesia relative to level of surgical stimulus
Vasopressor administration
Prolonged tourniquet time
In patients with pregnancy-induced hypertension
Acute drug intoxication (e.g., cocaine)
Drug withdrawal

PREVENTION

Treat preoperative hypertension adequately
    Continue preoperative administration of antihypertensive medications up to the time of surgery
        Consider holding angiotensin-converting enzyme inhibitor (ACEI) and angiotensin receptor blocker (ARB) on the day of surgery to reduce risk of intraoperative hypotension
    Consider postponing elective surgery if severe hypertension is present (e.g., systolic blood pressure [SBP] >200 mm Hg or diastolic blood pressure [DBP] >110 mm Hg)
    Postpone elective surgery if organ dysfunction is present (e.g., myocardial ischemia, congestive heart failure [CHF], neurologic dysfunction)
Consider arterial line for continuous BP monitoring
Consider TTE to assess myocardial ischemia or heart failure
Consider the use of clonidine as oral premedication
Avoid ketamine for induction of anesthesia in known hypertensive patients
Anticipate times of high levels of surgical stimulation and prophylactically increase the depth of anesthesia
Avoid hypervolemia (e.g., transurethral resection of the prostate [TURP] cases)

Carefully titrate vasoactive medications

Maintain oxygenation and ventilation at normal levels

Use BP monitoring equipment properly

Treat severe pain, hypoxemia, or bladder distention in the postoperative period

Minimize tubing between vasopressor infusion pump and patient and use carrier infusion to prevent accumulation of vasopressor in tubing being inadvertently bolused into patient

Consider using a separate IV for drug infusions

MANIFESTATIONS

Rise in, or high, arterial pressure (systolic, diastolic, or mean)

If hypertension is due to light anesthesia, the patient may exhibit

Tachypnea if breathing spontaneously

Tachycardia

Sweating

Tearing

Pupillary dilation

Movement

Bradycardia may occur as a result of baroreceptor activity, especially if the cause of hypertension is autonomic dysreflexia, raised ICP, or administration of vasopressor (e.g., phenylephrine)

SIMILAR EVENTS

Artifacts of BP measurement system

Motion artifact with NIBP device

Inappropriately small NIBP cuff

Faulty or inaccurately zeroed transducer

Transducer placed lower than the patient's heart

Resonance artifact of measurement

Drug administration error (see Event 63, Drug Administration Error)

MH (see Event 45, Malignant Hyperthermia)

Hypertensive disorders of pregnancy (see Event 88, Preeclampsia-Eclampsia)

Acute drug intoxication

Acute drug withdrawal

Thyrotoxicosis (see Event 49, Thyroid Storm)

Pheochromocytoma

Carcinoid syndrome

Raised ICP

Autonomic dysreflexia (see Event 17, Autonomic Dysreflexia)

MANAGEMENT

Verify that hypertension is real

If using a NIBP monitoring device

Repeat measurement

Check for artifact of NIBP system

Consider moving BP cuff to another site

Measure BP manually
If using an arterial line
  Check transducer height
  Zero arterial transducer
  Flush the arterial line
  Correlate with NIBP measurement
  Check that there are no kinks in the arterial line tubing

Check drug administration
If infusions of vasoactive drugs or IV anesthetics are being administered
  Check tubing from source to patient
  Check that infusion devices are set properly and the intended drugs are running at the desired rate
  Check the dosage calculations carefully
  Check the concentration of the medications being infused
  Check that the carrier IV line is running at an appropriate rate
  Check for IV disconnection or infiltration
If administering a volatile anesthetic
  Check that the vaporizer is set correctly
  Check the level of liquid anesthetic in the vaporizer
  Check the inspired concentration of anesthetic

Ensure adequate oxygenation and ventilation
Check ABGs if there is any question of hypoxemia or hypercarbia (see Event 10, Hypoxemia, and Event 32, Hypercarbia)

Assess depth of anesthesia
Assess clinical signs of anesthetic depth
Look for a new surgical stimulus
Increase anesthesia/analgesia as necessary
  Increase delivery of volatile or IV anesthetic
  Administer bolus of IV opioid
  Administer bolus of IV anesthetic
  If using a continuous regional anesthesia technique, administer additional local anesthetic via the catheter
  Ask surgeon to administer local anesthesia at surgical site
Consider use of processed EEG to assess depth of anesthesia
For isolated hypertension not resulting from an identifiable cause
  Decrease surgical stimulation (e.g., empty bladder in a patient with autonomic dysreflexia)
  Check for secondary manifestations of hypertension (tachycardia, ST-T wave changes [see Event 12, ST Segment Change])
  If additional treatment is necessary, consider
    Deepening the anesthetic
    β-Blockade (use with caution in patients with asthma/COPD)
      Labetalol IV, 5 to 10 mg bolus
      Esmolol IV, 10 to 50 mg bolus
      Metoprolol IV, 1 to 2 mg bolus
    Hydralazine IV, 2 to 4 mg bolus
    Nitroglycerine (NTG) IV infusion, 0.1 to 2 µg/kg/min
    Nitroprusside IV infusion, 0.1 to 3 µg/kg/min
    Calcium channel blockade

Verapamil IV, 2.5 mg increments

Diltiazem IV, loading dose 0.25 mg/kg over 2 min. If IV infusion is necessary, 10-25 mg/hr after IV bolus dose

Nicardipine IV infusion, 3 to 15 mg/hr

α-Blockade

Phentolamine IV, 0.5 to 1 mg (see Event 17, Autonomic Dysreflexia)

Review fluid management

If volume overload is likely, administer furosemide IV, 5 to 10 mg

Check for the presence of a distended bladder; place a urinary catheter if the bladder is distended

Raised ICP may require urgent therapy

Mannitol IV, 0.5 g/kg

Furosemide IV, 5 to 10 mg

Hyperventilation to partial pressure of carbon dioxide in arterial blood ($PaCO_2$) of 25 to 30 mm Hg

Rapid neurosurgical intervention

Exclude MH as a diagnosis (see Event 45, Malignant Hyperthermia)

COMPLICATIONS

Myocardial ischemia/infarction
Arrhythmias
CHF/pulmonary edema
Increased operative blood loss
Poor surgical visibility (e.g., endoscopic procedures)
Awareness (if insufficient anesthetic)
Raised ICP
Disruption of vascular suture lines
Cerebral hemorrhage (including ruptured aneurysm) or hypertensive encephalopathy

SUGGESTED READING

1. Levy JH. Management of systemic and pulmonary hypertension. Tex Heart Inst J 2005;32:467-71.
2. Paix AD, Runciman WB, Horan BF, Chapman MJ, Currie M. Crisis management during anaesthesia: hypertension. Qual Saf Health Care 2005;14:e12.
3. Howell SJ, Sear JW, Foex P. Hypertension, hypertensive heart disease and perioperative cardiac risk. Br J Anaesth 2004;92:570-84.

9   Hypotension

DEFINITION

Hypotension is a fall in arterial BP of more than 20% below baseline or an absolute value of SBP below 90 mm Hg or of MAP below 60 mm Hg.

ETIOLOGY

Decreased preload

Hypovolemia (e.g., hemorrhage including occult blood loss)

Surgical maneuvers restricting venous return
Elevated intrathoracic pressure (e.g., pneumothorax)
Patient position or gravid uterus
PE
Cardiac tamponade
Primary cardiac causes (e.g., diastolic dysfunction, valvular regurgitation)
Decreased contractility
Inotropic depressant drugs (e.g., anesthetic agents)
CHF (e.g., cardiomyopathy)
Myocardial ischemia/infarction
Hypoxemia
Valvular heart disease
Abrupt increase in afterload
Decreased systemic vascular resistance (SVR)
Drug effects (e.g., anesthetics, vasodilators)
Shock (e.g., sepsis, anaphylaxis, neurogenic)
Endocrine abnormalities (Addisonian crisis, hypothyroidism, hypoglycemia, after removal of pheochromocytoma)
Abrupt change in mechanical afterload
Arrhythmias
Tachycardia or irregular rhythm (loss of ventricular filling)
Bradycardia

TYPICAL SITUATIONS

After anesthetic induction and before surgical incision
Hypovolemia (e.g., trauma, chronic hypertension)
Neuraxial anesthesia
Surgery with major fluid shifts
Surgery on or near major vascular structures
Patients on ACEIs or ARBs
Patients with history of chronic amphetamine abuse
Patients with history of cardiovascular disease
Position other than supine (especially in obese patients)
Peritoneal insufflation
During arrhythmias

PREVENTION

Carefully assess cardiovascular status preoperatively, checking for
Patient history and fluid status
Increased HR or orthostatic hypotension
CVP or jugular venous filling
Preoperative hematocrit
Ensure adequate intravascular volume before induction of anesthesia
Consider fluid loading prior to induction of anesthesia or neuraxial blockade
Consider placing arterial line prior to induction of anesthesia in patients at high risk of intraoperative hypotension

Correlate invasive BP with NIBP early in case
Avoid high doses of anesthetic agents
Treat bradycardia early in patients with neuraxial blockade
Administer drugs slowly if hypotension is a known side effect (e.g., vancomycin)
Use appropriate doses of local anesthetics in single-shot regional techniques and carefully
    titrate local anesthetics in continuous regional techniques
Monitor surgical activities and track blood loss carefully
Consider holding ACEIs and ARBs prior to surgery

MANIFESTATIONS

Fall in or low BP (systolic, diastolic, or mean)
    NIBP cuff with low value or continually cycling
    Dampened or low arterial line waveform
Mental status changes (nausea and/or vomiting in conscious patient)
Weak or absent peripheral pulses
Decreased O_2 saturation or inability of pulse oximeter to obtain a satisfactory reading
Arrhythmias, including sinus tachycardia
Decreased ET CO_2
Decreased urine output
Diminished heart sounds
Skin mottling

SIMILAR EVENTS

Artifact of BP measurement system
    Motion artifact with NIBP device
    Incorrect size of NIBP cuff
    Faulty BP transducer
    Transducer placed higher than patient
    Loose connections on arterial line
Vasospasm of radial artery or subclavian stenosis
Lack of correlation of BPs on dependent and nondependent arms in patients in lateral decubitus
    position

MANAGEMENT

Rule out rapidly lethal, often missed causes of severe hypotension: hemorrhage (occult blood loss), anesthetic overdose, myocardial ischemia, hypertrophic obstructive cardiomyopathy, pneumothorax, auto-PEEP, anaphylaxis, and surgical causes (e.g., pneumoperitoneum, inferior vena cava [IVC] compression)

Ensure adequate oxygenation and ventilation
    Check the O_2 saturation
        Increase the FiO_2 if O_2 saturation is low or if hypotension is severe
    Auscultate breath sounds (see Event 35, Pneumothorax, Event 16, Anaphylactic and
        Anaphylactoid Reactions, and Event 29, Bronchospasm)
    Check airway pressure (see Event 7, High Peak Inspiratory Pressure)

Verify that the patient is hypotensive

    Repeat NIBP measurement once

    Flush arterial line if present

    Palpate pulse and check capnograph

    If no pulse, start CPR (see Event 2, Cardiac Arrest)

        Call for help and get crash cart with defibrillator

    If pulse is strong and other vital signs stable, consider artifact or transient

        Repeat NIBP measurement, ensuring nobody is leaning on cuff

        Measure at a different site (e.g., leg)

        Measure BP manually

        Re-zero the arterial line transducer

        Check that the transducer is at the correct level

        Ensure that the transducer is connected to the appropriate monitoring cable of the physiologic monitor

        Check the arterial line for any open or loose stopcocks or connections

Reduce or turn off any vasodilating drugs (including anesthetics)

If anaphylaxis is suspected, stop administration of possible antigen and administer epinephrine and IV fluids (see Event 16, Anaphylactic and Anaphylactoid Reactions)

Expand circulating blood volume

    Lift the patient's legs above the level of the heart or put the patient into the Trendelenburg position

    Administer IV fluids rapidly

        If history of CHF, use multiple small boluses and reevaluate frequently

    Use crystalloid, colloids, or blood for rapid volume expansion

    Ensure sufficient large-bore IV access if continued volume replacement is necessary

        Call for help

        Consider placement of IO line if peripheral IV access is difficult or not possible

    Communicate situation to surgeons

        Check for retractors causing venous compression

        Check for ongoing or occult blood loss

        Discuss need for additional expert surgical help or whether the surgical procedure should be terminated

Treat severe hypotension with vasopressors

    Ephedrine IV, 5 to 50 mg

    Phenylephrine IV, 50 to 200 μg

    Epinephrine IV, 10 to 100 μg

    Vasopressin IV, 1 to 4 units

    Repeat as necessary to maintain an acceptable BP

    Consider infusion of vasopressors with ongoing needs

    Consider infusion of methylene blue IV in cases of sepsis or hypotension secondary to ACEIs and ARBs

    Consider administration of IV steroid (see Event 38, Addisonian Crisis)

        Administer hydrocortisone IV, 100 mg bolus, repeat q8h

Elucidate and correct the underlying cause of hypotension

    Consider placement of an arterial line and urinary catheter if not present

    TEE or TTE to assess myocardial filling and function

    Consider placement of PA catheter for fluid management

    Check urine output, hematocrit, and fluid balance

Consider placing an arterial line into the central arterial circulation (usually the femoral artery), especially if overall assessment is consistent with a failure of the radial artery pressure to correlate with central arterial pressure

Check ABG and labs, including hemoglobin (Hgb), electrolytes, calcium, lactate, cardiac enzymes, type and cross (see Event 46, Metabolic Acidosis, and Event 13, The Septic Patient)

Evaluate myocardial status

Check the ECG and/or TEE/TTE for signs of ischemia (see Event 12, ST Segment Change)

COMPLICATIONS

Myocardial ischemia/infarction
Cerebral ischemia
Acute renal failure
CHF or pulmonary edema from excessive fluid administration
Hypertension from treatment of artifact or transient
Cardiac arrest

SUGGESTED READING

1. Bijker JB, van Klei WA, Vergouwe Y, et al. Intraoperative hypotension and 1-year mortality after noncardiac surgery. Anesthesiology 2009;111:1217-26.
2. Morris RW, Watterson LM, Westhorpe RN, Webb RK. Crisis management during anaesthesia: hypotension. Qual Saf Health Care 2005;14:e11.
3. Moitra V, Gabrielli A, Maccioli GA, O'Connor MF. Anesthesia advanced circulatory life support. Can J Anesth 2012;59:586-603.
4. Subramaniam B, Talmor D. Echocardiography for management of hypotension in the intensive care unit. Crit Care Med 2007;35:S401-7.
5. Pollard JB. Cardiac arrest during spinal anesthesia: common mechanisms and strategies for prevention. Anesth Analg 2001;92:252-6.

10   Hypoxemia

DEFINITION

A fall in O_2 saturation of more than 5%, an absolute value of O_2 saturation below 90%, or an absolute value of partial pressure of arterial oxygen (PaO_2) below 60 mm Hg

ETIOLOGY

Low FiO_2
    Relative (inadequate for the patient's condition)
    Absolute (problems delivering O_2 to the breathing circuit)
Inadequate alveolar ventilation
Ventilation/perfusion ($\dot{V}/\dot{Q}$) mismatch
Anatomic shunt
Excessive metabolic O_2 demand

Low cardiac output (CO)
Diffusion abnormality (usually chronic, not acute)

TYPICAL SITUATIONS

Inadequate ventilation from any cause
    Failure to maintain the airway during general or regional anesthesia, or during sedation
    Failure to ventilate adequately during general anesthesia (e.g., surgery with pneumoperitoneum)
    Morbid obesity
Patients with increased alveolar–arterial (A–a) gradient
    Preexisting lung disease
    Pulmonary edema
    Aspiration of gastric contents
    Atelectasis
    Pulmonary embolus
    One-lung ventilation
Patients at extremes of age are more likely to have anatomic and physiologic features or disease states that compromise oxygenation

PREVENTION

Perform a careful check of the anesthesia machine, O_2 analyzer, and alarms before use
Preoxygenate for 3 minutes with a goal of obtaining an ET $O_2 > 80\%$
    Alternatively, have patient take 10 large breaths
    Consider preoxygenating in reverse Trendelenburg, especially in patients with decreased functional residual capacity (FRC) (e.g., obese patients)
Monitor and adjust FiO_2 and ventilation as necessary to maintain patient oxygenation
Consider adding 5 cm H_2O PEEP during mechanical ventilation
Avoid prolonged spontaneous ventilation during general anesthesia in patients with lung disease or when the patient is not in the supine position
Evaluate the effect of positioning on the patient's cardiopulmonary function prior to incision (e.g., steep Trendelenburg during robotic prostatectomy)

MANIFESTATIONS

Decreased or low O_2 saturation measured by pulse oximetry is the cardinal sign of hypoxemia
Pulse oximetry may not function properly in the presence of
    Hypothermia
    Poor peripheral circulation
    Artifacts owing to electrocautery, motion, ambient lighting, poor contact, blue/black-based nail polish, or dyes (e.g., methylene blue, indigo carmine)
Cyanosis or dark blood in the surgical field
    Clinically detectable cyanosis corresponds to an arterial O_2 saturation of approximately 85%, requires 5 g of reduced Hgb, and may be masked by anemia
Under anesthesia, the circulatory and respiratory responses to hypoxemia are blunted by anesthetic agents
Late signs of hypoxemia include

Bradycardia
Myocardial arrhythmias/ischemia
Tachycardia
Hypotension
Cardiac arrest

SIMILAR EVENTS

Pulse oximeter artifact
Blood gas analysis of venous blood
Methemoglobinemia
Low CO

MANAGEMENT

Assume that low O_2 saturation indicates hypoxemia until proven otherwise
> Development of hypoxemia within 10 minutes of intubation must be assumed to be due to an esophageal intubation unless capnography demonstrates a persistent normal ET CO_2 waveform or the ETT can be clearly visualized passing through the vocal cords with direct or video-assisted laryngoscopy

Increase FiO_2 to 100%
> Use high O_2 flow to equilibrate the breathing circuit rapidly
> Verify that FiO_2 approaches 100%

Check that ventilation is adequate
> Check ET CO_2
>> Maintain tidal volumes (6 to 8 mL/kg predicted body weight) and adjust respiratory rate (RR) as indicated
> Consider the addition of 5 cm H_2O PEEP to breathing circuit to prevent atelectasis
> Check position of the ETT
>> Direct visualization of ETT cuff passing through the cords or visualization of tracheal rings and the carina via bronchoscopy
>> Adjust the position of the ETT if necessary
> Check PIP
>> High PIP (see Event 7, High Peak Inspiratory Pressure)
>>> Switch to hand ventilation to assess pulmonary compliance
>>> If cardiovascularly stable, hand ventilate with large tidal volumes to expand collapsed lung segments
>>> Auscultate breath sounds and assess symmetry of chest movement to rule out bronchospasm, endobronchial intubation, or pneumothorax (see Event 29, Bronchospasm, Event 30, Endobronchial Intubation, and Event 35, Pneumothorax)
>> Low PIP
>>> Check for leak (see Event 69, Major Leak in the Anesthesia Breathing Circuit)
>>> Auscultate breath sounds and assess symmetry of chest movement
> Consider asynchrony of the ventilator with patient's effort to breathe
>> Check level of neuromuscular blockade and redose muscle relaxant if indicated
> Obtain ABG and ask blood gas laboratory to perform co-oximetry if presence of carboxyhemoglobin or methemoglobin is suspected

10

Check vital signs
Verify function of the pulse oximeter
Do not fixate on oximeter function. Monitor the patient carefully while ruling out artifacts and transients
Correlate oximeter readings with activation of electrocautery
Check the probe position and consider changing the site of the probe (e.g., from finger to ear)
Shield the probe from ambient light
Assess adequacy of oximeter signal amplitude
Use a secondary or portable pulse oximeter to confirm readings
If situation does not resolve, look for conditions that increase venous admixture
Pulmonary aspiration of gastric contents (see Event 28, Aspiration of Gastric Contents)
Massive atelectasis/aspiration of foreign body
PE (see Event 21, Pulmonary Embolism)
Bronchospasm (see Event 29, Bronchospasm)
Anaphylaxis (see Event 16, Anaphylactic and Anaphylactoid Reactions)
Increased intracardiac shunting in congenital heart disease
Pleural effusion or worsening CHF (see Event 20, Pulmonary Edema)
Pneumothorax (see Event 35, Pneumothorax)
Check ETT for kink or obstruction by passing an ETT suction catheter
If catheter does not pass, rule out ETT kink, cuff herniation, or intraluminal obstruction
Perform aggressive pulmonary toilet
Suction ETT with suction catheter
Place 3 cc sterile saline in ETT to loosen thick secretions
Consider bronchoscopy to assist pulmonary toilet
Restore adequate circulating blood volume to maintain CO and Hgb levels
Rule out MH (see Event 45, Malignant Hyperthermia)
Inform surgeons if hypoxemia persists
Check for retractors causing impairment of ventilation
Have surgeons pause cementing or reaming of long bones if hypoxemia worsens
Release of pneumoperitoneum during laparoscopic surgery
Consider urgent return to the supine position (e.g., from prone, steep Trendelenburg, lithotomy), particularly if recent position change is thought to have impaired ventilation
Reinflate nonventilated lung during one lung ventilation (see Event 33, Hypoxemia during One Lung Ventilation)
Terminate surgery as soon as possible
Arrange for ICU transfer for postoperative care
In patients who have been extubated, consider hypoventilation secondary to residual neuromuscular blockade or opioid effect

COMPLICATIONS

Neurologic injury manifested as confusion, coma, delayed recovery from anesthesia
Arrhythmias
Hypotension
Bradycardia
Cardiac arrest

SUGGESTED READING

1. Szekely SM, Runciman WB, Webb RK, Ludbrook GL. Crisis management during anaesthesia: desaturation. Qual Saf Health Care 2005;14(3):e6:1-6.
2. Acute Respiratory Distress Syndrome Network. Ventilation with lower tidal volumes as compared with traditional tidal volumes for acute lung injury and the acute respiratory distress syndrome. New Engl J Med 2000;342:1301-8.

11 Operating Room Fire

DEFINITION

This event includes all fires in an OR except airway fires.

ETIOLOGY

An OR fire requires the presence of three simultaneous elements
   Oxidizer
   Ignition source
   Fuel source

TYPICAL SITUATIONS

Cases involving ignition sources
   Electrocautery
   Laser
   Fiberoptic or other light sources
High concentration of oxidizer (O_2 or N_2O) near an ignition source
   Head, neck, and chest surgery
Incorrect operation of ignition sources
Cases in which flammable (alcohol-based) surgical preparations or ointments are used
Flammable patient coverings (e.g., drapes and blankets)
Electrical faults that give rise to sparks

PREVENTION

Create institutional plan for management of OR fires
Drill and practice management of OR fires using simulation if feasible (otherwise via a walk-through drill)
Assess fire risk in **every** case
Consider using an LMA or ETT for head, neck, and chest surgery requiring moderate or deep sedation or in patients requiring an increased FiO_2
If open O_2 delivery must be used near an ignition source
   Start with the **lowest** O_2 concentration to maintain acceptable O_2 saturation
   Do not deliver 100% O_2 through nasal cannula or mask in high fire-risk cases
      Use an O_2 blender
      Use blended gas from the common gas outlet of the anesthesia machine
      Use blended gas from the patient circuit Y-connector

Use 5 to 10 L/min flow of air from the breathing circuit under the drapes to wash out excess O_2

Use alternative surgical modalities such as harmonic or bipolar scalpel to decrease ignition risk

Modify draping techniques to minimize accumulation of O_2 under the drapes

Perform routine maintenance of OR electrical equipment and remove from service if faults are detected

Allow flammable skin preparation solutions to fully dry before draping

Turn off ignition sources when not actively in use

Moisten gauze or other potential fuel sources when used near ignition source

For high-risk cases, prepare bowl of saline or water to use to extinguish a fire

Have an appropriate fire extinguisher in every OR

Use nonflammable patient coverings

MANIFESTATIONS

Smoke
Visible charring of drapes or OR linens
Visible flames or flashes
Palpable heat
Sparks from electrical equipment or OR lights
Explosion
Fire alarm

SIMILAR EVENTS

Fire elsewhere in the hospital
Smoke or smell from use of electrocautery
Steam pipe leak

MANAGEMENT

For management of airway fires, see Event 25, Airway Burn.

Immediately alert all personnel in the OR
Stop procedure
Stop flow of oxidizer
Remove drapes and all burning or flammable materials from patient
    May need to use fire extinguisher on burning drapes
Pour saline or water on patient, or use a CO_2 fire extinguisher (safe in wounds) at fire site
    Do not pour water on electrical equipment
If the fire continues
    Activate hospital fire alarm
    Continue to extinguish the fire if it is safe for you to do so
    Turn off and unplug any electrical equipment involved if safe to do so
    Use appropriate type of fire extinguisher
If the fire is not quickly controlled
    Evacuate the patient on the operating table, if possible

Notify staff in other ORs
After exiting, isolate the OR to contain smoke or fire
    Close the doors and any other openings into the OR
    Turn off piped gases (this could affect other ORs)
    Consider turning off air conditioning and ventilation to the affected OR or OR suite
Prepare to evacuate the entire OR suite
Continue to fight the fire with extinguishers or fire hose if it is safe to do so
Evaluate and treat injuries to the patient and OR personnel
    Check for burns, bleeding, or other injuries
    Maintain ventilation of paralyzed patients
        Use IV amnestic or anesthetic agents
    Monitor the patient with transport monitor
Replace damaged equipment, especially that needed for life support
Follow up
    Save suspect equipment or materials for investigation
    Report laser-triggered fires to laser safety committee
    There may be a statutory responsibility to report a fire to local, state, or federal agencies

COMPLICATIONS

Burns
Smoke inhalation
Light anesthesia and awareness of the patient while disconnected from inhalation anesthetics

SUGGESTED READING

1. Apfelbaum JL, Caplan RA, Barker SJ, et al. Practice advisory for the prevention and management of operating room fires: an updated report by the American Society of Anesthesiologists Task Force on operating room fires. Anesthesiology 2013;118:271-90.
2. ECRI Institute. New clinical guide to surgical fire prevention. Health Devices 2009;38:330.

12 ST Segment Change

DEFINITION

Elevation or depression of the ST segment of the ECG from the isoelectric level

ETIOLOGY

Inadequate coronary perfusion for a given myocardial O_2 demand
Acute myocardial ischemia or infarction
Myocardial contusion
Acute pericarditis
Electrolyte abnormalities (hypokalemia or hyperkalemia, hypercalcemia)
Head injury or raised ICP, including subarachnoid hemorrhage
Hypothermia (below 30° C)
Defibrillation injury of myocardium

Acute hypertensive crisis
Spontaneous coronary artery dissection (SCAD): usually in premenopausal women
Early repolarization (normal variant)

TYPICAL SITUATIONS

In patients with preexisting CAD or aortic stenosis
During any acute change in myocardial O_2 demand or delivery, including tachycardia,
    arrhythmias, hypertension, hypotension, hypoxemia, hemodilution, coronary spasm,
    coronary stent occlusion, coronary dissection, or coronary thrombus
After head or chest trauma
During vaginal delivery or cesarean section

PREVENTION

Carefully evaluate and optimize medical management in patients with CAD
        Continue β-blockade in patients on chronic β-blocker therapy
        Continue statin therapy perioperatively
        Management of antiplatelet therapy (e.g, aspirin, clopidogrel, etc.) in collaboration with
            surgical team
        Consider perioperative β-blockade in patients with cardiac risk factors
Carefully manage hemodynamics and hematocrit to optimize myocardial O_2 balance
Identify and evaluate preexisting ST segment abnormalities preoperatively
Run rhythm strip recording of ECG prior to induction of anesthesia for comparison
    during case

MANIFESTATIONS

Depression or elevation of ST segment from the isoelectric level
If the ST segment changes are due to myocardial ischemia, the following signs and symptoms
    may be present:
        Central chest pain radiating into the arms or throat
        Dyspnea
        Nausea and vomiting
        Altered level of consciousness or cognitive function
        Arrhythmias (PVCs, premature atrial contractions [PACs], atrial fibrillation [AF], VT
            or VF)
        Hypotension
        New or worsening mitral regurgitation
        Elevation of ventricular filling pressures
        V wave on PA wedge tracing
        Global or regional wall motion abnormalities on TEE or TTE
        The development of Q waves in the ECG

SIMILAR EVENTS

Artifact of ECG
        Improper electrode position on the patient

Alteration in position of heart relative to the electrodes owing to changes in patient position or surgical manipulation
Change in cardiac conduction from normal to abnormal pathway
Left ventricular hypertrophy
Drug effects
Ventricular pacing
Left ventricular aneurysm
Acute pericarditis
Acute PE
Hypercalcemia
Hyperkalemia

MANAGEMENT

All ST changes should be considered ischemic in origin until proven otherwise.

Verify ST segment changes
Evaluate electrode placement and ECG analysis settings
Evaluate multiple ECG leads on physiologic monitor
Review and compare previous ECGs and ST segment tracking data
Record rhythm strip from physiologic monitor
Consider obtaining a 12-lead ECG
Consider TEE or TTE to evaluate new regional wall motion abnormalities
Ensure adequate oxygenation and ventilation
Increase FiO_2 to 100%
Check pulse oximeter
Check capnograph
Check ABGs if there is any question of oxygenation or ventilation
Treat tachycardia and/or hypertension
Tachycardia is the most important determinant of increased myocardial O_2 demand; therefore decrease HR if possible but avoid hypotension
Increase the depth of anesthesia if appropriate
Consider β-blockade
Esmolol IV, 10 to 30 mg bolus, 50 to 300 µg/kg/min infusion
Labetolol IV 5 to 10 mg bolus, repeat as necessary (hold for hypotension)
Metoprolol IV, 1 to 5 mg bolus, repeat as necessary
Avoid β-blockade in patients that are hypotensive or have severely reduced ejection fraction. Use with caution if the patient has severe COPD or asthma
Treat hypertension
Nitroglycerin (NTG)
Sublingual (absorption uncertain, can cause hypotension)
Transdermal paste, 1 to 2 inches applied to the chest wall (slow onset)
IV infusion, 0.25 to 2 µg/kg/min (titrated to effect)
Do not administer when patients are hypotensive or have recently taken phosphodiesterase inhibitors
Calcium channel blockade
Diltiazem IV, loading dose 0.25 mg/kg over 2 min; if IV infusion is necessary, 10-25 mg/hr after IV bolus dose
Treat hypotension and/or bradycardia
Optimize circulating fluid volume

TEE or TTE to assess and optimize myocardial filling and function

Support myocardial contractility as needed using inotropic agents

Positive inotropes may increase myocardial O_2 demand and worsen ischemia

Ephedrine IV, 5 to 10 mg increments

Dobutamine IV infusion, 2.5 to 10 μg/kg/min (may cause hypotension through vasodilation)

Dopamine IV infusion, 2.5 to 10 μg/kg/min

Epinephrine IV infusion, 10 to 100 ng/kg/min

Avoid NTG and calcium channel blockade until hypotension or bradycardia are resolved

Consider combined use of phenylephrine and NTG infusions

Inform the surgeon

Discuss early termination of the surgical procedure

Discuss transfer to ICU for postoperative management

Discuss transfer to cardiac catheterization lab for possible percutaneous coronary intervention (PCI), including possible need for anticoagulation and antiplatelet therapy

If ST segment elevation myocardial infarction (STEMI) is suspected or there is no response to therapy, obtain stat cardiology consultation (see Event 15, Acute Coronary Syndrome)

If severe hypotension or cardiogenic shock, consider placement of intra-aortic balloon pump (IABP)

Send blood samples to laboratory for ABG, hematocrit, glucose, electrolytes, creatine kinase (CK) isoenzymes, troponin

Treat underlying causes of ST segment changes other than myocardial ischemia

COMPLICATIONS

MI

Arrhythmias

Cardiac arrest

SUGGESTED READING

1. Hollenberg SM, Parrillo JE. Myocardial ischemia. In: Hall JB, Schmidt GA, Wood LD, editors. Principles of critical care. 3rd ed. New York: McGraw-Hill; 2005, chapter 25.
2. Goldberger AL. Electrocardiography. In: Longo DL, Fauci AS, Kasper DL, et al, editors. Harrison's principles of internal medicine. 18th ed. New York: McGraw-Hill; 2012, chapter 228.
3. Skidmore Kimberly L, London MJ. Myocardial ischemia: monitoring to diagnose ischemia: how do I monitor therapy? Anesthesiol Clin North America 2001;19:651-72.
4. London MJ, Hur K, Schwartz GG, Henderson WG. Association of perioperative β-blockade with mortality and cardiovascular morbidity following major noncardiac surgery. JAMA 2013;309:1704-13.

13 The Septic Patient

DEFINITION

Sepsis is a systemic inflammatory response syndrome (SIRS) caused by severe infection.

ETIOLOGY

Overwhelming infection
   Pneumonia
   Abdominal infection
   Kidney infection
   Bloodstream infection

TYPICAL SITUATIONS

Patients at the extremes of age
Patients with compromised immune systems
Patients who require care in the ICU
   ICU patients have conduits for infection (e.g., CVP catheters, urinary catheters, ETTs)
Also can be associated with
   Surgical procedures (e.g., necrotizing fasciitis, lithotripsy)
   Pancreatitis
   Fulminant hepatic failure
   Patients on multiple antibiotics
   Toxic shock syndrome
   Anaphylaxis/anaphylactoid reactions
   Insect bites, transfusion reactions, heavy metal poisoning
   Contaminated IV solutions or medications

PREVENTION

Multidisciplinary quality improvement plans directed toward decreasing infections
   Wash hands before and after every patient contact
   Prevent central line associated bloodstream infections (CLABSI)
      Follow Centers for Disease Control recommendations for CVP placement
   Reduce duration of IV lipid and CVP line use
   Provide respiratory care to reduce the risk of ventilator-associated pneumonia (VAP)
      Prevent aspiration
         Elevate the head of the bed 30 to 40 degrees unless contraindicated
         Avoid gastric overdistention
         Avoid unplanned extubation and reintubation
         Use a cuffed ETT with in-line suctioning
      Minimize the duration of endotracheal intubation
         Daily assessments of readiness to wean
         Use weaning protocols
         Educate healthcare personnel about VAP
      Conduct active surveillance for VAP
      Use noninvasive ventilation when applicable
      Selective oral decontamination with oral chlorhexidine
      Methicillin-resistant *Staphylococcus aureus* (MRSA) screening and isolation of
         carriers
   Minimize use and duration of bladder catheters

Skin care assessment
  Follow wound care procedures
  Prevent pressure sores
  Administer peptic ulcer disease prophylaxis
Screen seriously ill patients for infection to allow early implementation of therapy
Implement and follow sepsis bundles (as described in Management Section)
Reassess antimicrobial regimens daily for potential de-escalation to prevent the development
  of bacterial resistance, to reduce drug toxicity, and to reduce costs

MANIFESTATIONS

Infection (either documented or suspected)
  General variables
    $T > 38°$ C or $< 36°$ C
    $HR > 90$/min
    Tachypnea
    Altered mental status
    Edema or positive fluid balance
    Hyperglycemia
  Inflammatory variables
    White blood cell (WBC) count >12,000 or <4000 cells/μL, >10% bands
    Increase in C-reactive protein
    Presence of procalcitonin in the blood
  Hemodynamic variables
    SBP <90, MAP <70, or DBP <40 mm Hg
    Venous oxygen saturation (SvO_2) >70%
    Cardiac index >3.5 L/min
  Organ dysfunction variables
    Hypoxemia
    Oliguria
    Increased creatinine
    Coagulopathy
    Ileus
    Thrombocytopenia
    Hyperbilirubinemia
  Tissue perfusion variables
    Increased lactate
    Poor capillary refill
    Skin mottling
SIRS may occur without evidence of infection and involves two or more of the following:
  Temp > 38° C or < 36° C
  HR > 90 beats/min
  Respiration rate > 20 breaths/min
  WBC count >12,000 or <4000 cells/μL, or >10% bands
Sepsis: SIRS in the presence of proven or suspected infection
Severe sepsis: acute, often multiple organ dysfunction syndrome (MODS) secondary to docu-
  mented or suspected infection

13

Septic shock: severe sepsis plus hypotension not reversed by fluid resuscitation (distributive shock)

In septic shock, high CO low SVR, hypotension, and regional blood flow redistribution lead to tissue hypoperfusion

MODS

Severe sepsis leading to multiple organ dysfunction

Mortality ranges from 30% to 100%

SIMILAR EVENTS

Hemorrhagic shock (e.g., polytrauma, GI bleed) (see Event 1, Acute Hemorrhage)

Acute MI (see Event 15, Acute Coronary Syndrome)

Stroke

Anaphylaxis (see Event 16, Anaphylactic or Anaphylactoid Reactions)

SCI

MANAGEMENT

Rapid diagnosis with appropriate therapy of sepsis improves outcome. Clear communication among clinicians in emergency medicine, anesthesia, surgery, internal medicine, and critical care is essential in the treatment of the septic patient.

Surviving Sepsis Campaign Bundles

To be completed within 3 hours:

Measure lactate level

Obtain blood cultures prior to administration of antibiotics

Administer broad spectrum antibiotics

Administer 30 mL/kg crystalloid for hypotension or lactate ≥4 mmol/L

To be completed within 6 hours:

Administer vasopressors for hypotension that does not respond to initial fluid resuscitation

In the event of persistent hypotension despite volume resuscitation (septic shock) or initial lactate ≥4 mmol/L

Continue to administer IV fluid and vasopressors until

MAP ≥65 mm Hg

CVP ≥8 mm Hg

Central $ScvO_2$ ≥70%

Urine output ≥0.5 mL/kg/hr

Normal serum lactate levels

Antimicrobial regimens can be complex and should be guided by appropriate infectious disease consultation

Antiviral therapy initiated as early as possible in patients with severe sepsis or septic shock of viral origin

Antimicrobial regimen should be reassessed daily for potential de-escalation

High procalcitonin levels are consistent with severe sepsis

Low or decreasing levels can be used to guide antimicrobial therapy

Determine and treat the source of sepsis

Once diagnosed, the intervention with the least physiologic insult should be considered (e.g., percutaneous rather than surgical drainage of an abscess)

Remove/replace intravascular catheters if they are a possible source of infection

Fluid Therapy of Severe Sepsis
>Crystalloids are the initial fluid of choice
>>Administer 30 mL/kg of crystalloid initially
>>Avoid use of hydroxyethyl starches
>>Large amounts of fluid may be needed
>Albumin can be added to the IV fluid regimen when patients require substantial amounts of crystalloids

Vasopressor Therapy of Severe Sepsis
>Norepinephrine IV infusion, 10 to 100 ng/kg/min
>Epinephrine IV infusion, 10 to 100 ng/kg/min, may be added to, and potentially substituted for, norepinephrine
>Vasopressin IV infusion, 0.03 units/min, can be added to norepinephrine to raise the MAP or decrease the norepinephrine dose
>Dopamine IV infusion, 2 to 10 µg/kg/min
>Phenylephrine is not recommended in the treatment of the septic patient except
>>Where norepinephrine is associated with serious arrhythmias
>>Where CO is known to be high and BP persistently low
>>As salvage therapy when other agents (e.g., vasopressin) have failed to achieve MAP target
>All patients requiring vasopressors should have an arterial catheter placed

Corticosteroids
>Systemic corticosteroids are not indicated if patient is resuscitatable with IV fluid and vasopressor administration
>>If the patient has been fluid resuscitated but remains hypotensive, consider hydrocortisone IV, 200 mg/day (see Event 38, Addisonian Crisis)
>>Taper corticosteroids when vasopressors are no longer required

Blood Product Administration
>In the absence of myocardial ischemia, severe hypoxemia, or acute hemorrhage, RBCs should be transfused when Hgb concentration decreases to <7.0 g/dL to achieve Hgb concentration of 7.0 to 9.0 g/dL in adults
>Administer platelets
>>Prophylactically when counts are <10 K/µL
>>If the patient has a significant risk of bleeding and platelet count <20 K/µL
>>If the patient is actively bleeding or undergoing surgery or an invasive procedure and has a platelet count <50 K/µL

Glucose Control
>Monitor glucose levels every 1 to 2 hours and treat hyperglycemia with IV insulin infusion
>Target glucose levels 140 to 180 mg/dL

SUGGESTED READING

1. NIH Sepsis Fact Sheet. Available from: http://www.nigms.nih.gov/Publications/factsheet_sepsis.htm. [accessed 03.07.13].
2. Dellinger RP, Levy ML, Opal S, et al. Surviving Sepsis Campaign: international guidelines for management of severe sepsis and septic shock—2012. Crit Care Med 2013;41:580-637.
3. Levy MM, Dellinger RP, Townsend SR, et al. The Surviving Sepsis Campaign: results of an international guideline-based performance improvement program targeting severe sepsis. Crit Care Med 2010;38:367-74.
4. Wacker C, Prkno A, Brunkhorst FM, Schlattmann P. Procalcitonin as a diagnostic marker for sepsis: a systematic review and meta-analysis. Lancet Infect Dis 2013;13:426-35.

14 The Trauma Patient

DEFINITION

Trauma patients have severe, life-threatening injuries that affect multiple organ systems and that frequently result in the immediate need for life-saving resuscitative, airway, and surgical intervention.

ETIOLOGY

Motor vehicle accidents (MVAs)
Penetrating injuries
    Gunshot wounds
    Knife or other stab wounds
Falls
Crush injuries
Central nervous system (CNS) injuries
    Blunt trauma
    Acute acceleration or deceleration injuries

TYPICAL SITUATIONS

MVAs
Gunshot wounds
Workplace accidents
Falls
Abuse (children, elderly, domestic violence)

PREVENTION

There are 60 million injuries annually in the United States, and trauma is the leading cause of death among children, adolescents, and young adults. Prevention of trauma is a public health issue of enormous importance.

Trauma centers should have the following immediately available at all times
    An OR
    Fully functional anesthesia workstation
    Appropriate staff
    Drugs and resuscitative equipment
    Transfusion services
Systematic and coordinated training of the entire team for the management of the trauma patient improves emergency response and patient survival
    Preassign roles to anesthesiology, surgery, and nursing team members
    Use simulation to drill and practice responses to the trauma patient
    Team meetings at the start of shifts will enhance role clarity and the team's ability to manage critical patients

MANIFESTATIONS

Stat call to the trauma bay or ED
Patient presentation is variable and depends on the type and extent of injury and mode of transportation to the ED
Evaluate the patient's vital signs and expect the trauma patient to be unstable
Hypotension, hypertension, tachycardia, bradycardia
Oxygenation and ventilation problems
Pain
Alteration in mental status

SIMILAR EVENTS

Major medical or surgical emergencies (e.g., ruptured abdominal aortic aneurysm)

MANAGEMENT

The acute resuscitation of patients with serious medical and surgical emergencies will often follow these guidelines, although, strictly speaking, they are not all "trauma" patients.

All arriving team members responding to a trauma call should clearly state their role
Preparation of trauma bay prior to patient arrival
Trauma bay equipment
Provider barrier equipment
Surgical gowns
Eye protection
Gloves
Masks
Lead x-ray gowns
Crash cart with defibrillator
Airway equipment
Self-inflating bag and mask attached to a high flow O_2 source
Confirm suction is functional
Check airway equipment (oral airway, ETT, laryngoscope with different blades)
Video-assisted laryngoscope for difficult airway
SGA and bougie for possible difficult airway
ET CO_2 monitor
Equipment for surgical airway (e.g., cricothyrotomy kit)
Anesthesia workstation—checked and ready if available
Most patients will need to be transported to a trauma OR for emergency surgical care beyond the initial resuscitation
IV equipment
Rapid infuser device and tubing
IV and IO start kits
Medications
Induction agent (e.g., ketamine, etomidate, propofol)
Paralytic (e.g., succinylcholine unless contraindicated)
Vasopressors (epinephrine, ephedrine, phenylephrine)
Trauma service may receive advance warning of incoming casualties (there may be multiple trauma victims)

Establish if the patient is in cardiac arrest

Initiate BLS/ACLS/pediatric advanced life support (PALS)/advanced trauma life support (ATLS) if patient is in cardiac arrest (see Event 2, Cardiac Arrest, and Event 94, Cardiac Arrest in the Pediatric Patient)

Anesthesiology role

If patient is able to communicate

Obtain brief history and physical (including allergies)

Assess patient's visible injuries, especially any near the airway that may make airway management difficult

Ensure adequate oxygenation and ventilation; check O_2 saturation

Evaluate the patient's ability to protect the airway

Assess level of consciousness

Emergency induction of anesthesia and intubation of trauma patients is often necessary

Get additional anesthesia help if a difficult intubation is anticipated

Preoxygenate while the trauma team places monitors

Assume that the patient has a full stomach and may have ingested substances of abuse

Reduce or eliminate induction dose of anesthetic based on vital signs and patient comorbidities

Perform a RSI with cricoid pressure

Consider video-assisted laryngoscopy as primary choice for intubation

Assign a member of the trauma team to apply manual in-line stabilization of the neck

Manipulate or release cricoid pressure if unable to intubate the trachea (see Event 3, Difficult Tracheal Intubation)

Provide anesthesia to the patient, balancing risk of awareness with hemodynamic stability

Administer IV fluid and vasopressors in accordance with patient hemodynamics and blood loss

Assess the need for additional IVs, arterial line, or CVP access and assist in their placement

Assess the patient's pain level

Treat with small doses of short-acting opioids

Balance risk of pain with hemodynamic stability

Hypovolemic patients may become hypotensive with small doses of opioids

Nursing service role

Apply basic monitors and measure vital signs

Communicate these to anesthesia and surgery team

HR

BP

O_2 saturation

Insert bilateral, large-bore IVs (e.g., 14 or 16 g)

Assist anesthesia team with managing airway and obtaining other IV access and special monitoring

Assist surgeons with surgical airway, chest tube placement, laparotomy, or other procedures as necessary

Act as timekeeper to track events of the resuscitation, including medication administration, defibrillation, etc.

Ensure that blood, blood products, and a rapid infuser system are available

Consider activating MTP, if available

Trauma surgery role

    Ensure that the primary survey is completed and resuscitation begins (ABCDE of ATLS)

    Airway maintenance with cervical spine precautions

    Breathing and ventilation

        Recognize and treat tension pneumothorax, massive hemothorax, flail chest, cardiac tamponade, etc.

    Circulation with control of hemorrhage

        Recognize hypovolemic shock and initiate transfusion

        Control bleeding

    Disability (neurologic assessment)

        Establish level of consciousness, pupil size and reaction to light, lateralizing signs, and SCI level

    Exposure and environmental control

        Expose the patient so a complete examination can be performed

        Prevent hypothermia

    If asked, be ready to place a surgical airway

    If asked, be ready to provide IV or IO access

    Once primary survey is complete, resuscitation efforts are established, and patient is stabilized, proceed to the next stage

    Perform the secondary survey

        Comprehensively evaluate the patient's injuries

            Identify sites of potential internal injuries looking for abdominal bruising and distention, flail chest, pneumothorax, head injury (Glasgow Coma Scale)

        Make critical decisions about the patient's immediate resuscitative and diagnostic needs

            Abdominal taps, chest tube placement, laparotomy, aortic clamping, or other procedures, FAST examination

            Assess need for transfer to computed tomography (CT) for scans, interventional radiology (IR) for procedures, or OR for surgery

        Request necessary consultations from other surgical services

Be prepared to call for additional help (anesthesia, surgery, nursing)

COMMUNICATION BETWEEN TEAM MEMBERS IS CRUCIAL: It may be difficult to keep track of and comprehend the complex and changing issues and the numerous tasks that must be accomplished.

    Clear, closed-loop communication within the trauma team is essential.

Be prepared to transport the patient to CT, IR, or OR

If the patient requires transportation to the main OR

    A second anesthesia team should prepare the OR for emergency surgery. See Event 4, Emergent (Crash) Induction of Anesthesia

        Warm the room to maintain the patient's core temperature >35° C

        Prepare for massive resuscitation

            Crystalloid and blood products

            CVP line

            Ultrasound machine for line placement

            Rapid infuser devices available

        Confirm that the blood bank has activated the MTP or that blood is available

OR management of massive hemorrhage (see Event 1, Acute Hemorrhage)

Prepare for acidosis and further hemorrhage

COMPLICATIONS

Aspiration of gastric contents
Difficult intubation
Awareness under anesthesia
Massive hemorrhage
Coagulopathy
Pulmonary edema
Multisystem organ failure
TRALI
Sepsis
Cardiac arrest
Death

SUGGESTED READING

1. Gray LD, Morris CG. The principles and conduct of anaesthesia for, emergency surgery. Anaesthesia 2013;68(Suppl. 1):14-29.
2. Varon AJ, Smith CE, editors. Essentials of trauma anesthesia. Cambridge, Mass: Cambridge University Press; 2012.
3. Diez C, Varon AJ. Airway management and initial resuscitation of the trauma patient. Curr Opin Crit Care 2009;15:542-7.
4. Advanced Trauma Life Support (ATLS) for doctors: student manual with DVD. 8th ed. Chicago: American College of Surgeons; 2008.

14

Chapter 6

Cardiovascular Events
JOHANNES STEYN and JOHANNES DORFLING

---

15 Acute Coronary Syndrome

DEFINITION

Acute coronary syndrome (ACS) is an acute imbalance between myocardial O_2 supply and demand that leads to ischemia and infarction. ACS is classified as being unstable angina, non–ST segment elevation myocardial infarction (NSTEMI), or STEMI.

ETIOLOGY

Total or subtotal coronary artery occlusion

    Primary ACS results from coronary artery occlusion
        Plaque disruption with thrombus formation
        Coronary vasospasm from endothelial dysfunction or drug ingestion (e.g., cocaine, serotonin receptor agonists)
        Coronary artery embolism
        Coronary artery dissection
        Aortic dissection
    Secondary ACS results from
        Increased myocardial O_2 demand
        Decreased myocardial O_2 supply

TYPICAL SITUATIONS

Patients with known CAD or risk factors for atherosclerosis (males, hypertension, hyperlipidemia, diabetes, peripheral vascular disease, smoking, family history of CAD)

Increased myocardial O_2 demand
    Tachycardia, fever, severe hypertension, or thyrotoxicosis
Decreased myocardial O_2 supply
    Systemic hypotension, hypoxemia, or anemia
Miscellaneous factors (e.g., polyarteritis nodosa, Kawasaki disease)

PREVENTION

Evaluate myocardial function and reserve and optimize medical therapy prior to surgery
    Modify cardiac risk factors if possible
    Optimize β-blocker and statin therapy
    Manage antiplatelet therapy (e.g., aspirin, clopidogrel) in collaboration with surgical team
        Patients with coronary stents on antiplatelet therapy require comanagement with cardiologist and surgeon
            Patients may require "bridging therapy" (e.g., eptifibatide and heparin) to reduce risk of perioperative stent thrombosis

15

Avoid elective anesthesia and surgery in patients with unstable angina or with a history of MI in the previous 6 months

Optimize hemodynamics and hematocrit during anesthesia

Maintain myocardial O_2 supply

Prevent increases in myocardial O_2 demand

Revascularization (CABG or PCI) prior to elective surgery is not usually recommended

Consult cardiology and cardiac surgery

MANIFESTATIONS

In awake patients

Chest pain, pressure, or discomfort radiating to arm and jaw

Women, diabetics, and the elderly may exhibit atypical chest pain (e.g., epigastric pain, sharp pain, fatigue, or dyspnea) or no symptoms at all

Nausea, diaphoresis, palpitations, syncope

Cardiac arrest

Electrocardiogram

ST segment elevation or depression

Conduction abnormalities (e.g., left bundle branch block or complete atrioventricular block)

Peaked T-waves

Progression to inverted T-waves and development of Q-waves

Arrhythmias including PVCs, VT, or VF

Cardiac biomarkers

Increase in troponin I, troponin T, and CK-MB isoenzyme

Diagnosis of MI requires presence of ECG changes or symptoms, because other conditions may be responsible for elevated cardiac biomarkers

Hemodynamic abnormalities

Hypotension

Tachycardia

Bradycardia

New regional wall motion abnormality on TEE or TTE

Elevation of filling pressures (CVP, PCWP)

Criteria required for diagnosis of MI

Symptoms of ischemia

ECG changes

ST segment changes

Q-waves

New left bundle branch block

Evidence of new regional wall motion abnormality

Detection of rise and/or fall of cardiac biomarkers including

Troponin I

Troponin T

CK-MB

SIMILAR EVENTS

PE (see Event 21, Pulmonary Embolism)

Esophageal spasm, costochondritis, acute abdomen

Primary pulmonary pathology (e.g., pneumonia, pulmonary infarction)
Acute aortic dissection
Nonischemic ST segment or T-wave changes (see Event 12, ST Segment Change)
ECG artifact
  Improper electrode placement
  Changes in patient position or surgical manipulation may alter position of heart relative
    to the electrodes

MANAGEMENT

Inform the surgeon
Confirm diagnosis by evaluating available leads on ECG monitor
Ensure adequate oxygenation and ventilation
Optimize hemodynamics—improve myocardial O_2 supply while decreasing demand
  Treat hypotension with vasopressors and IV fluids to increase DBP
    Phenylephrine IV bolus, 50 to 200 μg
    Phenylephrine IV infusion, 10 to 100 μg/min
    Optimize circulating blood volume
  Treat tachycardia
    Assure adequate depth of anesthesia
    Administer β-blockers in the absence of evidence of heart failure
      Esmolol IV, 10 to 30 mg
      Esmolol IV infusion, 25 to 200 μg/kg/min
      Metoprolol IV, 1 to 5 mg
    Calcium channel blockers
      Diltiazem IV, 0.15 to 0.25 mg/kg load, then 5 to 15 mg/hr
Improve collateral myocardial blood flow and decrease myocardial wall stress
  Administer nitroglycerin IV, 0.2 to 2 μg/kg/min
    Do not administer when patients are hypotensive or have recently taken phosphodi-
      esterase inhibitors
Draw labs
  ABG, HCT, electrolytes, cardiac biomarkers
Consider additional monitoring
  Arterial line, CVP line, TEE
Administer aspirin (PO, NGT, or PR) 325 mg
Treat arrhythmias according to ACLS protocol (see Event 19, Nonlethal Ventricular Arrhythmias)
In case of STEMI
  Obtain stat interventional cardiology consult and alert cardiac catheterization laboratory of
    your concerns for management
  Terminate surgery as soon as possible and prepare patient for transport to cardiac cath-
    eterization lab
  Evaluate and treat cardiogenic shock
    Consider treating with vasopressors and/or ionotropes to improve end-organ perfusion
      Dopamine IV infusion, 2 to 10 μg/kg/min
      Norepinephrine IV infusion, 10 to 100 ng/kg/min
    Consider mechanical support with IABP or percutaneous left ventricular assist de-
      vice (LVAD) for patients not responding to pharmacologic support

Consider antiplatelet therapy and anticoagulant therapy
>Weigh risk of bleeding from recent surgery against benefit of improved mortality from ACS; requires joint discussion with cardiologist and surgeon

Request ICU bed for postoperative care

COMPLICATIONS

Heart failure

Arrhythmias

Cardiac arrest

Thromboembolic complications

Papillary muscle dysfunction or rupture

Rupture of the interventricular septum or the ventricular wall

SUGGESTED READING

1. Antman EM, Anbe DT, Armstrong PW, et al. ACC/AHA guidelines for the management of patients with ST-elevation myocardial infarction: a report of the American College of Cardiology/American Heart Association Task Force on Practice Guidelines (committee to revise the 1999 guidelines for the management of patients with acute myocardial infarction). Circulation 2004;110:e82-e292.
2. Anderson JL, Adams CD, Antman EM, et al. ACC/AHA 2007 guidelines for the management of patients with unstable angina/non-ST-Elevation myocardial infarction: a report of the American College of Cardiology/American Heart Association Task Force on Practice Guidelines (writing committee to revise the 2002 guidelines for the management of patients with unstable angina/non-ST-elevation myocardial infarction) developed in collaboration with the American College of Emergency Physicians, the Society for Cardiovascular Angiography and Interventions, and the Society of Thoracic Surgeons endorsed by the American Association of Cardiovascular and Pulmonary Rehabilitation and the Society for Academic Emergency Medicine. J Am Coll Cardiol 2007;50:e1-e157.
3. Thiele H, Sick P, Boudriot E, et al. Randomized comparison of intra-aortic balloon support with a percutaneous left ventricular assist device in patients with revascularized acute myocardial infarction complicated by cardiogenic shock. Eur Heart J 2005;26:1276-83.
4. Eagle KA, Guyton RA, Davidoff R, et al. ACC/AHA 2004 guideline update for coronary artery bypass graft surgery: a report of the American College of Cardiology/American Heart Association Task Force on Practice Guidelines (committee to update the 1999 guidelines for coronary artery bypass graft surgery). Circulation 2004;110:e340-e437.

16   Anaphylactic and Anaphylactoid Reactions

DEFINITION

Anaphylactic and anaphylactoid reactions are serious allergic reactions that are rapid in onset and may cause death.

Anaphylactic reaction (immunologic) involves antigen and IgE antibodies; requires previous sensitization to the antigen

Anaphylactoid reaction (nonimmunologic) mediated primarily by histamine; may occur with the first exposure to a triggering agent

Complement activation may follow both immunologic and nonimmunologic reactions

ETIOLOGY

Administration or exposure to an agent that the patient has been sensitized to by prior exposure, with production of antigen-specific IgE (anaphylactic reaction)
Allergic reaction to agent requiring no previous exposure (anaphylactoid reaction)

TYPICAL SITUATIONS

The true incidence is unknown, but is estimated at 1 in 10,000 to 1 in 20,000 anesthetic procedures. Approximately 1500 deaths occur each year in the United States from anaphylaxis in all settings.

In patients with a known allergy or sensitivity to a specific agent or with conditions making a
reaction to an agent more likely
  Allergic reactions to protamine are more likely in patients with fish allergy, prior protamine administration, or after treatment with protamine-zinc insulin
  Patients with a history of allergy to nondrug allergens have a higher risk of anaphylaxis
    during anesthesia
After exposure to substances that can trigger anaphylactic or anaphylactoid reactions
  Neuromuscular blocking drugs (60% of anesthesia-related anaphylaxis)
  Latex (20% of anesthesia-related anaphylaxis)
  Antibiotics (15% of anesthesia-related anaphylaxis, with penicillins and cephalosporins
    responsible for 70% of antibiotic induced anaphylaxis)
  Opioids
  Amino-ester local anesthetic agents
  Blood and blood products
  Iodinated contrast material
  Chlorhexidine preparation solutions
  Individuals with frequent latex exposure
    Health care workers
    Patients who have undergone multiple surgical procedures
    Patients who require intermittent bladder catheterization
      SCI patients
      Chronic care patients

PREVENTION

Avoid agents to which the patient has a documented allergy
Minimize the use of latex products in health care (in the United States many institutions have
  replaced most products with latex-free versions)
If there is a history of latex allergy, establish a latex-free environment
  Avoid contact with or manipulation of latex devices
  Use nonlatex surgical gloves
  Use syringe/stopcock or unidirectional valves for injecting medications
  Do not insert a needle through any multiple-dose vial with a natural rubber stopper
    Take the top of the vial completely off
    Use medication from a glass ampule, if available
  Use glass syringes with glass plunger or plastic syringes with known non-latex plungers.
    (Check manufacturer for materials used.)

Obtain a careful history of previous allergic reactions, atopy, asthma, or significant latex exposure

Avoid transfusion of blood or blood products whenever possible

    Check the identity of the patient and blood products carefully prior to transfusion

If a specific drug must be administered to a patient known to be at risk of an allergic reaction, administer prophylaxis

    Corticosteroids

        Dexamethasone IV, 20 mg, or methylprednisolone IV, 100 mg

    H_1 antagonist

        Diphenhydramine IV, 25 to 50 mg

    Administer a test dose of drug

Obtain a consultation from an allergist if a critical allergy must be defined

MANIFESTATIONS

Anaphylaxis has the potential for acute onset with catastrophic consequences. Severe hypotension, increased PIP, and hypoxemia are the most common initial signs but need not be present simultaneously.

Cardiovascular

    The awake patient may complain of dizziness or lose consciousness

    Severe hypotension

    Bradycardia—may be initial sign

    Arrhythmias

    Cardiac arrest

Respiratory

    The awake patient may complain of dyspnea or chest tightness

    Hypoxemia

    Decreased lung compliance

    Severe bronchospasm

Cutaneous—may be obscured by surgical drapes

    Flushing, hives, urticaria, pruritus

Swelling of mucosal membranes, conjunctiva, lips, tongue, and uvula

SIMILAR EVENTS

Anesthetic overdose (see Event 72, Volatile Anesthetic Overdose)

Pulmonary edema (see Event 20, Pulmonary Edema)

Hypotension from other causes (see Event 9, Hypotension)

ACS (see Event 15, Acute Coronary Syndrome)

Cardiac tamponade (see Event 18, Cardiac Tamponade)

Venous air embolism (see Event 24, Venous Air or Gas Embolism)

Vasovagal reaction

Septic shock (see Event 13, The Septic Patient)

Drug administration error (see Event 63, Drug Administration Error)

Stridor (see Event 36, Postoperative Stridor)

PE (see Event 21, Pulmonary Embolism)

Aspiration of gastric contents (see Event 28, Aspiration of Gastric Contents)

Pneumothorax (see Event 35, Pneumothorax)

Bronchospasm (see Event 29, Bronchospasm)
Skin manifestations of drug reactions not associated with anaphylaxis
Transfusion reaction (see Event 50, Transfusion Reaction)
Fat embolism syndrome
Amniotic fluid embolism (see Event 81, Amniotic Fluid Embolism)

MANAGEMENT

Stop administration of any possible antigen
Retain blood products for analysis
Remove all latex-containing products from contact with the patient
Inform the surgeons and call for help
Check to see whether they have injected or instilled a substance into a body cavity
Consider aborting the surgical procedure if severe
Anaphylaxis may be biphasic and can recur after successful initial treatment
Ensure adequate oxygenation and ventilation
Administer 100% O_2
Intubate the trachea if not already intubated
The airway can rapidly become very edematous making intubation (or extubation) more difficult or impossible
Treat hypotension
Epinephrine is the drug of choice for treatment of anaphylaxis
For mild to moderate hypotension, administer epinephrine IV, 10 to 50 µg increments, and repeat as necessary with escalating doses
For cardiovascular collapse or cardiac arrest, administer epinephrine IV, 500 to 1000 µg boluses, and repeat as necessary (see Event 2, Cardiac Arrest)
Administer vasopressin IV, 10 to 40 U, in cases of anaphylactic shock resistant to catecholamines; in pulseless arrest, follow the ACLS pulseless arrest algorithm
Norepinephrine infusion may be required
Glucagon IV, 1 to 5 mg, may be useful in patients receiving β-blocker therapy who do not respond to epinephrine
Methylene blue IV, 10 to 50 mg, has been successfully used in catecholamine- and vasopressin-resistant anaphylaxis
Rapidly expand the circulating fluid volume
Place patient in Trendelenburg position
Immediate fluid needs may be massive (several liters of crystalloid)
Ensure adequate IV access
Decrease or stop administration of anesthetic agents if hypotension is severe
If bronchospasm is present
Administer bronchodilator
Albuterol metered dose inhaler (MDI), 5 to 10 puffs
Volatile anesthetics may be administered for bronchodilation if the patient is normotensive
Administer an H_1 and H_2 histamine antagonist
Diphenhydramine IV, 50 mg
Ranitidine IV, 50 mg
Administer corticosteroids
This is not helpful for the acute event, but may reduce risk of further episodes
Dexamethasone IV, 20 mg bolus, or methylprednisolone IV, 100 mg bolus

In the absence of any other cause, consider latex allergy

    Ensure all latex products in contact with the patient have been removed from the surgical field (double check whether these products do or do not contain latex)

        Surgical gloves

        Urinary catheter

        Medications drawn up through a latex stopper

    Place invasive monitors to help guide fluid and vasopressor management

        Arterial line

        CVP or PA catheter

        TTE or TEE

        Urinary catheter

    Obtain blood sample for measurement of mast cell tryptase within 2 hours of onset to confirm diagnosis of anaphylactic reaction

    Arrange admission to an ICU for postoperative management and observation

    Consider referring patient to an allergist on discharge from the hospital

COMPLICATIONS

Inability to intubate, ventilate, or oxygenate

Hypertension, tachycardia from vasopressors

ARDS

Renal failure

Cardiac arrest

Anoxic brain injury

Death

SUGGESTED READING

1. Dewachter P, Mouton-Faivre C, Emala CW. Anaphylaxis and anesthesia. Anesthesiology 2009;111:1141-50.
2. Harper NJ, Dixon T, Dugué P, et al. Working Party of the Association of Anaesthetists of Great Britain and Ireland. Suspected anaphylactic reactions associated with anaesthesia. Anaesthesia 2009;64:199-211.
3. Sampson HA, Muñoz-Furlong A, Bock SA, et al. Symposium on the definition and management of anaphylaxis: summary report. J Allergy Clin Immunol 2005;115:584-91.
4. Mertes PM, Malinovsky JM, Jouffroy L, et al. Reducing the risk of anaphylaxis during anesthesia: 2011 updated guidelines for clinical practice. J Investig Allergol Clin Immunol 2011;21:442-53.

17   Autonomic Dysreflexia

DEFINITION

Autonomic dysreflexia (AD) is a massive, unopposed, reflex sympathetic discharge triggered by a noxious stimulus below the level of a chronic SCI.

ETIOLOGY

Bladder or urinary tract distention (e.g., instrumentation, infection, or calculi of the urinary tract)

Lower GI tract stimulation (e.g., bowel distention from any cause)

Performance of a surgical procedure below the level of an SCI with inadequate anesthesia/analgesia

Skin stimulation (e.g., pressure sore, ingrown toenail, tight-fitting clothing)
Exposure to temperature extremes
Medications (e.g., nasal decongestants, sympathomimetic drugs, misoprostol)

TYPICAL SITUATIONS

In patients with SCI, usually at least 6 weeks after the injury
In patients whose level of SCI is at or above T6 (the higher and more complete the lesion, the
   higher the incidence)
During performance of urologic procedures such as bladder catheterization, cystoscopy, or
   cystometrography
In patients with disorders of the lower GI tract (e.g., fecal impaction, hemorrhoids, anal fissure)
During procedures involving the rectum or colon
During recovery from neuraxial, regional, or general anesthesia
During labor and delivery

PREVENTION

Obtain a thorough history from patients with SCI. They are often aware of some of the stimuli
   that will evoke this response
Avoid stimuli known to trigger AD if possible
Check the baseline BP for comparison with perioperative values
Consider preoperative prophylaxis of patients at risk of AD
      Clonidine 0.2 to 0.4 mg PO, preoperatively
      Nifedipine 10 mg SL, immediately preoperatively
      Phenoxybenzamine 10 mg PO, 3 times daily to maximum of 60 mg/day
      Prazosin 6 to 15 mg PO
Provide adequate regional or general anesthesia and postoperative analgesia for a surgical
   procedure

MANIFESTATIONS

Acute, paroxysmal onset of severe systolic and diastolic hypertension
      Normal BP in most SCI patients is low, so reference the change in BP to the patient's
         resting value
      Increased blood loss from surgical site
      Reflex bradycardia (tachycardia and arrhythmias may also occur)
Additional signs of sympathetic hyperreactivity
      Below the level of SCI: cool, pale skin; pilomotor erection; spastic muscle contraction
         and increased muscle tone; penile erection
      Above level of SCI: sweating, vasodilation and flushing of the skin, mydriasis, nasal and
         conjunctival congestion, eyelid retraction
If the patient is awake
      Severe pounding headache, blurred vision, nasal congestion, dyspnea, nausea, or anxiety

SIMILAR EVENTS

Light anesthesia
Vasopressor overdose

Preeclampsia/eclampsia in pregnant SCI patient (see Event 88, Preeclampsia and Eclampsia)
Intraoperative hypertension from other causes (see Event 8, Hypertension)
Pheochromocytoma
Migraine and cluster headaches

MANAGEMENT

Verify the BP; check for additional signs and symptoms of sympathetic hyperreactivity
Inform the surgeon and ask for the surgical stimulus to be stopped (e.g., drain bladder)
Place patient in reverse Trendelenburg position to facilitate venous pooling in lower extremities
If the patient is under general anesthesia

> Increase the depth of anesthesia
>> Increase the inspired concentration of volatile anesthetic
>> Administer additional opioid (e.g, fentanyl IV, 25 to 50 µg)
> If hypertension persists, administer drugs with rapid onset and short duration
>> Phentolamine 2 to 10 mg IV, titrated to effect
>> Sodium nitroprusside IV infusion, 0.2 to 1.0 µg/kg/min, titrated to effect with arterial line monitoring
> AD may occur during emergence and recovery

If the patient is awake

> For less severe hypertension:
>> NTG 0.4 mg/spray into oral cavity
>> Nitropaste 2%, 1 inch applied to the skin above the level of the SCI
>> Captopril 25 mg SL
>> Nifedipine 10 mg capsule, bitten and swallowed
> For severe elevation in BP:
>> Phentolamine 2 to 10 mg IV, titrated to effect
>> Sodium nitroprusside IV infusion, 0.2 to 2.0 µg/kg/min, titrated to effect with arterial line monitoring
> If AD resolves, continue with surgery (AD may recur)

If AD does not resolve with treatment

> **Abort surgery if possible**
> Place an additional peripheral IV or a CVP line to administer potent vasodilators
> Insert an arterial line if not already done

COMPLICATIONS

Myocardial ischemia or infarction
Pulmonary edema
Hypertensive encephalopathy or stroke
Atrial and ventricular arrhythmias, heart block
Seizures, coma, intracerebral or subarachnoid hemorrhage
Increased surgical blood loss
Hypotension secondary to therapy with vasodilators
Cardiac arrest

SUGGESTED READING

1. Hambly PR, Martin B. Anaesthesia for chronic spinal cord lesions. Anaesthesia 1998;53:273-89.
2. Krassioukov A, Warburton DE, Teasell R, Eng JJ. A systematic review of the management of autonomic dysreflexia after spinal cord injury. Arch Phys Med Rehabil 2009;90:682-95.
3. Milligan J, Lee J, McMillan C, Klassen H. Autonomic dysreflexia: recognizing a common serious condition in patients with spinal cord injury. Can Fam Physician 2012;58:831-5.
4. Skowronski E, Hartman K. Obstetric management following traumatic tetraplegia: case series and literature review. Aust N Z J Obstet Gynaecol 2008;48:485-91.
5. Blackmer J. Rehabilitation medicine: 1. Autonomic dysreflexia. CMAJ 2003;169:931-5.

18   Cardiac Tamponade

DEFINITION

Cardiac tamponade is the accumulation of blood, a blood clot, or fluid in the pericardial space, limiting ventricular filling and resulting in hemodynamic compromise.

ETIOLOGY

Bleeding after cardiac surgery
Coagulopathy
Cardiac perforation
Rheumatologic or autoimmune diseases
Pericardial malignancy or tumor metastasis
Pericardial infection, typically as a complication of sepsis
Chronic renal failure
Radiation-induced pericardial effusion

TYPICAL SITUATIONS

Idiopathic
Iatrogenic
    Post cardiac surgery
        Clots may cause tamponade even in the presence of an open pericardium and patent mediastinal drains
    Erosion of CVP catheter, especially through right atrial wall
    Invasive cardiac procedure
        PCI
        Electrophysiologic procedure
        Percutaneous valve repair/replacement
Trauma, including gun shot wounds (may be insidious in onset)
Malignancy
End-stage renal disease
Collagen vascular disease (e.g., systemic lupus erythematosus, scleroderma)
Post MI (myocardial rupture, consequences of anticoagulant or thrombolytic therapy)

Bacterial infection (e.g., tuberculosis)
Aortic dissection
Radiation therapy to the mediastinum

PREVENTION

Achieve and maintain hemostasis during and after cardiothoracic surgery
Treat coagulopathy
Place central lines and pacemaker leads carefully
> CVP catheter tip should be at the junction of the superior vena cava (SVC) and right atrium
> Obtain a CXR following placement to confirm the position of the CVP catheter tip when feasible
Treat and control underlying medical problems that predispose the patient to pericardial effusion
Perform pericardiocentesis of large pericardial effusion prior to surgery

MANIFESTATIONS

Beck triad (distant heart sounds, jugular venous distension, hypotension)
Tachycardia, decreased CO
Narrow pulse pressure, exaggeration of pulsus paradoxus
> Normal limit of pulsus paradoxus is a decrease in SBP on inspiration of less than 10 mm Hg
Equalization of cardiac diastolic filling pressures at a relatively high value (right atrial pressure, PA diastolic pressure, PA wedge pressure)
Dyspnea, orthopnea
Following cardiac surgery
> Consider tamponade in the differential diagnosis of any patient with low CO
> Increased drainage followed by decreased drainage from the mediastinal chest tube
Pericardial fluid visible on TEE or TTE in conjunction with
> Atrial and/or ventricular collapse
> Abnormal ventricular septal motion with respiration
> IVC plethora (i.e., lack of the normal inspiratory collapse of the IVC on TTE)
Low-amplitude ECG with ST changes and/or electrical alternans
Increased size and bottle shape of the cardiac silhouette on CXR

SIMILAR EVENTS

Congestive heart failure
Constrictive pericarditis
Exacerbation of asthma or COPD (see Event 29, Bronchospasm)
Hypovolemia
ACS (see Event 15, Acute Coronary Syndrome)
Acute aortic dissection
PE (see Event 21, Pulmonary Embolism)
Acute RV infarction

Tension pneumothorax (see Event 35, Pneumothorax)
Restrictive cardiomyopathy
Auto-PEEP

MANAGEMENT

The pericardium has low compliance, and the rate of fluid accumulation will determine the rapidity of onset of symptoms. Rapid accumulation of 150 to 200 mL of blood or fluid can critically compromise myocardial function.

Ensure adequate oxygenation and ventilation
　　Administer supplemental O_2 by nonrebreathing face mask
Expand and maintain the circulating fluid volume
　　Ensure adequate IV access
　　Place additional large-bore IV catheters as needed
　　Rapidly administer 250 to 500 mL crystalloid
Place invasive monitoring lines as indicated
　　Arterial line
　　CVP catheter for monitoring and drug administration
　　PA catheter for monitoring of cardiac filling pressures and CO
Support the circulation
　　Phenylephrine IV, 100 to 200 µg; may repeat and increase dose as needed
　　Epinephrine IV, 5 to 10 µg; may repeat and increase dose as needed
　　Vasopressin IV, 1 to 2 U; may repeat and increase dose as needed
　　Norepinephrine IV, 8 to 16 µg; may repeat and increase dose as needed
　　Commence infusions of vasopressors as needed
Confirm diagnosis with TEE or TTE
Consider CXR if patient is stable
Apply and connect external defibrillator pads
If the patient has had recent cardiothoracic surgery
　　Call for cardiac surgeon stat
　　Open the chest immediately to relieve the cardiac tamponade
　　Prepare the OR for possible mediastinal exploration
　　　　Notify nursing staff and perfusionist
If the patient has NOT had recent cardiothoracic surgery
　　Perform subxiphoid pericardiocentesis
　　　　This may remove enough fluid to temporarily improve the patient's condition prior to emergency surgery
　　　　A negative aspiration does not exclude cardiac tamponade
If cardiac tamponade is suspected and the patient is stable
Review the patient's history
Check coagulation status of the patient
　　PT and PTT
　　Platelet count
　　Platelet function
　　ACT
　　Thromboelastogram (TEG)
Monitor the patient using invasive techniques

Obtain CXR and TEE or TTE for diagnosis

Obtain consultation from a cardiologist and/or cardiothoracic surgeon for definitive treatment

Anesthetic management of the patient with cardiac tamponade

Hemodynamic goals are best described as keeping the patient fast (tachycardia), full (hypervolemia), and tight (increased SVR)

Maintain HR in the range of 90 to 140 bpm

Optimize filling pressures to compensate for the vasodilation that occurs with induction of anesthesia

Administer fluid bolus (250 to 500 mL crystalloid)

Consider femoral venous and arterial cannulation for emergent CPB if difficult surgical exposure is anticipated

Maintain spontaneous ventilation as long as possible, as it augments venous return and maintains CO

With positive pressure ventilation, use low airway pressure without PEEP to minimize decrease in venous return

Consider prepping and draping patient prior to induction of general anesthesia

For anesthesia, use drugs that do not decrease sympathetic output

Ketamine IV, 0.25 to 1 mg/kg

Should still anticipate hemodynamic compromise

Use succinylcholine IV, 1 to 2 mg/kg for intubation

Provide additional IV anesthesia as tolerated

Ketamine 10 to 20 mg

Fentanyl 25 to 50 μg

Midazolam 0.25 to 0.5 mg

Correct metabolic acidosis

Anticipate a rebound hypertensive response or return of normal hemodynamics after tamponade is relieved

Use additional anesthetic agents (e.g., volatile anesthetics)

COMPLICATIONS

Arrhythmias

Myocardial ischemia or infarction

Complications of pericardiocentesis

Pneumothorax, hemothorax

Laceration of heart or lungs

Infection

Cardiac arrest

SUGGESTED READING

1. Oliver WC, Mauermann WJ, Nuttall GA. Uncommon cardiac diseases. In: Kaplan JA, Reich DL, Savino JS, editors. Kaplan's cardiac anesthesia: the echo era. 6th ed. Philadelphia: Saunders; 2011, p. 710-3.
2. O'Connor CJ, Tuman KJ. The intraoperative management of patients with pericardial tamponade. Anesthesiol Clin 2010;28:87-96.
3. Grocott HP, Gulati H, Srinathan S, et al. Anesthesia and the patient with pericardial disease. Can J Anesth 2011;58:952-66.
4. Soler-Soler J, Sagrista-Sauleda J, Permanyer-Miralda G. Management of pericardial effusion. Heart 2001;86:235-40.
5. Spodick DH. Current concepts. Acute Cardiac Tamponade. NEJM 2003;349:684-90 Review article.

18

19   Nonlethal Ventricular Arrhythmias

DEFINITION

Nonlethal ventricular arrhythmias originate at the level of the ventricles and are characterized by a wide QRS complex (e.g., PVC, VT, and torsades de pointes)

ETIOLOGY

Abnormal automaticity of ventricular myocardium
Reentry mechanisms
Drug toxicity
R on T phenomenon (a PVC or a pacemaker spike occurring at the apex of the T wave, initiating VT)
Electrolyte abnormalities

TYPICAL SITUATIONS

PVCs are seen frequently in healthy people and are more likely to occur after tea, coffee, alcohol, tobacco, or emotional excitement

Patients with
    Myocardial ischemia or infarction
    Heart failure and cardiomyopathy
    Hypoxemia and/or hypercarbia
    Potassium and/or acid-base disturbance
    Hypomagnesemia
    Mitral valve prolapse
    Inappropriate depth of anesthesia for level of surgical stimulus
Mechanical stimulation of the heart
    Handling of the heart during cardiothoracic surgery
    Passage of a PA catheter through the RV
Acute hypertension and/or tachycardia
Acute hypotension and/or bradycardia
Drugs
    Digitalis toxicity
    Tricyclic antidepressant toxicity
    Aminophylline toxicity
    Antiarrhythmic drugs (quinidine, procainamide, disopyramide)
Hypothermia (core temperature less than 32°C)

PREVENTION

Recognize and treat preoperative ventricular arrhythmias
Correct electrolyte abnormalities
Identify patients taking drugs known to cause ventricular arrhythmias
Avoid/minimize mechanical stimulation of heart
Avoid/minimize hemodynamic abnormalities

MANIFESTATIONS

PVC
>   Wide QRS complex on ECG not preceded by a P wave
>>   PVCs may not produce ejection of blood into the aorta or a palpable pulse
>>   There is usually a compensatory pause between the PVC and the next normal beat

VT
>   A succession of three or more PVCs at a rate > 100 bpm
>>   Some VTs support adequate circulation and do not degenerate into lethal arrhythmias

Torsades de pointes
>   Paroxysms of polymorphic VT in which the QRS axis changes direction continuously, with a periodicity of 5 to 20 beats
>   Associated with prolonged QT-interval

SIMILAR EVENTS

ECG artifact
Supraventricular rhythm with aberrant conduction (see Event 23, Supraventricular Arrhythmias)
AV reentrant rhythms
Bundle branch blocks, especially in the presence of tachycardia
Paced rhythm

MANAGEMENT

19

Ensure adequate oxygenation and ventilation
Check the hemodynamic significance of the rhythm
>   Palpate the peripheral pulses
>   Check the BP
>   Examine the arterial waveform (if arterial line is present)

Measure and maintain normal body temperature
Maintain appropriate depth of anesthesia

If the arrhythmia causes significant hemodynamic impairment
>   Evaluate possible underlying etiologies
>>   Draw appropriate labs (e.g., ABG, electrolytes, CBC, cardiac enzymes)
>>   Obtain 12-lead ECG
>>   Consider TEE or TTE to evaluate cardiac function and possible ischemia

>   PVCs
>>   PVCs frequent enough to cause symptoms may be treated with β-blockers or antiarrhythmic agents (e.g., lidocaine, flecainide, amiodarone, sotalol)

VT
>   Hemodynamically unstable VT should be treated with unsynchronized electrical cardioversion (see Event 2, Cardiac Arrest)
>   Hemodynamically stable monomorphic VT
>>   Consider urgent synchronized electrical cardioversion because of the risk of developing hemodynamic instability or conversion to VF
>>>   Biphasic defibrillators: 200 J
>>>   Monophasic defibrillators: 360 J
>>   Pharmacologic therapy
>>>   Amiodarone slow IV bolus, 150 mg over 10 minutes, followed by 1 mg/min infusion for 6 hours

Lidocaine IV bolus, 1.5 mg/kg, followed by 1 to 4 mg/min infusion
Torsades de pointes
    If hemodynamically unstable, perform unsynchronized electrical cardioversion
        Biphasic defibrillators: 200 J
        Monophasic defibrillators: 360 J
    If hemodynamically stable
        Administer $MgSO_4$ IV, 2 g over 2 minutes
        Consider overdrive pacing (rate ~100 bpm)
        Consider isoproterenol IV infusion titrated to HR, ~100 bpm
        Consider phenytoin IV, 250 mg over 5 minutes
    Withdraw medications causing QT prolongation

COMPLICATIONS

Progression of nonlethal arrhythmia to lethal arrhythmia
Organ hypoperfusion
Side effects from therapy
    VF
    Hyperkalemia or cardiac arrest from rapid K^+ administration
    Lidocaine toxicity
    Hypotension from isoproterenol
Cardiac arrest

SUGGESTED READING

1. European Heart Rhythm Association, Heart Rhythm Society, Zipes DP, et al. ACC/AHA/ESC 2006 guidelines for management of patients with ventricular arrhythmias and the prevention of sudden cardiac death: a report of the American College of Cardiology/American Heart Association Task Force and the European Society of Cardiology Committee for Practice Guidelines (writing committee to develop guidelines for management of patients with ventricular arrhythmias and the prevention of sudden cardiac death). J Am Coll Cardiol 2006;48:e247-e346.
2. Lin D, Callans DJ. Nonsustained VT during exercise testing: causes and work-up. Am Coll Cardiol Curr J Rev 2003; Nov-Dec 57-60.
3. Bikkina M, Larson MG, Levy D. Prognostic implications of asymptomatic ventricular arrhythmias: the Framingham Heart Study. Ann Intern Med 1992;117:990-6.
4. Griffith MJ, Linker NJ, Garratt CJ, et al. Relative efficacy and safety of intravenous drugs for termination of sustained ventricular tachycardia. Lancet 1990;336:670-3.

---

20   Pulmonary Edema

DEFINITION

Pulmonary edema is the accumulation of fluid in the interstitium and alveoli of the lung.

ETIOLOGY

Cardiogenic pulmonary edema
    Caused by high pulmonary capillary hydrostatic pressure

Noncardiogenic pulmonary edema
> Caused by increased permeability of pulmonary capillary membranes, ARDS, or low capillary oncotic pressure

Negative pressure pulmonary edema
> Strong inspiratory efforts against an obstructed upper airway (laryngospasm, upper airway tumor, or foreign body)

Inadequate lymphatic clearance of normal or excessive interstitial and alveolar fluid

TYPICAL SITUATIONS

Cardiogenic pulmonary edema
> Myocardial dysfunction
>> Acute myocardial ischemia or infarction
>> Acute valvular dysfunction
>> Severe hypertension
> Fluid overload
>> In patients with CHF
>> In patients with renal insufficiency or renal failure
> With massive fluid resuscitation
>> May occur 2 to 3 days after surgery when fluids are mobilized
> With rapid fluid absorption (e.g., during TURP)

Noncardiogenic pulmonary edema (e.g., ARDS) secondary to
> Sepsis (most common in-hospital cause)
> Pneumonia (most common cause outside of the hospital)
> Pulmonary aspiration of gastric contents
> Trauma (e.g., bilateral lung contusions, massive tissue injury, smoke inhalation)
> Massive transfusion
> TRALI
> Medical causes (e.g., blood and hemopoietic stem cell transplant, acute pancreatitis, drug or alcohol overdose, opiate reversal with naloxone)
> Near-drowning
> Amniotic fluid embolism
> Post-CPB
> Post-pneumonectomy
> Neurogenic pulmonary edema (after major head trauma, stroke, subarachnoid or intracerebral hemorrhage, intracranial surgery)
> Reexpansion pulmonary edema (e.g., evacuation of large amount of fluid or air from pleural space)
> Reperfusion pulmonary edema (after lung transplantation)

PREVENTION

Optimize perioperative medical management
Monitor fluid replacement carefully
Use invasive hemodynamic monitoring in patients at risk of pulmonary edema or CHF
Monitor for signs of possible fluid absorption during TURP
Treat the underlying problem in ARDS

MANIFESTATIONS

Vital signs
    Hypotension, hypertension, tachycardia, and arrhythmias
Physical examination
    Fine crackles (rales) audible in the lung fields on auscultation
Pulmonary manifestations
    Decreased O_2 saturation
    Increased A–a gradient
    Serosanguinous pulmonary edema fluid in the ETT or under the face mask
    In the awake patient
        Dyspnea, "air hunger," and restlessness, even with normal O_2 saturation
        Hypoxemia may develop later
    In the mechanically ventilated patient
        Decreased lung compliance
        Increase in PIP during volume mode ventilation
        Decreased tidal volume during pressure mode ventilation
In patients with cardiogenic pulmonary edema
    Elevated cardiac filling pressures
        Jugular venous distention
        Increased CVP
        Increased PCWP
    CXR
        Increase in interstitial and alveolar fluid
        Cardiomegaly
        Increased pulmonary vascularity
        Perivascular cuffing
        Kerley B lines
        Interstitial infiltrate
        "White-out" of lung fields
In patients with noncardiogenic pulmonary edema
    Cardiac filling pressures are normal or decreased
    CXR
        Increased pulmonary vascularity
        Perivascular cuffing
        Kerley B lines
        Interstitial infiltrate
        "White-out" of lung fields

20

SIMILAR EVENTS

Bronchospasm (see Event 29, Bronchospasm)
Anaphylaxis (see Event 16, Anaphylactic and Anaphylactoid Reactions)
Endobronchial intubation (see Event 30, Endobronchial Intubation)
Kinked or obstructed ETT (see Event 7, High Peak Inspiratory Pressure)
Pneumothorax, tension pneumothorax (see Event 35, Pneumothorax)
Residual neuromuscular blockade
Drug administration error (see Event 63, Drug Administration Error)

MANAGEMENT

Increase FiO$_2$

Use high-flow nonrebreathing face mask

Assist ventilation if necessary with continuous positive airway pressure (CPAP) or bilevel positive airway pressure (BiPAP)

In intubated patients, deliver 100% O$_2$ and consider adding PEEP

Assess respiratory effort and adequacy of ventilation

Evaluate the patient looking for use of accessory muscles of respiration, tachypnea, hemodynamic compromise, altered mental status

Intubate the patient who is not already intubated if pulmonary edema persists in the presence of hypoxemia not responsive to supplementary O$_2$, altered mental status, or if respiratory failure is imminent

Check for pneumothorax (see Event 35, Pneumothorax)

In postoperative patients, consider residual neuromuscular blockade if respiratory effort is inadequate

Obtain an ABG, CXR, ECG

Assess myocardial function with TEE or TTE

For patients with cardiogenic pulmonary edema

Reduce the cardiac preload

Sit the awake patient upright

Position the anesthetized patient in the reverse Trendelenburg if not contraindicated by the surgical procedure or hypotension

Administer furosemide IV, 10 to 20 mg bolus (use an increased dose if the patient is already on diuretic therapy)

Consider placing a urinary catheter

Administer morphine IV, 2 mg increments (exercise caution in the spontaneously breathing patient to avoid respiratory depression)

Consider an infusion of NTG IV, 0.25 to 1 μg/kg/min unless the patient is hypotensive

Optimize myocardial contractility

Discontinue myocardial depressant drugs (e.g., volatile anesthetics) and replace with other agents

Place invasive hemodynamic monitors (arterial line, CVP, PA catheter)

Consider inotropic support

Dopamine, 3 to 10 μg/kg/min

Dobutamine, 5 to 10 μg/kg/min

Milrinone IV, 50 μg/kg loading dose (over 10 minutes), infusion of 0.375 to 0.75 μg/kg/min

Epinephrine 10 to 200 ng/kg/min

Consider use of IABP

For patients with noncardiogenic pulmonary edema

As above for cardiogenic pulmonary edema plus treat underlying cause

In the presence of bronchospasm, consider inhalation of nebulized β$_2$ agonists (see Event 29, Bronchospasm)

Terminate the surgical procedure as quickly as possible and make arrangements to transfer the patient to the ICU for further management

Obtain an urgent medical consultation as indicated by the clinical diagnosis

Consider extracorporeal membrane oxygenation (ECMO) in severe cases refractory to medical management

COMPLICATIONS

Hypovolemia and hypotension from overaggressive diuresis or reduction of preload
Electrolyte disturbances
Metabolic and/or respiratory acidosis
Cardiac arrest

SUGGESTED READING

1. Walkey AJ, Summer R, Ho V, Alkana P. Acute respiratory distress syndrome: epidemiology and management approaches. Clin Epidemiol 2012;4:159-69.
2. Krodel DJ, Bittner EA, Abdulnour R, et al. Case scenario: acute postoperative negative pressure pulmonary edema. Anesthesiology 2010;113:200-7.

21   Pulmonary Embolism

DEFINITION

Pulmonary embolism (PE) is a partial or complete obstruction of the pulmonary arterial circulation by substances originating elsewhere in the cardiovascular system.

ETIOLOGY

Substances that can cause a PE

> Blood clot
> Fat
> Amniotic fluid
> Gas
> Tumor

TYPICAL SITUATIONS

Deep venous thrombosis (DVT)
> Recent major surgery
> Elderly—risk increases exponentially with increasing age
> Malignancy (especially with metastatic disease)
> Postpartum
> History of previous DVT or venous insufficiency of the lower extremities
> Prolonged immobilization
> History of CHF or recent MI
> Thrombophilia (hypercoagulability or a prothrombotic state) following splenectomy with rebound thrombocytosis or polycythemia
> Obesity
Fat embolism
> Multiple fractures, long bone fractures, or pelvic fractures
> Reaming of bone marrow cavity
> High pressure injection into bone marrow cavity during total joint replacement

PREVENTION

Different recommendations are suggested for prophylaxis in patients at risk of developing DVT and vary with the perceived level of risk.

> Heparin SC, 5000 U, 1 to 2 hours before surgery and every 6 to 8 hours until the patient is ambulatory
>
> Enoxaparin SC, 30 to 40 mg twice a day
>
> Oral anticoagulants (e.g., warfarin, with the first dose given the day before surgery)
>> Monitor the level of anticoagulation with serial international normalized ratio (INR) measurements
>
> Graduated compression stockings (used alone these devices do not protect the high-risk patient)
>
> Intermittent pneumatic compression boots
>
> Have an IVC filter placed in patients at high risk of PE from DVT
>> When pharmacologic methods fail to prevent DVT
>> If anticoagulants are contraindicated

MANIFESTATIONS

Massive PE can present as severe hemodynamic decompensation or cardiac arrest (PEA or asystole).

If the patient is conscious
> Dyspnea, pleuritic chest pain, and hemoptysis
>
> Hypotension and tachycardia
>
> Hypoxemia or increased A–a gradient is usually present
>
> Fine crackles (rales), wheezes, or a pleural rub may be heard on auscultation of the chest
>
> The CXR is usually normal, but there may be a change in vessel diameter, vessel "cutoff," increased radiolucency in areas of hypoperfusion, atelectasis, and/or a pleural effusion

In the patient who is under general anesthesia
> Tachypnea if the patient is breathing spontaneously
>
> Hypotension and tachycardia
>
> Hypoxemia, increased A–a gradient, or cyanosis, even when breathing 100% O_2
>
> Decreased ET CO_2 (change is usually abrupt but depends on severity of embolism)
>
> Increased CVP and PA pressures
>
> Acute right heart failure
>
> ECG changes
>> Right heart strain, ST-T wave changes, bradycardia, PEA, asystole, $S_1Q_3T_3$ pattern, or new-onset right bundle branch block (RBBB)

Fat embolism
> Triad of hypoxemia, altered mental status, and petechial rash usually involving neck and upper body
>
> Thrombocytopenia
>
> Presents typically 24 to 72 hours after the insult
>
> Fat globules may be present in the urine, sputum, or retinal vessels

Amniotic fluid embolism (AFE)
> Typically occurring during or shortly after labor, characterized by cardiogenic shock, hypoxemia, respiratory failure, DIC, coma, and seizures

21

SIMILAR EVENTS

Hypoxemia from other causes (see Event 10, Hypoxemia)
Hypotension from other causes (see Event 9, Hypotension)
Increased dead space ventilation
Pulmonary hypertension
RV failure
Anaphylactic and anaphylactoid reactions (see Event 16, Anaphylactic and Anaphylactoid Reactions, Event 24, Venous Gas Embolism, and Event 81, Amniotic Fluid Embolism)

MANAGEMENT

The diagnosis of PE may be difficult during general anesthesia.

Ensure adequate oxygenation and ventilation
  Administer supplemental O_2
  For the nonintubated patient:
    Use a nonrebreathing face mask delivering 100% O_2
    Consider endotracheal intubation, mechanical ventilation, and PEEP
  For the intubated patient:
    Ventilate with 100% O_2
    Consider use of PEEP
  Perform ABG
    ET CO_2 measurements will not reliably indicate the adequacy of ventilation
Support the circulation
  Expand the circulating fluid volume
  Administer inotropic drugs by bolus or infusion
    Ephedrine IV, 5 to 20 mg, repeat as necessary
    Epinephrine IV, 10 to 50 µg, repeat as necessary
    Dopamine, dobutamine, milrinone, or epinephrine infusion (see Event 9, Hypotension)
  Place invasive monitors for diagnosis and management
    Arterial line
    TEE or TTE especially for evaluation of right heart function
    PA catheter (with mixed venous saturation and continuous CO monitoring, if available)
      If there is pulmonary hypertension with RV failure, consider using a NTG infusion, 0.25 to 1 µg/kg/min, as a pulmonary vasodilator
  If cardiac arrest is present
    Perform CPR (see Event 2, Cardiac Arrest)
    Consider emergency percutaneous CPB or ECMO
    Consider emergency pulmonary embolectomy
    Emergent consult with pulmonology or critical care expert to discuss treatment options
Establish the diagnosis
  Rule out other causes of hypoxemia, increased dead space ventilation, or hemodynamic compromise (see Event 10, Hypoxemia)
  Obtain a spiral CT scan, ventilation/perfusion ($\dot{V}/\dot{Q}$) scan, or a pulmonary angiogram

If pulmonary thromboembolism is confirmed

Emergent consult with pulmonology or critical care expert to discuss treatment options; advanced catheter-based therapies are emerging options for significant PE

Anticoagulation or thrombolytic therapy may prevent further embolization but may be contraindicated if there is an underlying bleeding site or recent surgical procedure

If anticoagulation is not contraindicated, administer heparin IV, 5000 U bolus, followed by a heparin infusion of 1000 U/hr, adjusted to maintain the aPTT at least twice normal

Insert an IVC filter in patients with recurrent PE who have received adequate anticoagulation or in patients in whom anticoagulation is contraindicated

COMPLICATIONS

Pulmonary infarction
Hemoptysis
Cardiac arrest
Hemorrhagic complications of anticoagulation therapy

SUGGESTED READING

1. Banks DA, Manecke GR, Maus TM, et al. Pulmonary thromboendarterectomy for chronic thromboembolic pulmonary hypertension. In: Kaplan JA, Reich DL, Savino JS, editors. Kaplan's cardiac anesthesia: the echo era. 6th ed. Philadelphia: Saunders, 2011, p. 769-76.
2. Agnelli G, Becattini C. Acute pulmonary embolism. N Engl J Med 2010;363:266-74.
3. Conde-Agudelo A, Romero R. Amniotic fluid embolism: an evidence-based review. Am J Obstet Gynecol 2009;201:e1-e13 (**Erratum in** Am J Obstet Gynecol 2010;202:92).
4. Konstantinides S. Acute pulmonary embolism. N Engl J Med 2008;359:2804-13.

22 Sinus Bradycardia

DEFINITION

Sinus bradycardia is a HR less than 60 bpm in an adult with the impulse formation originating in the sinoatrial node.

ETIOLOGY

Physiologic response in the absence of heart disease
    During normal sleep
    High level of physical fitness
    Heightened vagal activity
    Hypothermia
Pathologic response in the absence of heart disease
    Obstructive sleep apnea (OSA)
    Increased ICP (Cushing reflex)
    Hypothyroidism
    Hypoxemia
    Reflex response to hypertension
Drug effect
Pathologic response in the presence of heart disease

Sick sinus syndrome
Familial condition (e.g., pacemaker ion channel mutation)
Acute myocardial ischemia or infarction

TYPICAL SITUATIONS

Following administration of drugs that produce bradycardia
    Opioids (especially fentanyl, sufentanil)
    β-Adrenergic antagonists
    Calcium channel blockers
    Anticholinesterases
    α_2-Agonists (e.g., clonidine, dexmedetomidine)
During periods of vagal stimulation
    Traction on the eye or the peritoneum (including pneumoperitoneum)
    Laryngoscopy and intubation
    Bladder catheterization
Baroreceptor reflex during hypertensive episodes
During spinal or epidural anesthesia (block of cardiac accelerator fibers at levels T1-T4)
Electroconvulsive therapy
In the patient with acute myocardial ischemia or infarction

PREVENTION

Premedicate patients at risk of vagal responses with an anticholinergic agent
    Atropine IM, 0.4 mg (adults)
    Glycopyrrolate IM, 0.2 mg (adults)
During spinal or epidural anesthesia, treat bradycardia aggressively and early with atropine IV, 0.4 to 0.6 mg
    Bradycardia can rapidly progress to asystole in these patients
Vagal responses due to traction on the peritoneum or the extraocular muscles, or pressure on the carotid sinus, are not always avoidable
    Inform the surgeon of the bradycardia and ask him or her to release the pressure or traction
    Treat with atropine or glycopyrrolate IV and proceed with caution
    Repeat this sequence if necessary
Maintain normal plasma electrolyte levels

22

MANIFESTATIONS

Bradycardia may be well tolerated, particularly if it develops slowly. Acute onset of bradycardia is more likely to be symptomatic.

Slow HR
    ECG
    Pulse oximeter
    Arterial line
    Palpation of peripheral pulses
Hypotension
Junctional or idioventricular escape beats
In the conscious patient
    Nausea, vomiting
    Mental status change

SIMILAR EVENTS

Monitor artifact
    Failure of monitor to count QRS or pulse oximeter signal
    ECG lead disconnection or failure
    Oximeter probe displaced or failure
Dropped beats (second-degree AV heart block, Mobitz type I and type II)
Third-degree AV block
Pacemaker malfunction or failure
    Lead fracture
    Lead disconnection
    Inappropriate settings (e.g., output too low, sensitivity too high)
AF/flutter with poor perfusion or slow ventricular response

MANAGEMENT

Use aggressive treatment for bradycardic patients under spinal or epidural anesthesia, as it can progress rapidly to cardiac arrest without warning.

Verify bradycardia and assess its hemodynamic significance
    Check monitors of HR
    Check BP
    Check pulse oximeter
    Palpate a peripheral pulse
Scan the surgical field for operative causes
    If in response to surgical stimulus, alert surgeon to stop the precipitating stimulus
Notify the surgeon of the bradycardia
If bradycardia is associated with severe symptoms (profound hypotension, loss of consciousness, seizures), remove possible causes
Ensure adequate oxygenation and ventilation
    Deliver 100% O_2 and turn off all volatile anesthetics
    Manage the airway (patient may require intubation)
        Bradycardia is common in prolonged hypoxemia
Call for help
Treat with
    Atropine IV, 0.4 to 0.6 mg. Repeat every 3 to 5 minutes to total dose of 3 mg
    Dopamine IV infusion, 2 to 10 μg/kg/min
    Epinephrine IV, 10 μg bolus, repeat with escalating doses as necessary
    Commence an epinephrine infusion, 5 to 100 ng/kg/min, if necessary
    If bradycardia fails to resolve quickly with epinephrine boluses, initiate cardiac pacing
        Transcutaneous (newer defibrillators typically offer pacing function)
            Awake patient will probably need analgesia and sedation
        Transvenous (effective, but logistically difficult in an emergency)
        Commence CPR if necessary (see Event 2, Cardiac Arrest)
If bradycardia is associated with mild to moderate symptoms (modest decrease in BP, nausea, vomiting, or mild alteration in sensorium)
    Ephedrine IV, 5 to 10 mg increments, repeat as necessary
    Atropine IV, 0.4 mg, repeat as necessary
    Glycopyrrolate IV, 0.2 mg, repeat as necessary
If bradycardia is not associated with any obvious physiologic consequences
    Monitor the patient closely

COMPLICATIONS

Escape arrhythmias
Complications of pacemakers
Tachyarrhythmias and hypertension secondary to drug treatment
Cardiac arrest

SUGGESTED READING

1. Epstein AE, DiMarco JP, Ellenbogen KA, et al. ACC/AHA/HRS 2008 guidelines for device-based therapy of cardiac rhythm abnormalities: a report of the American College of Cardiology/American Heart Association Task Force on Practice Guidelines (writing committee to revise the ACC/AHA/NASPE 2002 guideline update for implantation of cardiac pacemakers and antiarrhythmia devices). Developed in collaboration with the American Association for Thoracic Surgery and Society of Thoracic Surgeons. Circulation 2008;117:e350-e408.
2. Stein R, Medeiros CM, Rosito GA, et al. Intrinsic sinus and atrioventricular node electrophysiologic adaptations in endurance athletes. J Am Coll Cardiol 2002;39:1033-8.
3. Neumar RW, Otto CW, Link MS, et al. Part 8: Adult advanced cardiovascular life support: 2010 American Heart Association guidelines for cardiopulmonary resuscitation and emergency cardiovascular care. Circulation 2010;122:S729-67.

23   Supraventricular Arrhythmias

DEFINITION

A supraventricular arrhythmia is an abnormal cardiac rhythm arising from a supraventricular source.

> Sinoatrial node (SA node)
> Atrium
> Atrioventricular node (AV node)

ETIOLOGY

Enhanced automaticity of supraventricular tissue (tachyarrhythmias)
Reentry
Reduced automaticity of supraventricular tissue (AV nodal rhythm)

TYPICAL SITUATIONS

Many atrial arrhythmias occur in patients with normal hearts
> During exercise
> After drinking coffee, tea, or alcohol
> Following smoking
> Pain or inadequate anesthesia
> Hypovolemia
> Anemia
> Fever
> Drug effects (e.g., epinephrine IV)
Acute myocardial ischemia or infarction

During or following pulmonary or cardiac surgery
Wolff-Parkinson-White syndrome or other cardiac disorders with accessory conduction pathways
Hypervolemia
Hypoxemia, hypercarbia, acidosis, alkalosis
Pyrexia
Electrolyte imbalance
Hypermetabolic states (e.g., hyperthyroidism, MH)
Acute or chronic pulmonary disease
PE
Valvular heart disease (e.g., mitral valve prolapse)
Pericarditis, myocarditis
OSA
Conditions causing catecholamine excess (pain, pheochromocytoma)
Autonomic reflexes

PREVENTION

Identify and treat patients with supraventricular arrhythmias preoperatively
Optimize medical therapy
Correct electrolyte abnormalities
Correct acidosis, alkalosis, hypoxemia, hypercarbia
Maintain adequate depth of anesthesia
Maintain euvolemia
Avoid hyperthermia

MANIFESTATIONS

If there is a rapid ventricular response, it may be difficult to determine the exact focus of the tachyarrhythmia.

Symptoms in the awake patient may include:
    Tachycardia
    Palpitations
    Syncope or presyncope
    Lightheadedness
    Diaphoresis
    Chest pain or discomfort
    Shortness of breath
    Hypotension
    Nausea and vomiting
    ECG abnormality

Sinus Tachycardia

    Impulse arises from the SA node
    Rate is greater than 100 bpm and may be as high as 170 bpm
    Most common arrhythmia in perioperative period

Sinus Arrhythmia

Impulse arises from the SA node at a variable rate of 60 to 100 bpm
PR intervals and QRS intervals are normal with a P/QRS ratio of 1:1
Rate commonly increases during inspiration and decreases during expiration

Atrial Escape Beats

Occur in setting of a long sinus pause or sinus arrest
Rate correlates with the automaticity of the atrial focus and is generally slower than the
   sinus rate
P-wave morphology differs from the sinus rhythm P-wave, and QRS complexes are normal

Atrial Premature Beats (APB)

Impulse is generated by an ectopic focus in the left or right atrium
P-wave is present but morphology differs from sinus rhythm P-wave
Impulse travels from the atria to the AV node and the PR interval may be shorter or longer
   than the sinus rhythm PR interval
At AV node, the impulse continues to the ventricular conduction system and also retro-
   grade to SA node, resetting the sinus pacemaker
Absence of compensatory pause

Wandering Atrial Pacemaker

Three or more ectopic foci within the atrium generate pulses with different P-wave morphologies
Rate is typically less than 100 bpm; when rate exceeds 100 bpm, the arrhythmia is known
   as multifocal atrial tachycardia
Rhythm is irregular
   May be confused with AF
      Difference from AF is clear P-waves (with differing morphologies) versus lack of
      P-waves in AF

Atrial Tachycardia (AT)

Atrial rate ranges from 100 to 250 bpm with variable ventricular response
Impulse may arise from a single focus (with a distinctive P-wave) or may be multifocal
   (with multiple P wave morphologies)
PR interval may vary in multifocal AT, and QRS complex typically remains normal
Multifocal AT commonly seen in patients with heart failure or COPD

Atrial Flutter

Regular, rapid atrial depolarizations with rates typically 300 bpm
Ventricular rate slower due to AV block (typically 2:1, up to 8:1)
Saw-tooth flutter waves (F-waves) are typically present
QRS complex typically remains normal and T-waves are lost in the F-waves

Atrial Fibrillation (AF)

Results from a rapid firing focus commonly arising from the pulmonary veins
Rapid and irregular contraction of the atria results in fibrillation
Ventricular rate may vary from 60 to 170 bpm
No P-waves evident on ECG

QRS complexes with normal configuration but with irregular rhythm

Loss of "atrial kick" may severely reduce CO and BP

Tendency to develop atrial thrombi may lead to pulmonary or systemic embolization

Atrioventricular Nodal Reentrant Tachycardia (AVNRT)

Reentrant tachycardia caused by AV nodal pathways

Regular fast rhythm (120 to 250 bpm)

P-waves might not be visible

Atrioventricular Reentrant Tachycardia (AVRT)

Reentrant tachycardia utilizing an accessory pathway between atria and ventricles (e.g., Wolff-Parkinson-White syndrome)

The most common type uses the AV node for antegrade conduction and accessory pathway for retrograde conduction (orthodromic conduction)

    QRS complex remains narrow

    Negative P-waves may be seen in the inferior leads

Less commonly, the accessory pathway conducts the antegrade impulse and the AV node conducts the retrograde impulse (antidromic conduction)

    QRS complexes are wide

    May be difficult to distinguish from VT

Junctional Rhythm

Results from an impulse generated from the AV node

When sinus node activity not suppressed, P-waves may be present and appear independent of QRS complexes (AV dissociation)

Sinus node activity may also be suppressed by retrograde atrial activation

Junctional tachycardia—ventricular rates greater than 100 bpm

Junctional escape rhythm—the SA node fails to generate an impulse with ventricular rates of 40 to 55 bpm

SIMILAR EVENTS

ECG artifact

Artificial pacing of right atrium

Other tachyarrhythmias

MANAGEMENT

Ensure adequate oxygenation and ventilation

Check the rhythm and BP

More likely SVT if

    Rate >150 bpm

    Sudden onset

    Irregular tachycardia is probably AF

If patient is UNSTABLE (systolic BP <80 mm Hg, "low" for patient, rapid BP decrease, or acute ischemia)

    Inform the team and call for help

    Obtain crash cart and defibrillator and place pads

23

Administer vasopressor (see Event 9, Hypotension)
Phenylephrine IV, 50 to 200 µg
Prepare to perform immediate synchronized cardioversion
If the patient is hemodynamically STABLE
Diagnose the arrhythmia
Palpate the peripheral pulses
Print rhythm strip from chart recorder, if available
Call for 12-lead ECG
Check multiple ECG leads on physiologic monitor to get the best atrial waveform
The diagnosis of a tachyarrhythmia may be easier if ventricular response rate can be slowed, which can be achieved with
Vagal maneuvers
Adenosine IV, 6 mg bolus
Phenylephrine IV, 25 to 50 µg bolus
Esmolol IV, 10 to 30 mg bolus
Treat the underlying rhythm and/or slow the ventricular response
Sinus tachycardia
Treat underlying cause of tachycardia including pain, inadequate anesthesia, hypovolemia, anemia, inflammation, and drug effects
Sinus arrhythmia, escape atrial beats, and atrial premature beats
No treatment indicated as long as the patient remains hemodynamically stable
Atrial tachycardia
Cardioversion generally ineffective
Withdraw possible precipitating agents (e.g., catecholamines)
In absence of left ventricular dysfunction, consider the use of
Verapamil IV, 2.5 to 5 mg, repeat as necessary q5min to maximum dose of 20 mg
Esmolol IV, 10 to 30 mg, repeat as necessary q3min to maximum dose of 100 mg
Esmolol infusion IV, 50 to 200 µg/kg/min
Amiodarone slow IV infusion, 150 mg over 10 minutes
In presence of left ventricular dysfunction, consider the use of
Amiodarone slow IV infusion, 150 mg over 10 minutes
Digoxin IV, 0.25 to 1.0 mg
Flecainide, propafenone, quinidine, and disopyramide are also effective but have a higher incidence of side effects
Atrial flutter and AF
Rate control
If hemodynamically unstable, immediate synchronized cardioversion
Narrow complex and regular—50 to 100 J
Narrow complex and irregular—120 to 200 J
If cardioversion is unsuccessful, perform synchronized cardioversion at a higher energy level
If hemodynamically stable, use medical management to slow conduction through AV node
If LV function preserved
Verapamil IV, 2.5 to 5 mg, repeat as necessary q5min to maximum dose of 20 mg
Esmolol IV, 10 to 30 mg, repeat as necessary q3min to maximum dose of 100 mg
Esmolol infusion IV, 50 to 200 µg/kg/min
If LV function impaired
Amiodarone slow IV infusion, 150 mg over 10 minutes

Digoxin IV, 0.25 to 1.0 mg
Rhythm control depends on the duration of the arrhythmia
Duration <48 hours
Electrical synchronized cardioversion is preferred
Pharmacologic cardioversion may be achieved with amiodarone or ibutilide
Duration >48 hours
Patients are at risk for developing a left atrial thrombus with systemic embolization
If hemodynamically stable, but would benefit from early cardioversion
Heparin should be started immediately
TEE to rule out presence of left atrial thrombus prior to synchronized cardioversion
AVRT and AVNRT
If hemodynamically unstable, immediate synchronized cardioversion
Narrow complex and regular—50 to 100 J
Narrow complex and irregular—120 to 200 J
If cardioversion is unsuccessful, perform synchronized cardioversion at a higher energy level
If hemodynamically stable
Vagal maneuvers or drugs to block conduction through the AV node and terminate reentrant arrhythmias
Carotid sinus massage
Valsalva maneuver
Adenosine IV, 6 mg bolus with flush and may repeat with 12 mg IV
Very fast onset and very short half-life; watch ECG during adenosine effect – if rhythm does not convert, the slower rate may allow better assessment of actual rhythm
Verapamil IV, 2.5 to 5 mg, repeat as necessary q5min to maximum dose of 20 mg
Esmolol IV, 10 to 30 mg, repeat as necessary q3min to maximum dose of 100 mg
Esmolol infusion IV, 50 to 200 μg/kg/min
Junctional tachycardia
Discontinue exogenous catecholamines
Electrical cardioversion is ineffective
Verapamil IV, 2.5 to 5 mg, repeat as necessary q5min to maximum dose of 20 mg
Esmolol IV, 10 to 30 mg, repeat as necessary q3min to maximum dose of 100 mg
Esmolol infusion IV, 50 to 200 μg/kg/min
Avoid using calcium channel blockade and β blockade together, which may cause profound bradycardia

It can be difficult to distinguish between VT and supraventricular tachyarrhythmias with aberrant conduction. If in doubt, treat as VT with cardioversion.

COMPLICATIONS

Organ hypoperfusion
Adverse drug reactions from therapy
Complications of cardioversion
Heart block
Conversion to a more dangerous rhythm (e.g., VF)
Pulmonary or systemic embolism (dislodged intracardiac thrombus)

SUGGESTED READING

1. Fuster V, Rydén LE, Cannom DS, et al. ACC/AHA/ESC 2006 guidelines for the management of patients with atrial fibrillation: a report of the American College of Cardiology/American Heart Association Task Force on Practice Guidelines and the European Society of Cardiology Committee for Practice Guidelines (writing committee to revise the 2001 guidelines for the management of patients with atrial fibrillation). Developed in collaboration with the European Heart Rhythm Association and the Heart Rhythm Society. Circulation 2006;114:e257-e354.
2. Kwaku KF, Josephson ME. Typical AVNRT – an update on mechanisms and therapy. Card Electrophysiol Rev 2002;6:414-21.
3. Blomström-Lundqvist C, Scheinman MM, Aliot EM, et al. ACC/AHA/ESC guidelines for the management of patients with supraventricular arrhythmias–executive summary: a report of the American College of Cardiology/American Heart Association Task Force on Practice Guidelines and the European Society of Cardiology Committee for Practice Guidelines (writing committee to develop guidelines for the management of patients with supraventricular arrhythmias). Circulation 2003;108:1871-909.
4. Ferguson JD, DiMarco JP. Contemporary management of paroxysmal supraventricular tachycardia. Circulation 2003;107:1096-9.
5. Chauhan VS, Krahn AD, Klein GJ, et al. Supraventricular tachycardia. Med Clin North Am 2001;85:193-223.
6. American Heart Association. Guidelines for cardiopulmonary resuscitation and emergency cardiovascular care. Part 7.3: management of symptomatic bradycardia and tachycardia. Circulation 2005;112:IV.67-77.

24 Venous Gas Embolism

DEFINITION

A venous gas embolism (VGE) occurs when air or other gas enters the venous circulation and travels to the right side of the heart or the pulmonary vessels.

24

ETIOLOGY

Entrainment of air into an open flowing vein or dural sinus
Infusion of air or other gas under pressure into a vein

TYPICAL SITUATIONS

Surgical procedures in which the operative site is above the level of the heart (e.g., sitting craniotomy, cesarean section during externalization of the uterus, shoulder arthroscopy, hip arthroplasty)
Surgical procedures requiring insufflation of gas (e.g., laparoscopic surgery)
Invasive procedures that expose an open vein to atmosphere during spontaneous ventilation (e.g., CVP placement or disconnection)
Any invasive procedure in which the patient is connected to a high-pressure gas source

PREVENTION

Avoid positioning the patient such that the surgical field or CVP cannulation site is above the level of the heart if possible
Mechanically ventilate the patient when the surgical field must be above the level of the heart
Place the patient in Trendelenburg during placement or removal of a CVP
   Maintain occlusive pressure on CVP decannulation sites for 5 minutes after bleeding has stopped, then place an occlusive dressing over the site

Remove all air from IV solution bags and lines (e.g., CPB cannulae, rapid infuser systems) prior to pressurized infusion

When there is a risk of VGE, maintain a high CVP with increased administration of IV fluids

Avoid administering N_2O to patients at risk of VGE

Consider placement of multiorifice CVP catheter in patients at high risk of VGE

MANIFESTATIONS

The manifestations are determined by the volume of gas embolized in relation to the size of the patient, the rate at which embolization occurs, and the rate at which the gas dissolves in the blood. Detection depends on the monitors in place at the time of the embolic event.

In the awake patient
  Coughing, dyspnea, bronchospasm, hypotension, altered mental status, and circulatory collapse
In the awake or anesthetized patient, manifestations will depend on the monitoring in place at the time of the event
  ECG changes
    Tachyarrhythmias are common
    Right heart strain pattern
    ST-T wave changes
  Hemodynamic changes
    Systemic hypotension secondary to decreased CO
    Increase in CVP due to mechanical obstruction and right heart failure
    Increase in PA pressure due to release of vasoactive inflammatory mediators
    A loud, coarse, continuous "mill wheel" murmur on auscultation
  Pulmonary signs and symptoms
    Crackles (rales) and wheezing
    Decreased ET CO_2
    Increased ET N_2; rarely measured (requires mass spectrometer or Raman scattering techniques)
    Decreased arterial O_2 saturation
  Central nervous system
    EEG changes may be caused by different mechanisms
      Cerebral hypoperfusion due to decreased CO
      Paradoxical embolism to the cerebral circulation through a patent foramen ovale (PFO)
  TEE
    Presence of air in cardiac chambers
    Detects as little as 0.02 mL/kg air in right heart
    Allows detection of intracardiac paradoxical embolism (most commonly due to a PFO)
  Precordial Doppler ultrasound
    VGE changes character and intensity of emitted sound
    Detects as little as 0.05 mL/kg of air in right heart
  Presence of gas bubble in the aspirate from a multiorifice CVP catheter
More than one means of detection should be used in cases at high risk for VGE

SIMILAR EVENTS

Myocardial ischemia (see Event 15, Acute Coronary Syndrome)
Brainstem retraction and ischemia

Nongas PE (see Event 21, Pulmonary Embolism and Event 81, Amniotic Fluid Embolism)
Other cause of hypotension (see Event 9, Hypotension)
Artifact on Doppler ultrasound device due to electrocautery, rapid fluid infusion, or movement
of the precordial probe
Entrainment of air into a respiratory gas analyzer

MANAGEMENT

Notify the surgeon immediately of a possible VGE
The surgeon should check for possible entry sites in the wound
The nurses should check surgical insufflation equipment
Turn off all pressurized gas sources
Call for help
Confirm the diagnosis
Check the ET CO_2 trend recording
Check the BP
Listen carefully to the precordial Doppler signal
Check TEE if in place
Listen for mill wheel murmur
Check PA pressures, if available
If multiorifice CVP catheter present, attempt to aspirate
Check the ET N_2, if available
Inspect for air in the aspirate
VGE may still be present if no air is aspirated
If gas embolism is confirmed
Attempt to aspirate gas from multiorifice CVP catheter again
The surgeons should flood the surgical field with saline or pack the wound with saline-
soaked sponges
Administer 100% O_2
Provide Valsalva maneuver by manual ventilation to prevent further air from entering the
heart and to reveal the vascular entry site to the surgeon
Infuse IV fluid rapidly
Use vasopressors and inotropes as needed to support the circulation (see Event 9,
Hypotension)
Reposition the patient, if feasible
First, tilt the operating table to lower the surgical site below the level of the heart
If possible, place patient in left-side-down position
Consider applying 5 cm H_2O PEEP
If hemodynamic compromise is severe
Perform CPR if cardiac arrest occurs (see Event 2, Cardiac Arrest)
Direct aspiration of air from the heart or great vessels via a thoracotomy may be necessary
Internal cardiac massage may be required
If VGE to cranial arterial system is suspected, consider emergency MRI and consider hyper-
baric O_2 therapy if available

COMPLICATIONS

Hypotension
Myocardial ischemia or infarction

Stroke
Paradoxical gas embolism to the arterial circulation
    PFO or other right-to-left shunt
    Massive VGE crossing the pulmonary capillaries to the arterial circulation
Pulmonary edema
Wound contamination from repositioning
Complications of thoracotomy and CPR
Cardiac arrest
Death

SUGGESTED READING

1. Archer DP, Pash MP, MacRae ME. Successful management of venous air embolism with inotropic support. Neuroanesth Intensive Care 2001;48:204-8.
2. Bithal PK, Pandia MP, Dash HH, et al. Comparative incidence of venous air embolism and associated hypotension in adults and children operated for neurosurgery in the sitting position. Eur J Anaesthesiol 2004;21:517-22.
3. Mirski MA, Lele AV, Fitzsimmons L, Young TJK. Diagnosis and treatment of vascular air embolism. Anesthesiology 2007;106:164-77.
4. Muth CM, Shanck E. Gas embolism. N Engl J Med 2000;342:476-82.
5. Schubert A, Deogaonkar A, Drummond JC. Precordial Doppler probe placement for optimal detection of venous air embolism during craniotomy. Anesth Analg 2006;102:1543-7.
6. Van Hulst RA, Klein J, Lachmann B. Gas embolism: pathophysiology and treatment. Clin Physiol Funct Imaging 2003;23:237-46.

24

Chapter 7
Pulmonary Events
GEOFFREY K. LIGHTHALL

---

25 Airway Burn

DEFINITION

Airway burn is thermal or chemical injury to the mucosa of the airway between the mouth and the alveoli.

ETIOLOGY

Inhalation of hot gases
    From breathing circuit
    Direct exposure to fire
    Exposure to smoke or toxic gases
Ignition of the ETT during laser surgery

TYPICAL SITUATIONS

Patients with acute burns
Laser surgery in the pharynx, the larynx, or the tracheobronchial tree
Tracheostomy using electrocautery
Rupture of ETT cuff, allowing escape of oxidizer from the lungs to the upper airway

25

PREVENTION

Assess fire risk in EVERY case
Hospital laser committee is responsible for monitoring laser safety-related issues
Safety training for hospital personnel working with lasers
Protect the ETT during laser airway surgery
    Use "laser-proof" ETT
    Fill ETT cuff with saline colored with methylene blue to create a visible marker for cuff puncture
Maintain a low FiO_2 (less than 30%) in air
    If higher FiO_2 is required to maintain an acceptable O_2 saturation
        Periodically oxygenate with a higher FiO_2, then decrease below 30% prior to recommencing with surgery
            Coordinate this with surgeons
            Allow a few minutes to wash out high FiO_2
    Consider aborting laser surgery if FiO_2 requirements are high
Use a cuffed ETT in surgery in and about the airway (e.g., tonsillectomy)
Surgeon should suction oropharynx prior to using electrocautery in the airway
During tracheostomy, enter the trachea with scalpel or scissors
Have a clamp available to occlude the ETT in case of ETT fire
Protect patient from exposure to OR fire or smoke

MANIFESTATIONS

Immediate manifestations
 Laser-ignited ETT fire
  Visible ignition or burning of the ETT
  Smell of burning, smoke, flames in the surgical field
  Fire may propagate into the breathing circuit
Later manifestations
 Airway edema or airway rupture
 Decreased O_2 saturation and PaO_2
 Decreased pulmonary compliance
 Pulmonary edema
 Bronchospasm
 Lung injury/ARDS
 Tracheal stenosis

SIMILAR EVENTS

Pulmonary edema from other causes (see Event 20, Pulmonary Edema)
Lung injury from other causes
Pneumonia
Bronchospasm (see Event 29, Bronchospasm)
Partial airway obstruction

MANAGEMENT

For laser-induced ETT fire
Stop the flow of O_2 to the ETT
 Clamp the ETT immediately
 Disconnect the patient from the breathing circuit
Pour saline or water into airway to extinguish burning material
Extubate the trachea
 Ventilate with 100% O_2 by bag valve mask
Reintubate the patient as soon as possible
 Rapid development of airway edema may make later reintubation difficult
  Consider use of tube exchanger and smaller ETT
 If reintubation is not possible, proceed to either cricothyrotomy or tracheostomy
Provide supportive care and mechanical ventilation
 Add PEEP as necessary to maintain oxygenation
 Consider administering high-dose steroids
  Methylprednisolone IV, 0.1 to 1 g
Immediate consultation with an otolaryngologist or a thoracic surgeon to evaluate the extent of the airway burn
 Fiberoptic bronchoscopy when the patient is stable
Impound any device thought to be defective for inspection by a biomedical engineer

COMPLICATIONS

Hypoxemia/hypercarbia
Inability to reintubate

Permanent pulmonary injury
    Pulmonary fibrosis
     Restrictive pulmonary disease
Tracheal stenosis
Pneumothorax
Pneumonia
Death

SUGGESTED READING

1. APSF fire prevention algorithm. Anesthesia Patient Safety Foundation Newsletter, Winter 2012;26(3):43. <http://www.apsf.org/newsletters/pdf/winter_2012.pdf> [accessed 22.08.13].
2. American Society of Anesthesiologists Task Force on Operating Room Fires. Practice advisory for the prevention and management of operating room fires. Anesthesiology 2013;118:1-12.
3. Smith LP, Roy S. Operating room fires in otolaryngology: risk factors and prevention. Am J Otolaryngol 2011;32:109-14.
4. Lai HC, Juang SE, Liu TJ, Ho WM. Fires of endotracheal tubes of three different materials during carbon dioxide laser surgery. Acta Anaesthesiol Sin 2002;40:47-51.

26 Airway Rupture

DEFINITION

Airway rupture includes traumatic perforation or disruption of any part of the airway.

ETIOLOGY

Mechanical or thermal energy rupturing airway walls
    Hyperextension of the neck combined with a direct blow to the unprotected trachea
    Penetrating injury of the chest or neck
    Erosion of the tracheobronchial wall by an ETT or tracheostomy cuff
    Aberrant entry of tracheostomy tube (e.g., during placement of percutaneous tracheostomy)

TYPICAL SITUATIONS

Following thoracic injury
    Blunt trauma in presence of a closed glottis
      Frequently no external evidence of injury
    Penetrating injury of the chest or neck
During placement of ETT with videolaryngoscopy
During laser surgery to the airway
During or following thoracic surgery
Associated with the use of a double-lumen ETT
With nasal intubation or instrumentation
Intubation of the airway with any rigid object
    During rigid or flexible bronchoscopy
    During placement of a metal ETT for laser surgery
    Stiff airway exchange catheters (e.g., bougie)
During attempts at jet ventilation

PREVENTION

Avoid excessive force during instrumentation of the airway
Avoid blind passage of ETT through oropharynx during videolaryngoscopy
Prewarm nasal ETT prior to placement
    Use nasal spray to vasoconstrict nasal mucosa
        Phenylephrine 1% spray
        Oxymetazoline 0.05% spray
        Cocaine 4% topical solution
    Use lubricated nasopharyngeal airways to dilate nasal passage prior to placing ETT
Do not allow the stylet to protrude beyond the tip of the ETT during intubation
Avoid overinflation of the ETT cuff or the endobronchial cuff of a double-lumen ETT
    Deflate endobronchial cuff on double-lumen ETT when lung separation is no longer required
Intermittently check the occlusion pressure of the ETT cuff(s)
    Especially in presence of N_2O
Maintain full relaxation of the patient during endoscopy, rigid bronchoscopy, and laser surgery of the airway
Assess depth of insertion of airway exchange catheters to avoid insertion beneath the carina

MANIFESTATIONS

Lacerations or partial rupture of the airway may easily be missed until some other event or a late complication demonstrates its presence (e.g., bronchial stenosis).

Rupture of nasopharynx
    Inability to pass ETT easily through the nasal cavity
    ETT not visible in the pharynx on direct laryngoscopy
    Blood or bloody secretions from nasopharynx or ETT
    Inability to ventilate through nasal ETT passed blindly
    Nasopharyngeal swelling and visible hematoma
Rupture of tracheobronchial tree
    Respiratory distress
        Dyspnea
        Hypoxemia
        Cyanosis
        Hemoptysis
    SC emphysema
    Mediastinal emphysema
    Pneumothorax
    CXR may be diagnostic
        Laryngeal or tracheal injuries are frequently associated with visible cervical, mediastinal, and SC air without accompanying pneumothorax
        Bronchial injury is associated with pneumomediastinum, with pneumothorax, and possibly with overlying rib fractures
        Rarely, CXR may show "fallen lung sign," in which the transected bronchus allows the lung to fall away from the mediastinum, not toward the mediastinum as in a pneumothorax
    Air leak from the site of a penetrating injury to the chest or neck
    Persistent air leak after placement of a chest tube is suggestive of bronchial rupture or bronchopleural fistula

26

Difficulty in establishing ventilation after intubation
> High PIP
> Decreased breath sounds

SIMILAR EVENTS

Other causes of airway obstruction
Pneumothorax (see Event 35, Pneumothorax)
High PIP (see Event 7, High Peak Inspiratory Pressure)
Hemoptysis (see Event 34, Massive Hemoptysis)
SC air

MANAGEMENT

Nasopharyngeal rupture
Orally intubate the trachea by direct laryngoscopy or videolaryngoscopy before removing nasal ETT
> If the ETT is removed first, severe hemorrhage may occur and make intubation difficult or impossible
> Obtain otolaryngology consult

Tracheobronchial tree rupture
Suspect airway rupture in major trauma cases with SC or mediastinal air, a pneumothorax, or other major abdominal, cervical, or thoracic injuries
Ensure adequate oxygenation and ventilation
If severe respiratory distress is present, manage the airway FIRST and assess site of rupture SECOND
> Intubate the trachea via direct laryngoscopy or videolaryngoscopy
> Carefully ventilate with 100% FiO_2
>> Assess ET CO_2 and bilateral chest expansion
> **If difficult airway is suspected** (see Event 3, Difficult Tracheal Intubation)
>> Prepare for awake fiberoptic intubation
>> Prepare for emergency surgical airway
>>> Stat surgery consult for cricothyrotomy or tracheostomy

Assess the site of airway rupture
> **Perform fiberoptic bronchoscopy in all cases of major thoracic trauma**
>> Will require an experienced bronchoscopist
>> Should be performed awake with topical anesthesia if feasible
>> May confirm the diagnosis and exact site of airway rupture
>> May allow aspirated material or secretions to be removed
>> **If tracheal rupture is diagnosed**
>>> Advance the ETT beyond the site of rupture if possible
>>> One lung ventilation may be required to maintain oxygenation
>>> Consider bronchial blocker or double-lumen ETT
>>> Repair the injury
>> **If bronchial rupture is diagnosed**
>>> Intubate under fiberoptic guidance
>>> Advance single-lumen ETT into unaffected bronchus or intubate the trachea and place a bronchial blocker into the affected side
>>> Double-lumen ETT may be necessary

26

Resuscitate the patient as necessary
    Diagnose and manage other injuries (see Event 14, The Trauma Patient)
    Exclude the presence of a pneumothorax (see Event 35, Pneumothorax)
If nonemergent intubation is required for bronchoscopy or surgery
    Treat as a known difficult intubation (see Event 3, Difficult Tracheal Intubation)
    Fiberoptic intubation with topical anesthesia is the method of choice
    Sedate the patient
        Fentanyl IV, 50 µg, repeat as necessary
        Midazolam IV, 0.5 mg, repeat as necessary
        Ketamine IV, 10 to 20 mg, repeat as necessary
        Dexmedetomidine infused at 0.1 to 0.7 µg/kg/hr
    Administer supplemental O_2 and, if necessary, manually ventilate with gentle breaths, avoiding high PIP
Surgical correction versus conservative management will depend on the location and extent of injury
    Plan management with ENT and thoracic surgeons
In patients with cervical injuries, consider performing fiberoptic bronchoscopy as the ETT is removed to identify tracheal injuries

COMPLICATIONS

Retropharyngeal abscess
Airway obstruction
Hypoxemia
Mediastinitis
Pneumonia distal to bronchial rupture
Tracheal or bronchial stenosis
Cardiac arrest

SUGGESTED READING

1. Minabres E, Burón J, Ballesteros MA, et al. Tracheal rupture after endotracheal intubation: a literature systematic review. Eur J Cardiothorac Surg 2009;35:1056-62.
2. Chow JL, Coady MA, Varner J, et al. Management of acute complete tracheal transection caused by nonpenetrating trauma: report of a case and review of the literature. J Cardiothorac Vasc Anesth 2004;18:475-8.
3. Mabry RL, Edens JW, Pearse L, Kelly JF, Harke H. Fatal airway injuries during Operation Enduring Freedom and Operation Iraqi Freedom. Prehosp Emerg Care 2010;14:272-7.
4. Cooper RM. Complications associated with the use of the GlideScope videolaryngoscope. Can J Anaesth 2007;54:54-7.
5. Fitzmaurice BG, Brodsky JB. Airway rupture from double-lumen tubes. J Cardiothorac Vasc Anesth 1999;13:322-9.

27 Anterior Mediastinal Mass

DEFINITION

An anterior mediastinal mass is a benign or malignant tumor found in the mediastinum anterior to the pericardium.

ETIOLOGY

Compression of vital structures within the chest
    Trachea or bronchi
    Heart and great vessels

TYPICAL SITUATIONS

Benign or malignant tumors
    Thymoma
    Teratoma
    Lymphomas
    Thyroid tumors
    Cysts of multiple origins
    Vascular malformations

PREVENTION

Carefully evaluate for signs and symptoms of symptomatic airway or vascular compression
    Intolerance of supine position
    Assess the effect on symptoms of changing patient position (e.g., right or left lateral)
    Obtain an anteroposterior (AP) and lateral CXR and CT scan of the thorax to evaluate
        mass
    There is questionable value of flow-volume loops in the upright and supine positions to
        evaluate dynamic compression of the airway in adults
Prepare for loss of airway or circulation during induction of anesthesia or intubation
    Have a rigid bronchoscope available
    Discuss the need for standby CPB or ECMO with surgeons

MANIFESTATIONS

Cardiac
    Chest pain or fullness, cough, syncopal symptoms and exercise intolerance
Pulmonary
    Dyspnea that might or might not be positional
Hoarseness
Dysphagia
Stridor
Systemic symptoms associated with malignancy
Upper extremity and facial/neck swelling (SVC syndrome)
Incidental finding on CXR or CT obtained for other reason
Intraoperative manifestations
    Inability to maintain a patent airway
    Difficulty in advancing an ETT
    Inability to ventilate through an ETT
    Hypoxemia
    Hypotension

SIMILAR EVENTS

Bronchospasm (see Event 29, Bronchospasm)
Epiglottitis (see Event 31, Epiglottitis [Supraglottitis])
Intrathoracic airway obstruction
    Tracheal or endobronchial tumor
Extrathoracic airway obstruction
      Foreign body, Ludwig angina, epiglottitis, postoperative hematoma from head/neck/carotid surgery
Stridor (see Event 36, Postoperative Stridor)

MANAGEMENT

Requires interdisciplinary approach with consultation with thoracic or general surgery, radiology, oncology, intensive care, and radiation oncology.

General principles
Obtain and examine imaging studies preoperatively
    AP and lateral CXR examination
    Thoracic CT scan
    TTE to evaluate for presence of pericardial effusion and other cardiac, systemic, or pulmonary vascular compression
Ensure adequate IV access
    In patients with SVC syndrome, place large-bore IV in lower extremity
Consider arterial line prior to procedure

Anesthesia management
    Local anesthesia may be adequate for biopsy, anterior mediastinoscopy, or CT-guided biopsy
    For asymptomatic adult patients
      IV induction and tracheal intubation
        Risk of airway obstruction and cardiovascular compromise is minimal in these patients
    For symptomatic adult patients
      Experienced bronchoscopist and rigid bronchoscope should be available prior to induction
      Consider the need for CPB or ECMO prior to induction
        Discuss options with cardiac surgery, cardiology, and perfusionist team
      Inhalation induction with sevoflurane maintaining spontaneous ventilation
        Assess the ability to ventilate prior to administering a short-acting muscle relaxant
          Intubate trachea with small ETT
        If unable to give positive pressure breaths, awaken the patient and reassess the situation

If airway obstruction occurs
    Check ETT position if intubated
    Attempt rigid bronchoscopy and ventilate via bronchoscope
    Prepare to institute emergency CPB or ECMO

If circulatory collapse occurs
    Change patient to lateral position
    If no response to change in position, proceed with immediate sternotomy (to relieve pressure on great vessels)

COMPLICATIONS

Hypoxemia
Inability to advance ETT into the trachea
Inability to ventilate the intubated patient
Airway trauma due to difficult intubation or rigid bronchoscopy
Postoperative stridor
Pulmonary edema due to excessive negative intrathoracic pressure
Cardiac arrest

SUGGESTED READING

1. Garey CL, Laituri CA, Valusek PA, St Peter SD, Snyder CL. Management of anterior mediastinal masses in children. Eur J Pediatr Surg 2011;21:310-21.
2. Slinger P, Karsli C. Management of the patient with a large anterior mediastinal mass: recurring myths. Curr Opin Anaesthesiol 2007;20:1-3.
3. Bechard P, Letourneau L, Lacasse Y, Cote D, Bussieres JS. Perioperative cardiorespiratory complications in adults with mediastinal mass: incidence and risk factors. Anesthesiology 2004;100:826-34, discussion 5A.
4. Hammer GB. Anaesthetic management for the child with a mediastinal mass. Paediatr Anaesth 2004;14:95-7.
5. Pompeo E, Tacconi F, Mineo TC. Awake video-assisted thoracoscopic biopsy in complex anterior mediastinal masses. Thorac Surg Clin 2010;20:225-33.

28 Aspiration of Gastric Contents

28

DEFINITION

Aspiration of gastric contents is inhalation of gastric contents into the tracheobronchial tree.

ETIOLOGY

Passive regurgitation or active vomiting of gastric contents in patients who are unable to protect their airway

TYPICAL SITUATIONS

Patients with a "full stomach" or raised intra-abdominal pressure
    Patients who are not NPO
    Patients who have acute pain or who are on opioids
    Bowel obstruction
    Gastroparesis (e.g., diabetic patients)
    Late pregnancy
    Acute alcohol intoxication
Patients with large amounts of gas in the stomach
    Prolonged positive pressure ventilation via mask or SGA
    Difficult tracheal intubation
Patients with an incompetent gastroesophageal junction
    Hiatal hernia
    Previous esophageal or gastric surgery

Obesity
> Patients who have had or are having bariatric surgery

Any patient with impaired laryngeal reflexes or cough
> Depressed level of consciousness
> Patients with residual neuromuscular blockade
> Topical anesthesia of the larynx or pharynx (e.g., upper gastrointestinal procedures under sedation)
> Chronic neurologic disease (e.g., patients with multiple sclerosis or stroke)
> Anatomic abnormalities in and around the larynx

Patients who have had ineffective cricoid pressure
Recently extubated patients in ICU or OR
During a cardiac arrest

PREVENTION

In patients at risk of aspiration of gastric contents
> Avoid general anesthesia if possible
> Delay nonemergent surgery as long as possible to allow the stomach to empty and to allow time for medications that assist gastric emptying and reduce gastric acidity to be effective
> Avoid depression of laryngeal reflexes (e.g., from excess sedation or topical anesthesia)
> Administer nonparticulate antacid immediately prior to induction of general anesthesia
>> Sodium citrate PO, 30 mL
> Administer H_2 antagonists at least 30 minutes prior to the induction of anesthesia
>> Famotidine IV, 20 mg
>> Ranitidine IV, 50 mg
> Administer metoclopramide IV, 10 mg, to stimulate gastric emptying

If general anesthesia is necessary
> Assess the patient's airway carefully prior to inducing general anesthesia
> Suction an in situ NGT prior to induction of general anesthesia
>> If a NGT is left in place, it may produce incompetence of the lower esophageal sphincter
>> There may still be gastric contents present even after suctioning an NGT
> Have a trained and experienced assistant apply cricoid pressure
>> Maintain cricoid pressure until the ETT position is confirmed (see Event 5, Esophageal Intubation)
> Intubate the trachea, inflate the ETT cuff, and confirm placement
> Patient is at risk for aspiration at the end of surgery
>> Apply NG suctioning prior to extubation
>> Extubate the patient only after recovery of protective laryngeal reflexes

Consider awake intubation
> Topical anesthesia of the larynx before securing the airway may ablate protective reflexes at a time that regurgitation or vomiting is likely to occur
> Fiberoptic intubation can be performed with the patient sitting, making regurgitation less likely
> Consider tracheostomy under local anesthesia if fiberoptic intubation is impossible and a difficult tracheal intubation is anticipated

MANIFESTATIONS

Gastric contents visualized in the oropharynx
Severe hypoxemia
Increased PIP
Bronchospasm
Copious tracheal secretions
Coughing, laryngospasm, rales, or chest retraction
Dyspnea, apnea, or hyperpnea
CXR findings
    Unremarkable in 15% to 20% of cases of aspiration
    Pneumonic infiltrates and atelectasis may be present

SIMILAR EVENTS

Hypoxemia from other causes (see Event 10, Hypoxemia)
Obstruction of the ETT
Bronchospasm from other causes (see Event 29, Bronchospasm)
Other causes of high PIP (see Event 7, High Peak Inspiratory Pressure)
Pneumonia
Pulmonary edema (see Event 20, Pulmonary Edema)
ARDS
PE (see Event 21, Pulmonary Embolism)

MANAGEMENT

If gastric contents are visible in the oropharynx or larynx
    Suction oropharynx with Yankauer suction tip
    Intubate the trachea
        Perform immediate tracheal suctioning prior to positive pressure ventilation
            Pass a suction catheter down the ETT
                Obtain a sample of the pulmonary aspirate for pH, Gram stain, and culture
                Do not make prolonged efforts at suctioning the trachea, especially if the
                    patient is desaturating
Ensure adequate oxygenation and ventilation
    Positive pressure ventilation with 100% FiO_2
    Add PEEP to maintain oxygenation
If particulate aspiration has occurred
    Lavage plus suctioning or bronchoscopy will be necessary to remove particulate material
        and to assess level of contamination
Cancel elective surgery and restrict emergency surgery to the minimum procedure consistent
    with safety
Provide supportive care
    Fluid management with crystalloid rather than colloid
    Administer H_2 blockers for stress ulcer prophylaxis
        Famotidine IV, 20 mg
        Ranitidine IV, 50 mg
    Perform intermittent pulmonary toilet (uninjured pulmonary cilia will continue to sweep
        particles and edema fluid to the bronchi)
        Large volume lavage via the ETT is usually not indicated

28

Consider the administration of antibiotics
> Choice of antibiotic should be based on the results of a Gram stain of the pulmonary aspirate
> Prophylaxis is indicated if there is a high likelihood of bacterial colonization of gastric contents (e.g., patients on H_2 antagonists and proton pump inhibitors and those with small or large bowel obstruction)

Steroids have not been shown to be of benefit during the period of acute hypoxemia and may impair the long-term healing process of the lung
Bronchodilators may be helpful in relieving large airway closure in less damaged areas of the lungs
Consider ECMO support if oxygenation cannot be maintained
Consider lung transplant

COMPLICATIONS

Pneumonia
ARDS
Sepsis
Barotrauma secondary to high PIP
Death

SUGGESTED READING

1. Marik PE. Aspiration pneumonitis and aspiration pneumonia. NEJM 2001;344:655-71.
2. Raghavendran K, Nemzek J, Napolitano LN, Knight PR. Aspiration-induced lung injury. Crit Care Med 2011;39:1-9.
3. American Society of Anesthesiologists 2011 practice guidelines for preoperative fasting and the use of pharmacologic agents to reduce the risk of pulmonary aspiration: application to healthy patients undergoing elective procedures. An updated report by the American Society of Anesthesiologists Committee on Standards and Practice Parameters. Anesthesiology 2011;114:495-511.

29 Bronchospasm

DEFINITION

Bronchospasm is a reversible narrowing of the medium and small airways because of smooth muscle contraction.

ETIOLOGY

Asthma
COPD with a reversible component of airway narrowing
Airway irritation (e.g., aspiration, bronchiolitis, upper respiratory infection [URI])
Medication side effects (e.g., allergy or anaphylaxis)

TYPICAL SITUATIONS

Patients with known asthma, COPD, or recent URI
Mechanical irritation of the airway
> Placement of oral or SGA
> Placement of ETT
> Endobronchial intubation

Chemical irritation of the airway
    Pungent anesthetic gases
    Soda lime dust
    Smoke inhalation
Carcinoid syndrome
Medications known to cause bronchospasm
    β_2-antagonists (labetalol, propanolol)
    Anticholinesterases
    Drug allergies (e.g., antibiotics, neuromuscular blockers, latex, adenosine, radiocontrast
        agents)
Aspiration of gastric contents
PE (fat, thrombus, amniotic fluid)

PREVENTION

Cancel elective surgery for patients who are actively in bronchospasm.
Avoid anesthesia and elective surgery when the patient is at risk of bronchospasm
    Acute URI
    Recent exacerbation of asthma or COPD
In patients with known asthma or COPD, optimize therapy with bronchodilators and/or
    systemic steroids prior to anesthesia
Administer bronchodilators on day of surgery
    Inhaled β_2-agonists prior to induction
        Albuterol MDI 4 to 8 puffs (90 μg/puff)
        Albuterol nebulizer solution 2.5 mg/3 mL
If it is necessary to proceed with surgery in patients with a known risk of bronchospasm
    Regional anesthesia will eliminate airway stimulation
    Consider SGA with general anesthesia
    Consider using ketamine IV, 1 to 2 mg/kg, for anesthetic induction
    Consider intraoperative ketamine infusion at 0.25 mg/kg/hr as an anesthetic adjuvant
Deepen anesthesia prior to intubation
    Administer additional propofol IV, 30 to 50 mg
    Lidocaine IV, 1 to 1.5 mg/kg, 1 to 3 minutes prior to intubation
    Ventilate with sevoflurane prior to intubation
Monitor flow-volume loops if available for early detection and treatment of bronchospasm

MANIFESTATIONS

Increased PIP
Audible wheezing, usually during exhalation
    If bronchospasm is severe, there may be an absence of wheezing or gas movement
Upward sloping of capnogram wave
    ET CO_2 may be absent or diminished depending on severity of bronchospasm
Decreased PaO_2 and O_2 saturation
Decreased tidal volume especially with pressure-controlled ventilation
Gradient between $PaCO_2$ and ET CO_2 will increase
Increased $PaCO_2$
Hypotension

SIMILAR EVENTS

Aspiration of gastric contents (see Event 28, Aspiration of Gastric Contents)
Kinked or obstructed ETT (see Event 7, High Peak Inspiratory Pressure)
Pneumothorax (see Event 35, Pneumothorax)
Aspiration of foreign body (usually unilateral wheeze vs. diffuse)
Amniotic fluid embolism (see Event 81, Amniotic Fluid Embolism)
Pulmonary edema (see Event 20, Pulmonary Edema)
PE (see Event 21, Pulmonary Embolism)
Endobronchial intubation (see Event 30, Endobronchial Intubation)
Anaphylaxis and anaphylactoid reactions (see Event 16, Anaphylactic and Anaphylactoid Reactions)
Air trapping

MANAGEMENT

Ensure adequate oxygenation and ventilation
  Increase FiO_2 to 100%
  Briefly ventilate the patient with reservoir bag
    Assess pulmonary compliance
    If hand ventilation will be an ongoing requirement, call for help
  Mechanically ventilate the patient
    Optimize RR and I:E ratio to avoid hyperinflation or auto-PEEP
Verify the diagnosis of bronchospasm
  Auscultate the chest
  Check ETT position
  Check patency of ETT
    Pass a suction catheter down the ETT
For mild bronchospasm
  Increase anesthetic depth with sevoflurane if the patient is not hypotensive
  Administer β_2-agonist to the lungs by MDI; repeat in 10 minutes if there is no response and no tachycardia
    A large dose of any aerosolized medication may be required when administered via the ETT
      Albuterol: initial dose, 4 to 8 metered puffs (90 μg/puff)
      Albuterol and ipratropium bromide combination therapy, initial dose, 8 metered puffs
For moderate to severe bronchospasm
  Institute measures as in mild bronchospasm
  Consider the possibility of silent aspiration of gastric contents
    Suction through the ETT and collect aspirate for analysis of pH
If bronchospasm does not resolve
  Inform the surgeon
  Administer β_2-agonist
    Albuterol MDI, initial dose 4 to 8 metered puffs (90 μg/puff) q20m
    Albuterol nebulized, 2.5 mg/3 mL q20m
  Institute IV bronchodilator therapy
    Epinephrine IV, 0.1 μg/kg bolus; infusion, 5 to 20 ng/kg/min, titrated to the pulse rate, BP, and bronchodilator response
    $MgSO_4$ IV, 2 g

29

Administer corticosteroids
　　Methylprednisolone IV, 125 mg bolus
Reassess ventilation
　　Avoid high PIP to minimize barotrauma
　　Alter tidal volume and I:E ratio to maintain oxygenation and minimize airway pressure, allowing permissive hypercapnia if necessary
　　Check for air trapping
　　　　Consider deepening volatile anesthetic or providing paralysis to improve patient-ventilator synchrony
Obtain a high-performance ventilator (such as an ICU ventilator)
　　Pulmonary compliance/resistance may exceed the performance envelope of the anesthesia workstation
Heliox may improve airflow in patients with severe bronchospasm
Stop the surgical procedure as soon as possible
Transfer patient to ICU for postoperative care if resolution is incomplete
If the patient is NOT intubated (e.g., bronchospasm in PACU)
　　Consider noninvasive ventilation CPAP or BiPAP
　　Bronchodilator therapy as previously stated
　　Evaluate for increased effort to breathe, fatigue, altered mental status, subjective distress, or hypercarbia
　　Intubate the trachea if treatment fails

COMPLICATIONS

Hypoxemia
Hypercarbia
Hypotension due to increased intrathoracic pressure
Arrhythmias
Barotrauma
Cardiac arrest

SUGGESTED READING

1. Fidkowski CW, Zheng H, Firth PG. The anesthetic considerations of tracheobronchial foreign bodies in children: a literature review of 12,979 cases. Anesth Analg 2010;111(4):1016-25.
2. Duggan M, Kavanagh BP. Perioperative modifications of respiratory function. Best Pract Res Clin Anaesthesiol 2010;24(2):145-55.
3. Woods BD, Sladen RN. Perioperative considerations for the patient with asthma and bronchospasm. Br J Anaesth 2009;103(Suppl. 1):i57-65.
4. Lazarus S. Emergency treatment of asthma. NEJM 2010;755-64.

30   Endobronchial Intubation

DEFINITION

Endobronchial intubation is the unintentional placement of the ETT in a mainstem or segmental bronchus, resulting in excessive ventilation of one lung or lung segment and hypoventilation of the other(s).

ETIOLOGY

ETT advanced too far during initial placement
Manipulation of the head or ETT after tracheal intubation
Mediastinal shift cephalad in the Trendelenburg position (robotic and pelvic laparoscopic surgery)
Aberrant tracheal/bronchial anatomy

TYPICAL SITUATIONS

Inadequate assessment of the insertion depth of the ETT during initial placement
>   Inexperienced anesthesia professional
>   Difficult intubation
>   ETT placed through a tracheostomy
>   Failure to check ETT position after change in patient position (e.g., steep Trendelenburg)

During certain types of surgery
>   Neurosurgery
>>   The head is frequently placed in a flexed or extended position; flexion can advance the ETT by up to 3 cm
>   ENT surgery (e.g., extubation and reintubation through a tracheostomy during laryngectomy)
>   Thoracic surgery
>>   Double-lumen ETT advanced too far
>>   Surgical manipulation of trachea and bronchi

Pediatric patients
>   Distance between the larynx and the carina is short

PREVENTION

Advance the ETT so that the cuff is just beyond the vocal cords
Carefully note the markings on the ETT at the teeth or gums after insertion
Secure the ETT firmly to the patient
Maintain security of the ETT when positioning the patient
Recheck the position of the ETT and auscultate breath sounds after positioning the patient
In patients who have a tracheostomy, advance the ETT so that the cuff is just beyond the tracheal stoma
>   Consider marking the ETT with an indelible pen at the entry point of the stoma

MANIFESTATIONS

Endobronchial intubation most commonly involves the ETT entering the right mainstem bronchus.
Increased PIP
Decreased breath sounds on the nonventilated side
Asymmetric chest movement with ventilation
Changes in oxygenation
> O_2 saturation may remain at or near 100% for several minutes after intubation, especially if the patient has been preoxygenated and ventilated with 100% O_2
>   Atelectasis occurs in the nonventilated lung increasing shunt fraction
> PaO_2 falls and patient desaturates as A–a gradient increases due to increasing shunt

Changes in ET CO_2
  ET CO_2 may increase, decrease, or remain unchanged depending on the $\dot{V}/\dot{Q}$ character-
    istics of the ventilated lung
Tidal volume may decrease if using pressure-controlled ventilation
Increase in shunt fraction may increase time lag to changes in volatile anesthetic concentration
Fiberoptic bronchoscopy
  The carina is not visualized distal to the tip of the ETT
    The division between segmental bronchi may resemble the carina
The tip of the ETT may be visualized at or below the level of the carina on a CXR
Lack of pleural sliding when comparing nonventilated to ventilated lung on TTE

SIMILAR EVENTS

Kinked or obstructed ETT (see Event 7, High Peak Inspiratory Pressure)
Pneumothorax (see Event 35, Pneumothorax)
Bronchospasm (see Event 29, Bronchospasm)
Lobar or segmental atelectasis or collapse
PE (see Event 21, Pulmonary Embolism)

MANAGEMENT

Ensure adequate oxygenation and ventilation
  If the patient desaturates, increase the FiO_2 to 100%
Auscultate both sides of chest for symmetry of breath sounds
  Auscultate in multiple zones including the axilla
  Breath sounds are often difficult to hear and may not be diagnostic of endobronchial intubation
  Manual ventilation with the anesthesia circuit will allow assessment of compliance while
    also auscultating breath sounds
Inspect the ETT
  Check that the insertion depth of the ETT is appropriate and has not changed since placement
  Palpate the intraoral part of the ETT for kinks
  If the ETT is visible in the surgical field, ask the surgeon to check ETT depth and to
    check for kinks
Ensure the patency of the ETT
  Pass a suction catheter down the ETT to rule out obstruction
If endobronchial intubation is diagnosed
  Suction secretions from oropharynx
  Deflate the cuff and pull back the ETT cautiously
    Be prepared to reintubate the trachea
  Auscultate the chest for symmetric breath sounds
  Check the PIP
  Resecure the ETT
  Consider laryngoscopy (regular or video) to ensure correct placement of ETT
Perform fiberoptic bronchoscopy if endobronchial intubation remains in the differential diagnosis
If the patient was difficult to intubate
  Place fiberoptic bronchoscope through ETT, deflate cuff, and withdraw carefully, identi-
    fying bronchial and tracheal anatomy while looking for tracheal rings
    Recheck ETT position, assessing distance above the carina
    Visualization of right upper lobe takeoff can help differentiate the carina
    Obtain a CXR

COMPLICATIONS

Hypoxemia
Hypercarbia
Atelectasis
Pneumonia of the atelectatic lung or segment
Barotrauma to the hyperventilated lung
Accidental extubation while correcting problem

SUGGESTED READING

1. Blaivas M, Tsung JW. Point-of-care sonographic detection of left endobronchial main stem intubation and obstruction versus endotracheal intubation. J Ultrasound Med 2008;27:785-9.

31   Epiglottitis (Supraglottitis)

DEFINITION

Epiglottitis (supraglottitis) is an infection of the epiglottis and supraglottic structures (epiglottis, arytenoid cartilage mucosa, and aryepiglottic folds).

ETIOLOGY

Bacterial infection
    Streptococcus pneumoniae
    Haemophilus influenzae type B
    Group A streptococci
    Staphylococcal organisms, including methicillin-resistant *Staphylococcus aureus*
Viral infection
    Parainfluenza virus
Immunocompromised hosts
    Pseudomonas, Candida

TYPICAL SITUATIONS

Children 3 to 5 years of age that have not been vaccinated against *H. influenzae* type B
Middle-aged adults
Increased prevalence in winter months
Secondary bacterial infection following a viral infection

PREVENTION

Ensure that infants receive prophylactic vaccination against *H. influenzae*
Recognize and treat the infection early, before significant airway compromise occurs

MANIFESTATIONS

A convenient mnemonic consists of the "four D's": dysphagia, dysphonia, dyspnea, and drooling.

Abrupt presentation of symptoms of severe infection
- Respiratory distress (dyspnea)
- Toxic appearance
- Tachycardia, flushing, and prostration
- High fever
- Severe sore throat
- Dysphagia
- Dysphonia
- Stridor

Drooling

Laryngeal tenderness to external palpation

Leukocytosis with neutrophilia

Lateral radiograph of the neck may show the "thumb sign" at the level of the epiglottis (indicative of epiglottitis)

Classic pediatric position: sitting bolt upright, leaning forward in a sniffing position

SIMILAR EVENTS

Postoperative stridor (see Event 36, Postoperative Stridor)

Retropharyngeal abscess

Submandibular abscess (Ludwig angina)

Uvular edema from traumatic intraoperative suctioning

Prevertebral soft tissue infection

Parotid infection

Angioedema (ACEI, C1 esterase deficiency)

Tonsillitis

Laryngotracheitis
- Diphtheria

Foreign body

MANAGEMENT

Early recognition of patients who may have epiglottitis is crucial. Urgent or emergent airway control (including emergent tracheostomy or cricothyroidotomy) may be required even before definitive diagnosis is established. Interdisciplinary management should involve otolaryngologists, anesthesiologists, and infectious disease consultants.

Administer supplemental O_2

Establish IV access
- In children, only if this can be done without exacerbating airway compromise

If the patient is not in extremis, confirm the diagnosis
- **Obtain a lateral and AP radiograph of the neck**
  - The patient should be attended continuously by personnel with appropriate airway management skills
  - In adults, consider evaluation by an otolaryngologist (i.e., nasal endoscopy or indirect mirror to visualize the epiglottis)

Secure the airway in the OR if the patient requires immediate airway management or following a radiologic or endoscopic diagnosis of epiglottitis

Protocol for Securing the Airway in the Patient with Epiglottitis

Surgeon must be present in the OR in case emergent surgical airway is required

    Surgical equipment must be opened and ready for use

    Mark anatomical features of neck (cricothyroid membrane)

Check that all anesthetic and surgical equipment is in place and is functioning correctly

    Laryngoscopes

    ETTs (including much smaller than normal sizes)

    Suction equipment

    Monitoring equipment

    Rigid bronchoscope

    Tracheostomy set

Administer glycopyrrolate IV (at age appropriate dose)

Induce general anesthesia by inhalation of sevoflurane and 100% O_2 with the patient in the sitting position

When the patient loses consciousness

    Maintain spontaneous ventilation

    Begin CPAP (5 to 10 cm H_2O)

    Change the patient's position from sitting to supine

    Establish IV access if not already present

Establish an adequate depth of anesthesia for laryngoscopy, as judged by

    Expired concentration of volatile anesthetic

    BP and HR response to general anesthesia

    Regular quiet diaphragmatic breathing

Consider lidocaine IV, 1 mg/kg, prior to laryngoscopy

Perform direct laryngoscopy to assess the ease of intubation

Establish an appropriate depth of anesthesia for intubation

Intubate the trachea by direct laryngoscopy using either an oral or nasal ETT one half to one size (0.5 to 1 mm internal diameter) smaller than normal

Once the airway is secure, draw blood cultures and administer broad-spectrum antibiotics

If the airway is lost during inhalation induction or attempts at intubation, move rapidly to establish a surgical airway (cricothyroidotomy or tracheostomy)

The patient may need to remain intubated for the next 24 to 48 hours in the ICU, although there is some evidence that two doses of antibiotics with a short (e.g., 6-hour) course of invasive airway support may be efficacious.

COMPLICATIONS

Systemic infection with the organism causing the epiglottitis

Secondary infection of neighboring structures (including lung, mediastinum, meninges, and perivertebral space)

Abscess or cyst at site of infection

Hypoxemia

Hypercarbia

Negative pressure pulmonary edema

Postextubation stridor

SUGGESTED READING

1. Shah RK, Stocks C. Epiglottitis in the United States: national trends, variances, prognosis, and management. Laryngoscope 2010;120:1256-62.
2. Isakson M, Hugosson S. Acute epiglottitis: epidemiology and *Streptococcus pneumoniae* serotype distribution in adults. J Laryngol Otol 2011;125:390-3.

32 Hypercarbia

DEFINITION

Hypercarbia is an abnormally high level of CO_2 in the blood or end-tidal gas.

ETIOLOGY

Increased production or decreased elimination of CO_2
Exogenous sources of CO_2 (insufflation gas)
Exhausted CO_2 absorbent
Compensatory mechanism for metabolic alkalosis

TYPICAL SITUATIONS

Increased production of CO_2
    Shivering
    Pyrexia, sepsis
    MH
    Neuroleptic malignant syndrome
    Thyrotoxicosis
    Parenteral nutrition with high glucose loads
Decreased elimination
    Central nervous system depression by drugs or disease
    Airway obstruction
    Mechanical failure of ETT, breathing circuit, or ventilator
    Neuromuscular disorders or residual effects of muscle relaxants
    Pain-induced decrease in tidal volume
    Respiratory muscle fatigue
    Altered lung mechanics
    Myxedema coma
    Pulmonary embolus
    ARDS, COPD
    Low CO states
    Cardiac arrest
Insufflation gas (laparoscopic and robotic surgery)
Exhausted CO_2 absorbent

PREVENTION

Use appropriate ventilator settings during mechanical ventilation
    6 to 8 mL/kg tidal volume
    8 to 14 breaths/min (adults)
Avoid excessive doses or combinations of respiratory depressant drugs
Set alarms on ventilator and capnograph to warn of hypoventilation
Monitor ET CO_2 levels for both inspired and expired concentrations
Anticipate need for increased elimination during laparoscopic and robotic procedures by increasing the RR
Carefully monitor patients who have received neuraxial opioids

MANIFESTATIONS

Increased ET CO_2

Clinical signs of hypercarbia (may be masked by general anesthesia)

    Sympathetic nervous system stimulation

        Hypertension

        Tachycardia

        PVCs

    Tachypnea in spontaneously ventilating patient

    Semiparalyzed patient may try to overbreathe the ventilator

    Peripheral vasodilation

Failure to awaken secondary to the anesthetic effect of increased $PaCO_2$

SIMILAR EVENTS

Physiologic increase in arterial $PaCO_2$ to 45 to 47 mm Hg during sleep

Capnograph artifact

MANAGEMENT

Temporary and mild hypercarbia ($PaCO_2$ of 45 to 50 mm Hg) during anesthesia is common if the patient is ventilating spontaneously.

Ensure adequate oxygenation

    If the O_2 saturation is low or decreasing, increase the FiO_2

Ensure adequate ventilation

    If the patient is ventilating spontaneously

        Ensure a patent airway, with mechanical aids if necessary

        Reduce the depth of anesthesia

        Consider use of reversal agents (e.g., naloxone, flumazenil) if appropriate

        Intubate the trachea and begin mechanical ventilation if hypercarbia or hypoxemia cannot be reversed

    If the patient is being mechanically ventilated

        Increase the minute ventilation

        Check for a malfunction in the ventilator or a major leak in the anesthesia breathing circuit (see Event 71, Ventilator Failure, and Event 69, Major Leak in the Anesthesia Breathing Circuit)

        Attempt to ventilate patient with alternate device (self-inflating bag, etc.) using current CO_2 monitoring system

Check the inspired CO_2 level; the presence of more than 1 to 2 mm Hg inspired CO_2 indicates rebreathing of CO_2 due to

    Exhausted CO_2 absorbent in CO_2 absorber

    Change the CO_2 absorbent

        Increase the fresh gas flow to convert the circle system to a semiopen system

    Incompetent valve in breathing circuit (see Event 61, Circle System Valve Stuck Open)

    Administration of exogenous CO_2

Obtain an ABG to confirm hypercarbia

Look for causes of increased CO_2 production

    Sepsis

    Pyrexia

    MH (CO_2 production will increase dramatically)

For hypercarbia in the early postoperative period

    Maintain controlled ventilation until adequate spontaneous ventilation can be sustained

        If the ETT is still in place, do not remove it

            Assist ventilation as necessary

        If the trachea has been extubated

            Assist ventilation with bag valve mask

            Maintain patency of the airway

            Consider CPAP or BiPAP

            Reintubate the trachea if necessary

    Use a nerve stimulator to ensure adequate reversal of neuromuscular blockade (see Event 56, Postoperative Failure to Breathe)

        Check the patient's ability to sustain head lift for more than 5 seconds

        If reversal of neuromuscular blockade is incomplete

            Administer additional neostigmine to a maximum dose of $70\,\mu g/kg$

            Maintain mechanical ventilation until reversal of neuromuscular blockade is ensured

    Reverse respiratory depressant drugs

        Antagonize opioid effect with naloxone IV, $40\,\mu g$ increments

        Antagonize benzodiazepine effect with flumazenil IV, 0.1 mg increments

    Check for syringe or ampule swaps (see Event 63, Drug Administration Error)

COMPLICATIONS

Hypertension and tachycardia
Pulmonary hypertension, right heart failure
Hypoxemia
Arrhythmias
Cardiac arrest

SUGGESTED READING

1. Kavanagh BP, Laffey JG. Hypercapnia: permissive and therapeutic. Minerva Anesthesiol 2006;72:567-76.
2. Hanson CW, Barshall BE, Frasch HF, Marchall C. Causes of hypercarbia with oxygen therapy in patients with chronic obstructive pulmonary disease. Crit Care Med 1996;24:23-8.
3. Brockwell RC, Andrews JJ. Complications of inhaled anesthesia delivery systems. Anesthesiol Clin North America 2002;20:539-54.

33 Hypoxemia During One-Lung Ventilation

DEFINITION

Hypoxemia during one-lung ventilation is a fall in O_2 saturation of more than 5%, an absolute value of O_2 saturation below 90%, or a PaO_2 below 60 mm Hg.

ETIOLOGY

Failure of lung isolation technique
Atelectasis
Occlusion of bronchus by secretions or blood

Intrinsic lung disease

Pulmonary shunt

Impairment of hypoxic pulmonary vasoconstriction (HPV) caused by vasodilators or volatile
anesthetics

TYPICAL SITUATIONS

Thoracotomy for lung or heart surgery

Video-assisted thoracoscopic surgery

Esophagectomy

Anterior thoracic spine surgery

PREVENTION

Identify patients with increased risk of intraoperative hypoxemia

Optimize pulmonary function before and during anesthesia

Avoid or minimize use of vasodilators

Avoid volatile anesthetic concentrations > 1 MAC

Maintain adequate muscle relaxation

Adjust FiO_2 to maintain oxygenation

Administer PEEP (5 to 7 cm H_2O) to the ventilated lung

MANIFESTATIONS

Decrease in O_2 saturation

Decrease in PaO_2 below 100 mm Hg

SIMILAR EVENTS

Mucus plug

Atelectasis

Endobronchial intubation (see Event 30, Endobronchial Intubation)

Pneumothorax (see Event 35, Pneumothorax)

Pulmonary edema/ARDS (see Event 20, Pulmonary Edema)

Pulse oximeter artifact

MANAGEMENT

Increase FiO_2 to 100% and notify surgeon

Assess isolation of the lung

Ensure that endobronchial and tracheal cuffs are inflated

Perform bronchoscopy to check position of double-lumen ETT

Endobronchial cuff of a left-sided double-lumen ETT should be just visible in the
left mainstem bronchus when looking down tracheal lumen (for a right-sided
double-lumen ETT, the endobronchial cuff position requires special placement of
the ETT to allow ventilation of right upper lobe bronchus)

Adjust ETT position if necessary

Suction airway secretions or blood

Alleviate any kinks in double-lumen ETT
Optimize ventilation of dependent lung
  Perform recruitment maneuver by giving large tidal volume breaths with inspiratory hold
    This may cause hypotension
  Institute or increase PEEP up to 10 cm H_2O
  Inspect ET CO_2 tracing for upsloping expiratory phase
    Adjust ventilatory rate and/or I:E ratio if needed
    Consider inhaled bronchodilator therapy (see Event 29, Bronchospasm)
Insufflate O_2 to nonventilated lung and reassess oxygenation
Apply CPAP (2 to 5 cm H_2O) to the nonventilated lung
If hypoxemia is profound, ventilate both lungs with 100% O_2
Discuss with surgeons whether or not to clamp the PA to decrease shunt
Preserve HPV
  Discontinue IV vasodilator infusions
  Keep volatile anesthetic dose < 1 MAC
Evaluate for low CO state
  Perform TEE
  Inspect arterial waveform for pulse pressure variability
    Administer fluid, vasopressor, inotrope, or blood as guided by above
Consider discontinuing surgery if patient remains unstable
Inhaled nitric oxide or epoprostenol can be considered but are not widely available

COMPLICATIONS

Hypoxemia
Hypoventilation (atelectasis, hypercarbia)
Barotrauma
Hypotension
Pulmonary hypertension and RV failure
Cardiac arrest

SUGGESTED READING

1. Karzai W, Schwarzkopf K. Hypoxemia during one-lung ventilation: prediction, prevention, and treatment. Anesthesiology 2009;110:1402-11.
2. Lohser J. Evidence-based management of one-lung ventilation. Anesthesiol Clin 2008;26:241-72.

34 Massive Hemoptysis

DEFINITION

Massive hemoptysis is expectoration of >600 mL of blood in 24 hours.

ETIOLOGY

Pulmonary infection
Pulmonary neoplasm
Surgery or biopsy of airway structures

Vascular malformations
Erosion of a tracheostomy tube into the vascular system
Pulmonary venous congestion from cardiovascular disease
Tissue necrosis from PE
Chronic pulmonary disease (e.g., bronchiectasis, cystic fibrosis)
Coagulopathy

TYPICAL SITUATIONS

Thoracic trauma or surgery
Endobronchial ultrasound-guided biopsy
Pulmonary infection
    Tuberculosis
    Aspergilloma
    Lung abscess
Pulmonary neoplasm
    Bronchogenic or metastatic carcinoma
    Endobronchial polyp
Coagulopathy
Pulmonary infarction
Mitral stenosis and/or pulmonary hypertension
Diffuse alveolar hemorrhage following bone marrow transplant
Tracheo-innominate fistula in a patient with tracheostomy
Rupture of the PA by the balloon of a PA catheter
Atheromatous or mycotic aneurysms of the thoracic aorta, or previous repair of an aneurysm
    of the thoracic aorta

34

PREVENTION

Prepare for the possibility of massive hemoptysis during thoracic or intrabronchial procedures
Avoid overinflation and persistent wedging of PA catheter

MANIFESTATIONS

Coughing or vomiting of blood
Blood in the ETT of the anesthetized patient that does not clear with suctioning
Hypoxemia
Hypercarbia
Hypotension
Bronchospasm

SIMILAR EVENTS

Hemorrhage from oral cavity or nasopharynx
Hematemesis
Fulminant pulmonary edema (see Event 20, Pulmonary Edema)

MANAGEMENT

Distinguishing between hemoptysis or hematemesis can be difficult.

Administer 100% O$_2$ by nonrebreather face mask, with anesthesia circuit, self-inflating bag, or nonrebreather circuit

Call for help (e.g., anesthesiology, thoracic surgery, pulmonology, and IR)

Establish large-bore IV access

Send blood sample for type and crossmatch, CBC, and PT/aPTT

Give IV fluids and vasopressors as necessary (see Event 9, Hypotension)

Consider placement of invasive monitors when adequate help arrives (e.g., arterial line and CVP line)

Call for difficult airway cart and rigid bronchoscope

If the side of pulmonary hemorrhage is known, place patient in lateral position with "bleeding side" down to prevent cross-aspiration of blood to the "good" lung

Intubate the patient if there is respiratory distress

  Intubation will likely be difficult and should be done by most experienced person; if the situation allows wait for help and relevant backup equipment

  Wear personal protective equipment (gown, gloves, face shield, glasses)

  Have suction available and turned on

  If success with RSI and intubation is questionable, attempt awake intubation via conventional or video laryngoscopy (may be difficult due to blood in airway)

    Topical anesthesia may not be very effective

  Perform RSI and orotracheal intubation

    Etomidate IV, 0.2 to 0.3 mg/kg, or ketamine IV, 0.5 to 2.0 mg/kg

    Succinylcholine IV, 1.5 to 2 mg/kg

    Large single-lumen ETT versus double-lumen ETT

      Single-lumen ETT probably easier to place and allows for flexible bronchoscopy, suctioning, and possible placement of bronchial blocker

      Double-lumen ETT may allow better and earlier lung isolation and protection from contamination, but may be much more difficult to place than single-lumen ETT

  If intubation is unsuccessful, perform rigid bronchoscopy to establish the airway

  Once the patient is intubated

    Suction the ETT

    If hypotension is not present, carefully sedate the patient to minimize cough and reduce the rate of hemorrhage

      Fentanyl IV, 25 to 50 μg q3min

      Midazolam IV, 0.5 to 1 mg q5min

When intubated with a single-lumen ETT

If the ETT fills with blood and ventilation is impossible

  Push the single-lumen ETT into the trachea as far as possible to perform deliberate endobronchial intubation

    The ETT *may* be guided down the left mainstem bronchus by turning the patient's head during intubation (right ear to right shoulder), or turning the tube 90 degrees toward the left side and inserting until resistance is felt

    If the right mainstem bronchus is intubated, the upper lobe bronchus may be obstructed

  If the ETT goes down the *bleeding* side

    Place a Fogarty catheter through a Bodai connector down the ETT to occlude the bronchus, then withdraw the ETT into the trachea

    If this fails, attempt to reposition the ETT into the nonbleeding bronchus

If the ETT goes down the *nonbleeding* side
>Suction the ETT to remove residual blood

If changing from a single-lumen ETT to a double-lumen ETT
>With significant hemoptysis, this tube change can be difficult and risks losing the airway entirely
>
>Administer muscle relaxant
>
>Place an airway exchange catheter, making sure it is long enough
>
>Remove the single-lumen ETT and reintubate the trachea with the double-lumen ETT
>>The use of direct laryngoscopy during this procedure will help double-lumen ETT placement through the larynx
>
>Passing the double-lumen ETT blindly over the guide can be difficult

Ventilate with 100% FiO$_2$
>Monitor oxygenation via pulse oximetry and repeated ABGs
>
>Avoid high airway pressures if possible to avoid air embolism

Prepare for and administer massive transfusion if necessary (see Event 1, Acute Hemorrhage)

In consultation with thoracic surgeon, pulmonologist, and an interventional radiologist
>Bronchoscopy may be the most appropriate and easiest first step for diagnosis
>
>CXR may identify the likely site of bleeding
>
>High-resolution CT scan is the most efficient means of localizing bleeding, identifying the cause, and guiding treatment
>
>Arteriography or bronchography are indicated if the bleeding is not catastrophic

Control the bleeding
>Correct any coagulopathy
>
>Interventional radiologist may be able to embolize bronchial, pulmonary, and/or intercostal arteries
>
>Interventional pulmonary procedures include
>>Endobronchial infusions of procoagulants
>>
>>Laser photocoagulation
>>
>>Topical vasoconstrictors and ice-cold saline instillation
>>
>>Occlusion of the bronchus leading to the bleeding site with a Fogarty balloon catheter or Arndt endobronchial blocker
>
>Emergency thoracotomy
>>Should be reserved for those patients with adequate lung function in whom the site of hemorrhage can be identified and who continue to suffer massive hemoptysis

COMPLICATIONS

Aspiration pneumonitis

Hypoxemia

Systemic air embolism from mechanical ventilation

Atelectasis

Hypotension

Prolonged intubation

Cardiac arrest

SUGGESTED READING

1. Maguire MF, Berry CB, Gellett L, Berrisford RG. Catastrophic haemoptysis during rigid bronchoscopy: a discussion of treatment options to salvage patients during catastrophic haemoptysis at rigid bronchoscopy. Interact Cardiovasc Thorac Surg 2004;3:222-5.
2. Ong TH, Eng P. Massive hemoptysis requiring intensive care. Intensive Care Med 2003;29:317-20.
3. Garwood S, Strange C, Sahn S. Massive hemoptysis. In: Parrillo JP, Dellinger RP, editors. Critical care medicine. Philadelphia: Mosby; 2008. p. 929-48.

35   Pneumothorax

DEFINITION

Pneumothorax is the presence of gas in the pleural space.

ETIOLOGY

Connection from the atmosphere to the pleural cavity
Rupture of an alveolus, emphysematous bulla, or bronchus into the pleural cavity

TYPICAL SITUATIONS

Following CVP line placement
    Subclavian or internal jugular approach
Regional nerve blocks
    Intercostal or paravertebral blocks
    Supraclavicular or infraclavicular brachial plexus block
    Stellate ganglion block
Procedures or surgery in close proximity to the pleural cavity
    Percutaneous, transpulmonary, or transbronchial needle biopsy of the lung
    Pleurocentesis
    Nephrectomy, splenectomy, esophageal, or laparoscopic surgery
    Bronchoscopy, mediastinoscopy, or esophagoscopy
    Percutaneous liver biopsy and other interventional procedures
Spontaneous pneumothorax in patients with or without bullous disease of the lungs
Barotrauma from ventilation of the lungs with a high PIP
    Excessive tidal volume
    Expiratory obstruction of the breathing circuit
    Ball valve effects in trachea or bronchus due to tumor or endobronchial cuff of double-
        lumen ETT
    Parenchymal lung disease
Chest trauma
    Penetrating injuries to the chest
    Blast trauma
    Rib fractures (e.g., trauma, including CPR)
        Injury does not have to be acute
Transport of patients with chest tubes receiving inadequate suction

PREVENTION

Identify patients at risk of pneumothorax
Avoid N_2O if there is a significant risk of pneumothorax
Increase vigilance during procedures and surgery on or near the pleural space
Place CVP lines carefully
    Use ultrasound guidance when placing CVP lines
    Delay CVP line placement if possible until patient receives adequate fluid resuscitation

Place femoral CVP lines in patients with tenuous pulmonary status or in patients that need to remain upright

Avoid the subclavian approach immediately before general anesthesia or if the patient is being mechanically ventilated

If the subclavian approach is used, consider obtaining a CXR to rule out pneumothorax before proceeding with surgery

Initial CXR may not show a pneumothorax if air accumulates slowly

Take care when using a double-lumen ETT

Do not overinflate the endobronchial cuff

Verify correct placement of the double-lumen ETT by auscultation and fiberoptic bronchoscopy after changes in the patient's position

MANIFESTATIONS

Pneumothorax is difficult to diagnose during general anesthesia because signs and symptoms are variable.

In the awake patient
Cough, tachypnea, and dyspnea
Hypoxemia, cyanosis
Tachycardia
Chest pain
In the anesthetized patient
Hypoxemia
Hypercarbia
High PIP with decreased pulmonary compliance
Ventilator alarms indicating low minute and tidal volumes, and high PIP
Hypotension, tachycardia
Asymmetric breath sounds, hyperresonant percussion over the affected hemithorax
TTE examination
More accurate and sensitive than CXR but more likely to detect clinically insignificant pneumothorax
Signs of pneumothorax when comparing two sides of lung
Loss of sliding pleura and "comet tails"
SC emphysema of the oropharynx, face, or neck
Tracheal deviation from the midline
Neck veins may appear distended
Bulging hemidiaphragm may be visible during abdominal surgery
Characteristic CXR examination results
Loss of lung markings
Visible edge of the partially collapsed lung
Deviation of the mediastinum away from the pneumothorax
In the supine position, CXR will not demonstrate the classic hyperlucent hemithorax
Air outlining the mediastinum or a basilar deep sulcus may be the only indication of pneumothorax.

SIMILAR EVENTS

Obstructed ETT (see Event 7, High Peak Inspiratory Pressure)
Endobronchial intubation (see Event 30, Endobronchial Intubation)

Bronchospasm (see Event 29, Bronchospasm)
Aspiration of gastric contents (see Event 28, Aspiration of Gastric Contents)
Expiratory valve or pop-off valve stuck in the closed position (see Event 59, Circle System Expiratory Valve Stuck Closed, and Event 70, Pop-Off Valve Failure)
Pulmonary edema (see Event 20, Pulmonary Edema)
Air embolism may occur with pulmonary trauma (see Event 24, Venous Gas Embolism)
Auto-PEEP

MANAGEMENT

Increase FiO$_2$ to 100%
    Turn off N$_2$O if in use
Confirm the diagnosis of pneumothorax
    Auscultate the chest
    Percuss the chest if possible
    Look and feel for tracheal deviation
    If time allows, obtain CXR
    Perform TTE examination (may take time to obtain equipment and/or expertise)
    Rule out endobronchial intubation, obstructed ETT, and valve malfunction on anesthesia workstation
Communication between surgical and anesthesia teams is critical for early diagnosis and treatment
Assess BP and HR
If significant hypotension is present without another probable etiology, treat for possible tension pneumothorax (may be lifesaving)
    Support the circulation
        Give IV fluid bolus
        Administer vasopressors or inotropic drugs (see Event 9, Hypotension)
            Drug and IV fluid effect may be delayed if a tension pneumothorax compromises venous return
        Decrease or discontinue inhaled anesthetics
    Insert a large-bore IV catheter into the pleural space (needle thoracostomy) on the side with decreased breath sounds or hyperresonant percussion
        Insert just cephalad to rib body to avoid the neurovascular bundle
        Insert either in the second intercostal space, midclavicular line, or in the fourth intercostal space, midaxillary line
        If tension pneumothorax is relieved, a "hiss" may be heard
        Hemodynamic improvement may occur after catheter insertion
            Evacuation of air with a small IV catheter may be diagnostic but may not completely relieve a tension pneumothorax
        Place a chest tube or Heimlich valve following needle thoracostomy, whether positive for air or not
    Consider the possibility of bilateral pneumothoraces
If a bronchopleural fistula (air leak) is noted after placement of chest tube
    Increase fresh gas flow into the anesthesia circuit
    Increase minute ventilation to maintain normocarbia
    Consider placing a double-lumen ETT or bronchial blocker to allow ventilation of the nonaffected lung
    Consider high-frequency jet ventilation if available

COMPLICATIONS

Hypoxemia
Hypotension
Arrhythmias
Venous or arterial gas embolism
Cardiac arrest (PEA or asystole)

SUGGESTED READING

1. Ueda K, Ahmed W, Ross AF. Intraoperative pneumothorax identified with transthoracic ultrasound. Anesthesiology 2011;115:653-5.
2. Jalli R, Sefidbakht S, Jafari SH. Value of ultrasound in diagnosis of pneumothorax: a prospective study. Emerg Radiol 2013;20:131-4.
3. On-line video describing method of evaluating for pneumothorax by trans thoracic ultrasound, <http://www.sonosite.com/education/learning-center/58/1425> [accessed 22.08.13].

36   Postoperative Stridor

DEFINITION

Postoperative stridor is a harsh, high-pitched inspiratory sound caused by airway obstruction.

ETIOLOGY

Laryngospasm (persistent coaptation of the vocal cords)
Laryngeal edema
Paralysis of one or both vocal cords
Obstruction or compression of the airway by a mass

TYPICAL SITUATIONS

Laryngospasm
    Following extubation during emergence from anesthesia
    Secretions on or near the larynx (e.g., blood)
    Recent URI
    Hypocalcemia from parathyroid removal (24 to 48 hours following surgery)
Laryngeal edema
    Laryngeal surgery or instrumentation
    Major fluid resuscitation
    Positional (e.g., prone surgery, prolonged Trendelenburg position, especially with laparoscopic/robotic surgery)
    Hematoma or swelling secondary to lymphatic obstruction following neck surgery (e.g., anterior cervical spine or carotid artery surgery)
    In parturients, following prolonged second stage of labor, worse with preeclampsia and eclampsia
Paralysis of vocal cord
    Injury to recurrent laryngeal nerve following cervical or thoracic surgery

Inadequate reversal of muscle relaxants
Pathology involving the recurrent laryngeal nerve (e.g., metastatic bronchial carcinoma)
Mass, secretions, blood, or fluid in the upper airway
Recent URI
Following airway surgery (e.g., panendoscopy or tonsillectomy)
Trauma from instrumentation (e.g., NGT, TEE probe, prolonged laryngoscopy)
Secretions in a heavy smoker
Preexisting airway pathology
Retained surgical pack
Vocal cord polyp or laryngeal tumor

PREVENTION

Administer prophylactic steroids to minimize airway edema following trauma or instrumentation, or before surgery of the airway
Consider delaying extubation if there is significant facial edema following surgery; recover in upright position until edema resolves
Ensure full reversal of neuromuscular blockade
Carefully suction secretions from the upper airway before extubation and as necessary afterward
   Consider prophylactic antisialogogue (glycopyrrolate IV, 0.2 to 0.4 mg) prior to airway surgery
Remove all foreign bodies from the airway at the end of surgery
Extubate the trachea when the patient is awake or when anesthesia is deep enough to ablate airway reflexes
Maintain the patency of the airway as necessary after extubation

MANIFESTATIONS

Noisy, high-pitched inspiratory sound
Reduced inspiratory volume
Retraction of the chest or neck during inspiration accompanied by use of the accessory muscles of respiration
Restlessness and dyspnea that are aggravated by increasing respiratory efforts or attempts to cough up secretions
Hypoxemia and cyanosis
Increasing ET CO_2 and $PaCO_2$

SIMILAR EVENTS

Airway obstruction from other causes
Bronchospasm (see Event 29, Bronchospasm)
Epiglottitis (see Event 31, Epiglottitis [Supraglottitis])
Anterior mediastinal mass (see Event 27, Anterior Mediastinal Mass)
Intrathoracic airway obstruction
Anxiety reaction

MANAGEMENT

Administer 100% O_2
Suction the oropharynx to remove secretions

Assist ventilation with CPAP

Use anesthesia breathing circuit or nonrebreather (Mapleson) circuit

Administer a small dose of succinylcholine IV, 0.3 mg/kg, or IM, 0.6 mg/kg, and continue mask ventilation with CPAP

Call respiratory therapy to assist management

Set up for noninvasive ventilatory support (e.g., BiPAP, CPAP)

Consider nebulized racemic epinephrine, 1 mg of a 1:1000 solution (1 mL) in 5 mL of saline, repeated every 30 minutes

Monitor for tachycardia and hypertension

Administer Heliox (helium concentration between 50% and 70%) if available

Consider dexmedetomidine IV (0.2 to 0.5 µg/kg/hr) for anxiolysis

Provide airway support maneuvers if level of consciousness is depressed

Jaw thrust

Oral or nasal airway

Check adequacy of the reversal of neuromuscular blockade, administer additional anticholinesterase if necessary (see Event 56, Postoperative Failure to Breathe)

Consider reversal of opioids and benzodiazepines in presence of depressed consciousness (see Event 56, Postoperative Failure to Breathe)

If stridor does not resolve, respiratory distress continues, or hypoxemia develops

Call for help

Prepare for emergency reintubation

Prepare for surgical airway (e.g., cricothyrotomy)

Treatment of specific underlying situations

Following neck surgery

Call for the surgeon immediately

Remove any dressings from the wound

If a hematoma is found, cut the wound sutures

This will require subsequent surgical exploration of the wound for hemostasis and reclosure

Reintubate the trachea if there is no immediate improvement in the patient's airway

Intubation may be difficult because of airway edema

Prepare for difficult tracheal intubation (see Event 3, Difficult Tracheal Intubation)

Perform intubation in the OR if the patient is stable

Use a smaller ETT than was used in original surgery

Following airway surgery

Call for the surgeon immediately

Administer steroids

Dexamethasone IV, 8 to 20 mg

Consider nebulized racemic epinephrine, 1 mg of a 1:1000 solution (1 mL) in 5 mL of saline, repeated every 30 minutes

Monitor for tachycardia and hypertension

Consider the possibility of retained gauze, throat packs, or other foreign body in the airway

Prepare for direct examination of the airway and/or reintubation

COMPLICATIONS

Hypoxemia

Inability to reintubate

Airway trauma due to difficult intubation

Aspiration of gastric contents
Pulmonary edema due to excessive negative intrathoracic pressure
Contamination of surgical wounds opened to relieve pressure in the neck
Cardiac arrest

SUGGESTED READING

1. Bharti N. Dexmedetomidine for the treatment of severe postoperative functional stridor. Anaesth Intensive Care 2012;40:354-5.

37   Unplanned Extubation

DEFINITION

An unplanned extubation is any unplanned dislodgement or removal of the ETT (or other SGA device) from the airway.

ETIOLOGY

Mechanical traction on the breathing circuit, ETT, or SGA
Inadequately secured airway device
Poor fit (e.g., RAE ETT in large adults)
Self-extubation

TYPICAL SITUATIONS

When the patient's position is changed
> Moving the operating table relative to the anesthesia workstation (e.g., turning table 180 degrees)
> Moving the patient from one bed or table to another
> Moving the patient into a surgical position (e.g., lithotomy, prone)

Repositioning of the head and neck during surgery
When manipulating the anesthesia breathing circuit hoses or surgical drapes
Taking adhesive surgical drapes down at the end of the case
When attempting to reposition an ETT
During placement or removal of a NGT or TEE probe
When repositioning fluoroscope during surgery

PREVENTION

Secure the ETT following placement
> Prepare the skin with benzoin solution and let dry
> Tape the ETT to the skin securely
> Note the markings of the ETT at the gums or teeth
> Avoid attaching the ETT to the operating table or other devices
> Add extension hoses to the breathing circuit or move OR table to minimize pulling on breathing circuit
> Consider administering glycopyrrolate IV, 0.2 mg, prior to turning to the prone position to prevent drooling loosening the adhesive tape

Special care is necessary for patients with facial hair

Hold the ETT securely in place or disconnect from the breathing circuit as the patient's position is changed

Check ETT after positioning the patient

Reconnect the ETT and turn on the ventilator after completing patient movement

Use properly sized RAE ETT

Hold the ETT in place during procedures such as fiberoptic bronchoscopy or direct laryngoscopy

If the patient is in the lateral or prone position, be prepared to move the patient into the supine position should reintubation become necessary

Avoid placing surgical drapes on ETT or tape holding ETT in place

MANIFESTATIONS

Major leak in the anesthesia breathing circuit
    The leak may develop slowly, as the extubation may not be complete
    The ventilator bellows collapses or the reservoir bag does not move
    The smell of volatile anesthetic may be apparent
    Sounds of a gas leak may be heard
    Low pressure, volume, or apnea alarms may sound
    An excessive amount of air in the ETT cuff may be required to achieve a seal
Decreased or zero PIP
Decreased or zero expiratory gas flow measured by spirometry
Decreased or no ET CO_2
On laryngoscopy, ETT may be visualized outside the trachea
Gastric distention may occur
Late signs of hypoventilation
    Hypoxemia
    Hypercarbia

SIMILAR EVENTS

ETT cuff rupture

Disconnection or other major leak in the anesthesia breathing circuit or anesthesia workstation (see Event 69, Major Leak in the Anesthesia Breathing Circuit)

Loss of O_2 pipeline supply (see Event 68, Loss of Pipeline Oxygen)

Ventilator failure (see Event 71, Ventilator Failure)

MANAGEMENT

Confirm the diagnosis
    Determine whether signs are due to unplanned extubation, disconnect, or other problem
        Check for disconnect of the breathing circuit and reconnect if present
    Switch to manual ventilation
        Feel the compliance of the lungs and anesthesia breathing circuit
        Check ET CO_2 and oxygenation
    If the head of bed is 90 to 180 degrees away, call for help as correction of the problem may require two people
    Palpate the pilot balloon of the ETT to ensure cuff is inflated
        Place more air into cuff and reassess with manual ventilation

Compensate for any leak in the anesthesia breathing circuit

Administer 100% O_2 and increase fresh gas flow

Inform the surgeon

If necessary, clear the access to the airway

If the airway is in or near the surgical field, halt the surgery and cover the wound with a sterile drape

Perform a direct or video-assisted laryngoscopy to determine the position of the ETT

Reposition or replace the ETT into the trachea

Consider using airway exchange catheter or fiberoptic bronchoscope to reposition ETT

Place bougie through ETT if tip is in the larynx but tube will not pass into the trachea

If repositioning or reintubation of ETT is not easily accomplished

Mask ventilate the patient with 100% FiO_2 if O_2 saturation is less than 95%

Place an SGA if mask ventilation is difficult or immediate reintubation is not possible

If intubation is necessary, consider intubating through the SGA or use an intubating LMA

If O_2 saturation improves, attempt reintubation and have contingency plans

Video-assisted laryngoscopy, direct laryngoscopy, fiberoptic bronchoscopy, surgical airway

If oxygenation cannot be maintained, move aggressively to cricothyrotomy (see Event 3, Difficult Tracheal Intubation)

If the patient is in the prone or lateral position

Call for help

Bring gurney into the room for possible repositioning

If the patient's O_2 saturation is lower than 95% or there is no ET CO_2 waveform

Move patient emergently to the supine position for mask ventilation and reintubation

If the patient's O_2 saturation is higher than 95% and there is an ET CO_2 waveform

Continue to ventilate manually with small tidal volumes and low airway pressures

Consider fiberoptic bronchoscopy to confirm the diagnosis and to reposition the ETT

If the preceding fails, move patient to the supine position for mask ventilation and reintubation

If the patient was difficult to intubate at the beginning of the case

Call for help

Position the patient supine

Mask ventilate with 100% FiO_2

Assemble the equipment needed for a difficult intubation (see Event 3, Difficult Tracheal Intubation)

Contingency plans include SGA, video-assisted laryngoscopy, direct laryngoscopy, fiberoptic bronchoscopy, surgical airway

Consider terminating the surgery and awakening the patient

COMPLICATIONS

Aspiration of gastric contents

Airway trauma from repeated instrumentation

Esophageal intubation

Contamination of the surgical wound

Disconnection or accidental removal of monitoring lines or sensor monitors during repositioning of the patient

Hypoxemia

Cardiac arrest

Chapter 8
Metabolic Events
GREGORY H. BOTZ

---

38 Addisonian Crisis (Acute Adrenal Insufficiency)

DEFINITION

Addisonian crisis, or acute adrenal insufficiency, is a relative or absolute deficiency of adrenal corticosteroid hormones resulting in hemodynamic or other compromise.

ETIOLOGY

Primary adrenal insufficiency (Addison disease)
Secondary adrenal insufficiency (pituitary disease)
Failure of hormone synthesis
    Etomidate inhibits adrenal corticosteroid synthesis (should be used with caution in critically ill patients)

TYPICAL SITUATIONS

Patients who have primary or secondary adrenal insufficiency
Abrupt termination of steroid therapy
Patients with a recent history of steroid therapy who are stressed by major surgery or perioperative infections
Septic patients unresponsive to vasopressor therapy

PREVENTION

Administer preoperative corticosteroids to any patient who has received adrenal suppressive doses of corticosteroids (more than 5 mg/day, for more than 3 weeks, of prednisone or equivalent) within the year prior to surgery
    Major surgery or stress:
        Hydrocortisone IV, 100 mg prior to induction of anesthesia, followed by 200 to 300 mg/day in divided doses
    Minor surgery or stress:
        Hydrocortisone IV, 50 mg prior to induction of anesthesia, followed by 100 to 200 mg/day in divided doses
Identify patients with primary or secondary adrenal insufficiency
Have a high index of suspicion for adrenal insufficiency in patients with significant systemic diseases that are often treated with corticosteroids (e.g., connective tissue diseases, asthma)
Careful communication with patients to identify steroid use before surgery

MANIFESTATIONS

Onset may be acute or delayed to the postoperative period.
Hypotension or shock refractory to treatment with fluids and vasopressors
Hyponatremia, hyperkalemia, and hypoglycemia
Nausea and vomiting

SIMILAR EVENTS

Septic shock (see Event 13, The Septic Patient)
Anaphylaxis (see Event 16, Anaphylactic and Anaphylactoid Reactions)
Hypotension secondary to other etiologies (see Event 9, Hypotension)
Patients on antihypertensive medications (e.g., ACEI)

MANAGEMENT

If hypotension or cardiovascular collapse occurs in the patient at risk of adrenal insufficiency
    Rapidly expand circulating fluid volume (crystalloid and/or colloid)
    Administer hydrocortisone IV, 100 mg bolus, repeat q8 h
    Replace Na^+ using normal saline (NS)
    Replace K^+ if hypokalemic (see Event 42, Hypokalemia)
    Administer dextrose to correct hypoglycemia if present (see Event 41, Hypoglycemia)
    Hemodynamic support with vasopressors, inotropes as necessary
        Ephedrine IV, 5 to 20 mg, escalate as necessary
        Phenylephrine IV, 100 to 200 µg, escalate as necessary
        Epinephrine IV, 5 to 20 µg, escalate as necessary
    Identify and treat underlying causes of adrenal insufficiency if possible
Ensure that other more likely etiologies of hypotension and shock are not responsible for hypotension
    Hypovolemia (see Event 1, Acute Hemorrhage, and Event 9, Hypotension)
    Anesthetic or drug overdose (see Event 72, Volatile Anesthetic Overdose)
    Primary cardiovascular impairment (see Event 15, Acute Coronary Syndrome, and Event 20, Pulmonary Edema)
    High intrathoracic pressure (see Event 7, High Peak Inspiratory Pressure)
    Anaphylaxis (see Event 16, Anaphylactic and Anaphylactoid Reactions)
If no response to hydrocortisone and IV fluid administration
    TEE or TTE to assess myocardial filling and function
Laboratory studies
    Plasma electrolytes and glucose
    Baseline cortisol and adrenocorticotropic hormone (ACTH) levels (ideally draw before administering hydrocortisone, but if hypotension is life-threatening, do not delay therapy)
Suspect adrenal crisis in older patients who remain vasopressor dependent after surgical procedures despite adequate volume resuscitation

38

COMPLICATIONS

Refractory hypotension
Organ hypoperfusion/dysfunction
Cardiac arrest
Complications of steroid therapy (e.g., hyperglycemia)

SUGGESTED READING

1. Schwartz JJ, Akhtar S, Rosenbaum SH. Endocrine function. In: Barash PG, Cullen BF, Stoelting RK, Calahan M, Stock MC, editors. Clinical anesthesia. 6th ed. Philadelphia: Lippincott Williams & Wilkins; 2009. p. 1289-91.
2. Coursin DB, Wood KE. Corticosteroid supplementation for adrenal insufficiency. JAMA 2002;287:236-40.
3. Jung C, Inder WJ. Management of adrenal insufficiency during the stress of medical illness and surgery. Med J Aust 2008;188:409-13.
4. Connery LE, Coursin DB. Assessment and therapy of selected endocrine disorders. Anesthesiol Clin North Am 2004;22:93-123.

39   Diabetic Ketoacidosis

DEFINITION

Diabetic ketoacidosis (DKA) is a metabolic acidosis associated with hyperglycemia and high levels of ketoacids in the blood and urine of the diabetic patient.

ETIOLOGY

An absolute or relative deficiency of insulin, causing mobilization and oxidation of fatty acids with resulting production of ketoacids

TYPICAL SITUATIONS

In patients with insulin-dependent diabetes mellitus
When an appropriate insulin dose has been administered but the patient's insulin requirements are increased because of
> Trauma
> Concurrent infection
> Excessive fluid losses or inadequate fluid intake
> Increased catabolic stress
An absolute deficiency of insulin
> Inadequate insulin dose administered
> Delayed absorption of SC insulin due to poor peripheral perfusion

PREVENTION

Prevention of DKA, rather than prevention of hyperglycemia, is the primary aim of surgical care of the diabetic patient.
Identify insulin-dependent patients preoperatively and optimize therapy
> The appropriate perioperative insulin regimen must be based on prior insulin requirements, the patient's history, the timing of surgery, and frequent measurements of blood glucose
>> Most insulin-dependent patients should receive some insulin on the day of surgery
>> Maintain euglycemia or mild hyperglycemia during anesthesia and surgery; the goal is 100 to 180 mg/dL
>> Treat infections early and aggressively with antibiotics
>> Replace fluid losses or treat dehydration aggressively

MANIFESTATIONS

The conscious patient may complain of nausea, vomiting, hunger, abdominal pain, sweating, or demonstrate confusion and/or altered level of consciousness
Hypovolemia
Hypotension
Tachycardia
Metabolic acidosis with increased anion gap
Hyperventilation (Kussmaul breathing) to compensate for metabolic acidosis
Polyuria or oliguria depending on the patient's underlying fluid volume status

SIMILAR EVENTS

Other forms of metabolic acidosis (see Event 46, Metabolic Acidosis)
Hyperosmolar hyperglycemic nonketotic syndrome
Hypovolemia from other causes (see Event 9, Hypotension)
Abdominal pain from other causes
Hyperglycemia from other causes

MANAGEMENT

Confirm the diagnosis
  Obtain blood and urine samples for
    ABGs
    Serum glucose
    Serum ketoacids
    Serum lactate
    Serum electrolytes (including PO_4^{3-}, Mg^{2+})
    Serum creatinine and BUN
    Plasma osmolality
    CBC with differential
    Urine ketoacids
    Troponin
    Blood cultures
Ensure adequate oxygenation and ventilation
  Intubate the trachea if the patient is obtunded or if respiratory distress is present
Expand the circulating fluid volume
  Administer 500 to 1000 mL of crystalloid
  Additional fluid administration should be based on the patient's response
    Average fluid deficit is 3 to 6 L
    If the patient has CAD, CHF, or renal failure, place an arterial line and consider a CVP catheter to assess/monitor filling pressures and fluid responsiveness, and to guide fluid management
Begin insulin therapy
  Administer regular insulin IV, 10 units
  Initiate an IV infusion of regular insulin at 5 to 10 units/hr
  Avoid SC insulin administration as absorption through this route is variable

39

Administer NaHCO₃ only for profound acidosis (pH below 7.1) (see Event 46, Metabolic Acidosis)

Repeat measurements of serum glucose, electrolytes, and ABGs q1-2h until the values normalize

> When blood glucose reaches 250 to 300 mg/dL
>> Consider adding glucose to IV solutions
>> Reduce insulin infusion rate, but continue infusion until anion gap normalizes
> Replace K⁺ deficit once urine output is ensured (see Event 42, Hypokalemia)
>> Most patients with DKA have a large total body K⁺ deficit

Replace PO₄³⁻, Mg²⁺ as indicated by laboratory measurements

Treat underlying etiology (infection, sepsis, MI, etc.)

Consult an internist or endocrinologist to assist in the patient's perioperative management

Consider briefly delaying urgent surgery to adequately resuscitate the patient

Cancel elective procedure

COMPLICATIONS

Hypotension

Hypoglycemia

Hypokalemia

Hyperkalemia

Pulmonary edema

Thrombotic events

SUGGESTED READING

1. Schwartz JJ, Akhtar S, Rosenbaum SH. Endocrine function. In: Barash PG, Cullen BF, Stoelting RK, Calahan M, Stock MC, editors. Clinical anesthesia. 6th ed. Philadelphia: Lippincott Williams & Wilkins; 2009. p. 1300.
2. Kitabchi AE, Umpierrez GE, Miles JM, Fisher JN. Hyperglycemic crises in adult patients with diabetes. Diabetes Care 2009;32:1335-43.
3. Dagogo-Jack S, George MM, Alberti K. Management of diabetes mellitus in surgical patients. Diabetes Spectrum 2002;15:44-8.

---

40 Hyperkalemia

DEFINITION

Hyperkalemia is a serum K⁺ level >5.5 mEq/L.

ETIOLOGY

Excessive intake

> Excessive parenteral or oral K⁺ supplements
> Massive blood transfusion
> Administration of hyperkalemic cardioplegia solution

Inadequate excretion of K⁺

> Renal failure
> Adrenal insufficiency
> K⁺-sparing diuretics
> Administration of ACEIs (indirectly reduces the secretion of aldosterone)

Shift of K$^+$ from the tissues to the plasma
>   Extensive tissue damage (muscle crushing injury, hemolysis, internal bleeding)
>   Administration of succinylcholine (in patients with renal failure, acute SCI, upper motor neuron disorders, prolonged immobilization, or severe burn injury)
>   Respiratory or metabolic acidosis
>   Acute release of K$^+$ into the plasma from transplanted organs with a high K$^+$ content
>   Hyperkalemic periodic paralysis
>   MH
>   Pseudohyperkalemia usually secondary to mechanical trauma caused by venipuncture

TYPICAL SITUATIONS

Major trauma
Aortic cross-clamp release
Cardiac and transplant surgery
During IV K$^+$ replacement
Renal failure patients, with or without ongoing renal dialysis
Burn victims
Patients receiving massive transfusion
Rarely in patients receiving epsilon-aminocaproic acid

PREVENTION

Use appropriate K$^+$ replacement protocols for at-risk patients
Avoid succinylcholine in patients susceptible to excessive K$^+$ release
Measure serum K$^+$ concentration frequently in patients at risk for hyperkalemia
Use continuous ECG monitoring
Administer K$^+$ supplements carefully; replace only to physiologic levels
Avoid metabolic or respiratory acidosis
Dialyze hyperkalemic renal failure patients preoperatively
Administer blood products via an appropriate blood-warming device to avoid hemolysis and hyperkalemia

MANIFESTATIONS

ECG abnormalities and arrhythmias usually seen after serum K$^+$ is above 6.5 mEq/L
>   Tall, peaked T waves
>   Prolonged PR interval, loss of P waves, or atrial asystole
>   Complete heart block
>   Widened QRS complex
>   Sine wave-type ventricular arrhythmia
>   VF or asystole
>   If serum K$^+$ rises rapidly, the first sign may be VF or asystole
Skeletal muscle weakness

SIMILAR EVENTS

Sample handling error
>   Blood sample hemolysis with poor venipuncture technique
>   In vitro hemolysis in the laboratory

Patients with thrombocytosis or leukocytosis
Transient rise following succinylcholine administration

MANAGEMENT

If ECG changes after induction of anesthesia suggest hyperkalemia
  Hyperventilate the patient
  Administer $CaCl_2$ 10% IV, 500 to 1000 mg
Stop administration of any K^+ containing solutions
  IV K^+ replacement
  LR IV solution (contains 4.0 mEq/L)
  PRBCs
Confirm diagnosis by STAT serum K^+ measurement
If moderate or severe hyperkalemia (serum K^+ greater than 6.0 mEq/L)
  Increase the blood pH
    Hyperventilate the patient unless contraindicated
    Administer $NaHCO_3$ IV, 50 to 150 mEq
    Draw blood for an ABG measurement
    Treat underlying metabolic acidosis, if present
  Administer $CaCl_2$ 10% IV, 500 to 1000 mg
  Administer dextrose 50% IV, 50 g, and regular insulin IV, 10 units
  Administer inhaled β2-agonist
    Albuterol MDI, 6 to 10 puffs
  Force a diuresis
    Increase fluid administration
    Administer loop diuretics IV (e.g., furosemide IV, 5 to 20 mg)
    Patient may require a urinary catheter
  Obtain emergent nephrologist or internist consultation to institute emergency peritoneal
    dialysis or hemodialysis
Mild hyperkalemia (serum K^+ less than 6.0 mEq/L)
  Monitor trend in serum K^+ every 1 to 2 hours and treat aggressively if symptoms persist
    or levels increase
  Administer cation exchange resins by rectal or oral routes

COMPLICATIONS

Arrhythmias
VF
Complications of therapy
  Hypokalemia
  Alkalosis
  Hyperosmolality
  Hypoglycemia or hyperglycemia
  Dialysis-related problems (vascular access, heparin-related)

SUGGESTED READING

1. Prough DS, Funston JS, Svensen CH, Wolf SW. Fluids, electrolytes and acid–base physiology. In: Barash PG, Cullen BF, Stoelting RK, Calahan M, Stock MC, editors. Clinical anesthesia. 6th ed. Philadelphia: Lippincott Williams & Wilkins; 2009. p. 313-4.
2. Strom S. Hyperkalemia. In: Roizen MF, Fleisher LA, editors. Essence of anesthesia practice. 3rd ed. Philadelphia: Saunders; 2010. p. 190.

3. Elliott MJ, Ronksley PE, Clase CM, Ahmed SB, Hemmelgarn BR. Management of patients with acute hyperkalemia. CMAJ 2010;182:1631-5.
4. Weisberg LS. Management of severe hyperkalemia. Crit Care Med 2008;36:3246-51.

41 Hypoglycemia

DEFINITION

Hypoglycemia is a blood glucose level of <70 mg/dL.

ETIOLOGY

Underproduction of glucose
Overutilization of glucose
Impaired gluconeogenesis

TYPICAL SITUATIONS

Patients who have inadequate glucose intake
  Chronic starvation
  Preoperative fasting
  Discontinuation of hyperalimentation
Patients who have metabolic diseases
  Hormone deficiencies
  Enzyme deficiency in the glycogenic pathway
  Acquired liver disease
Patients taking drugs that alter glucose metabolism
  Oral hypoglycemic agents
  Alcohol
  Propranolol
  Salicylates
Patients with excessive circulating insulin
  Insulin administration
  Insulinoma
  Newborn infants of diabetic mothers
"Dumping syndrome" following upper GI surgery

PREVENTION

Identify and treat patients at risk of hypoglycemia preoperatively
  Optimize the patient's metabolic status prior to surgery
  Measure serum glucose frequently in these patients
Establish a preoperative infusion of a glucose-containing solution in diabetic patients who are receiving insulin
  Reduce the patient's daily insulin dose on the day of surgery

Do not administer oral hypoglycemic agents on the morning of surgery

Continue hyperalimentation in the perioperative period or replace it with a 10% dextrose solution

MANIFESTATIONS

Hypoglycemia can be masked by general anesthesia or β*-blockade.*

CNS
    In the awake patient:
        Altered mental status, irritability, tremulousness
        Headache
        Lethargy
        Seizures
    In the anesthetized patient:
        Seizures
        Failure to awaken from general anesthesia
Sympathetic nervous system stimulation
    Hypertension
    Sweating
    Tachycardia
Cardiovascular collapse is a late sign of hypoglycemia

SIMILAR EVENTS

Light anesthesia

Hypoxemia (see Event 10, Hypoxemia)

TURP syndrome (see Event 43, Hyponatremia and Hypo-osmolality)

Seizures from other causes (see Event 57, Seizures)

Failure to awaken from general anesthesia due to other causes (see Event 55, Postoperative Alteration in Mental Status)

MANAGEMENT

Confirm the diagnosis
    Measure blood glucose level STAT
Treat suspected or known hypoglycemia
    Therapy for hypoglycemia carries little risk, whereas failure to treat hypoglycemia may be catastrophic
    Administer dextrose 50% IV, 1 mL/kg bolus, while waiting for clinical laboratory results
    Start a dextrose 10% IV infusion at 1 to 2 mL/kg/hr
Stop or reduce administration of insulin or other drugs that lower blood glucose levels
Monitor serum glucose frequently
Correct underlying metabolic problems
If there is no response to 50% dextrose IV, consider other etiologies for CNS manifestations

COMPLICATIONS

CNS injury
Cardiac arrest
Hyperglycemia and hyperosmolality from excessive glucose administration

SUGGESTED READING

1. Schwartz JJ, Akhtar S, Rosenbaum SH. Endocrine function. In: Barash PG, Cullen BF, Stoelting RK, Calahan M, Stock MC, editors. Clinical anesthesia. 6th ed. Philadelphia: Lippincott Williams & Wilkins; 2009. p. 1300.
2. Smiley DD, Umpierrez GE. Perioperative glucose control in the diabetic or nondiabetic patient. South Med J 2006;99:580-9.
3. Lipshutz AKM, Gropper MA. Perioperative glycemic control: an evidence-based review. Anesthesiology 2009;110:408-21.

42   Hypokalemia

DEFINITION

Hypokalemia is a plasma K^+ concentration of <3.0 mEq/L.

ETIOLOGY

GI deficiency or loss
    Deficient dietary intake
    NG suction
    GI loss caused by diarrhea, iliostomy drainage, or vomiting
Renal loss
    Diuretic therapy
    Excess mineralocorticoid or glucocorticoid effect
    Renal tubular diseases
    Mg^{2+} depletion
Cellular shifts
    Metabolic or respiratory alkalosis
    Insulin effect
    Hypokalemic periodic paralysis
    Hyperaldosteronism
    β_2-agonists and α-adrenergic antagonists enhance cellular K^+ entry

TYPICAL SITUATIONS

Acute hypokalemia presents a greater threat to patient safety than chronic hypokalemia.
Patients with diarrhea, vomiting, or preparation for large bowel surgery
Patients receiving diuretics, particularly loop diuretics
Following cardiac surgery
Following treatment of hyperkalemia
Hyperventilation
Increased availability of insulin
Elevated β-adrenergic stimulation (e.g., after administration of albuterol and dobutamine)

PREVENTION

Replacement of K^+ for patients receiving K^+-wasting diuretics
IV replacement of fluids and electrolytes during cathartic preparation for bowel surgery
Monitor serum K^+ and replace as necessary during and after CPB
Avoid hypomagnesemia
Avoid conditions that reduce serum K^+ acutely
    Hyperventilation
    Metabolic alkalosis
    β_2-adrenergic stimulation

MANIFESTATIONS

Serum K^+ less than 3.0 mEq/L
Cardiac
    ECG abnormalities (unusual until serum K^+ is less than 3.5 mEq/L)
        PVCs
        T-wave flattening or inversion
        Increased U-wave amplitude
        ST segment depression
        Tachycardia
        Digitalis toxicity may worsen significantly if combined with hypokalemia
    AV arrhythmias
        Cardiac conduction defects
        Cardiac arrest
Neuromuscular
    Increased sensitivity to neuromuscular blocking drugs
    Skeletal muscle weakness causing
        Respiratory failure
        Paralysis
    Decreased activity of the GI system, with paralytic ileus
Renal
    Polyuria
    Metabolic alkalosis

SIMILAR EVENTS

Laboratory error
Arrhythmias from other causes
Inadequate reversal of nondepolarizing muscle relaxants
Other causes of ST-T wave abnormalities (see Event 12, ST Segment Change)

MANAGEMENT

If serum K^+ is greater than 3.0 mEq/L and there are no ECG changes, carefully consider whether or not to proceed with elective surgery prior to K^+ replacement.

Postpone elective surgery and use oral K^+ replacement if serum K^+ is less than 3.0 mEq/L
    Oral replacement 20 to 80 mEq/day

For urgent or emergent surgery, if serum K⁺ is less than 3.0 mEq/L, or if the patient is symptomatic

Replace K⁺ by the IV route to achieve a serum K⁺ of at least 3.5 mEq/L before anesthesia induction

> Monitor the ECG during the infusion (see Event 40, Hyperkalemia)
> Administer through a CVP line, if possible
> Infuse no faster than 10 mEq/30 min, except for treatment of life-threatening ventricular arrhythmias in a patient known to be severely hypokalemic
> Prevent K⁺ from accumulating in the IV tubing or blood-warming devices
> Measure serum K⁺ hourly during rapid administration of K⁺

In the hypokalemic patient

> Be sure that muscle relaxants are fully reversed and that the patient has recovered appropriate neuromuscular function before the trachea is extubated
> Measure ABGs if neuromuscular function is slow to recover following surgery

COMPLICATIONS

Residual neuromuscular blockade

Hyperkalemia, myocardial arrhythmias, or cardiac arrest from excessive K⁺ replacement

Pain or thrombophlebitis at IV site from K⁺ replacement through a peripheral IV

SUGGESTED READING

1. Prough DS, Funston JS, Svensen CH, Wolf SW. Fluids, electrolytes and acid–base physiology. In: Barash PG, Cullen BF, Stoelting RK, Calahan M, Stock MC, editors. Clinical anesthesia. 6th ed. Philadelphia: Lippincott Williams & Wilkins; 2009. p. 311-3.
2. Gennari FJ. Hypokalemia. N Engl J Med 1998;339:451-8.
3. Sladen RN. Anesthetic considerations for the patient with renal failure. Anesthesiol Clin North America 2000;18:863-82.

---

43   Hyponatremia and Hypo-osmolality

DEFINITION

Hyponatremia is an abnormally low serum Na⁺ (<130 mEq/L). Hypo-osmolality is an abnormally low serum osmolality (<270 mOsm/L).

ETIOLOGY

Hemodilution

Decreased renal free water clearance

Pseudohyponatremia (low serum Na⁺ with normal or elevated osmolality)

TYPICAL SITUATIONS

Cystoscopic surgery

> Absorption of hypotonic irrigation fluid into the prostatic venous channels
> Hyperglycinemia secondary to the use of glycine-containing irrigation fluid (usually pseudohyponatremia as the serum osmolality may be near normal)

Infusion of hypotonic IV fluids, especially D5W
Impaired mechanisms of renal free water excretion
 Chronic renal failure
 Administration of drugs
  Oxytocin
  Nonsteroidal anti-inflammatory drugs (NSAIDs)
  Thiazide diuretics
 Decreased renal blood flow associated with major surgery
 Syndrome of inappropriate secretion of antidiuretic hormone (SIADH)
Psychogenic polydipsia
Patients with metabolic abnormalities causing pseudohyponatremia
 Hyperglycemia
 Hyperproteinemia
 Hyperlipidemia

PREVENTION

During TURP surgery
 Use bipolar (instead of monopolar) resection systems (allows NS as irrigant)
 Avoid using sterile water as the irrigation fluid
 Minimize resection time and consider staged procedure if large resection is necessary
 Achieve adequate venous sinus hemostasis
 Avoid high irrigation pressures (adjust height of irrigation fluid)
Avoid hypotonic fluid replacement
Check Na^+ levels frequently in
 Patients with chronic renal failure
 Patients undergoing prolonged TURP
 Patients receiving drugs that can cause hyponatremia

43

MANIFESTATIONS

Decrease in serum Na^+ concentration
In the awake patient:
 Restlessness, disorientation
 Visual disturbances
 Nausea, vomiting
 Altered mental status
In any patient:
 Preseizure irritability
 Seizures
Signs and symptoms of circulating fluid volume overload
 Tachycardia or bradycardia
 Hypertension
 Increased CVP
 Decreased O_2 saturation
 Dyspnea
 Crackles on auscultation of the lungs
Pulmonary or laryngeal edema
Intravascular hemolysis

SIMILAR EVENTS

Anxiety during regional anesthesia
Hypoxemia from other causes (see Event 10, Hypoxemia)
Altered mental status as a result of
    Sedative drugs
    Delirium
    Organic brain syndrome
Myocardial ischemia, infarction (see Event 15, Acute Coronary Syndrome)

MANAGEMENT

These management guidelines apply to monopolar TURP surgery. Use of bipolar resection systems in TURP surgery has been shown to decrease the incidence of hyponatremia because isotonic saline can be used as the irrigant.

Inform the surgeon of the problem
Replace sterile water irrigation fluid with a glycine-containing irrigation solution, which has
    a nearly normal osmolality
        Advise the surgeon to discontinue prostatic resection, achieve hemostasis, and terminate
            the procedure as soon as possible
        Consider changing to bipolar resection for remainder of procedure
Ensure adequate oxygenation and ventilation
    Administer supplemental O_2, as necessary
    If pulmonary or laryngeal edema develops, call for help
        Laryngeal edema can make airway management and intubation extremely difficult
        Consider early intubation
Send blood to the laboratory for STAT serum Na^+ and serum osmolality
    If serum Na^+ is low but osmolality is normal or near normal, pseudohyponatremia is most
        likely cause
        Glycine may be an unmeasured osmolar compound
        Hyperglycinemia may cause symptoms similar to those of true hyponatremia
Reduce the bladder irrigation fluid pressure by decreasing the height of the fluid
If there are signs of circulating fluid volume overload
    Decrease IV fluid rate or blood transfusion to a minimum
    Administer furosemide IV, 5 to 20 mg bolus
**Treat hyponatremia if the patient is symptomatic or if there is true hyponatremia with a
serum Na^+ less than 120 mEq/L**
    Administer furosemide IV, 5 to 20 mg bolus, if the patient is not hypotensive
    Switch IV fluids to NS for slow restoration of normal Na^+ concentration
    Consider administering a vasopressin receptor antagonist (e.g., conivaptan, 20 mg IV
        load over 30 minutes, then 20 mg/day IV infusion for 48 hours)
    Do not use hypertonic saline unless the patient is markedly symptomatic or has very low
        serum Na^+ **and** low serum osmolality
        3% hypertonic saline 1.5 to 2 mL/kg (~100 mL) over 10 minutes, may repeat twice
        Hypertonic saline may produce significant hypervolemia and neurologic injury
Monitor CVP or PCWP if clinically indicated
    If pulmonary edema is present (see Event 20, Pulmonary Edema)
    If the patient has a history of CAD or CHF
    If there are ST-T wave changes on the ECG

43

COMPLICATIONS

Hyperosmolality secondary to use of hypertonic saline
Cerebral edema
Central pontine myelinolysis or diffuse cerebral demyelination secondary to too rapid restoration of serum Na$^+$

SUGGESTED READING

1. Stafford-Smith M, Shaw A, George R, Muir H. The renal system and anesthesia for urologic surgery. In: Barash PG, Cullen BF, Stoelting RK, Calahan M, Stock MC, editors. Clinical anesthesia. 6th ed. Philadelphia: Lippincott Williams & Wilkins; 2009. p. 1351, 1365-66.
2. Gowrishankar M, Lin SH, Mallie JP, Oh MS, Halperin ML. Acute hyponatremia in the perioperative period: insights into its pathophysiology and recommendations for management. Clin Nephrol 1998;50:352-60.
3. Schrier RW, Bansal S. Diagnosis and management of hyponatremia in acute illness. Curr Opin Crit Care 2008;14:627-34.
4. Issa MM. Technological advances in transurethral resection of the prostate: bipolar vs. monopolar TURP. J Endourol 2008;22:1587-95.

---

44 Hypothermia

DEFINITION

Hypothermia is a core body temperature below 35° C during the perioperative period.

ETIOLOGY

Preexisting hypothermia
Depression of metabolic heat production by anesthesia
Increased heat loss to the environment
 Radiation
 Conduction
 Convection
 Evaporation
Infusion of large volumes of cold RBCs or IV solutions

TYPICAL SITUATIONS

Cool OR
Significant portions of the patient's body exposed to the air
Use of cold or room-temperature fluids
 Skin preparation solutions
 Irrigation fluids
 IV fluids or blood
Ventilation of the lungs with cool, dry gas through an ETT
When the abdominal or thoracic cavity is open
 Large amount of evaporative heat loss
During pediatric surgery (high ratio of body surface area to weight)
Direct contact between the patient and the operating table

Prolonged surgical cases
Trauma cases
Following environmental exposure or near-drowning

PREVENTION

Increase OR temperature to at least 21° C
Provide a local warm environment for the patient
  Forced-air warming device
  Prewarm OR table
  Circulation of heated water through hydrogel pads applied to the back (able to adhere to large surface areas)
  Other warming devices
Cover exposed areas of the patient whenever possible including the head as it is 18% of the body surface area
Warm all IV fluids, blood products, and irrigation fluids
Use passive or active breathing circuit humidification
Minimize exposure of viscera to the air
Use reflective blankets to minimize convective and radiative loss
Use warming lights for infants and neonates during preparation for anesthesia and surgery

MANIFESTATIONS

Body temperature is lower than normal
Shivering in the unparalyzed or awake patient
Cutaneous vasoconstriction, piloerection
Decreased level of consciousness, reduced anesthetic requirement
Bradycardia
If hypothermia is severe (body temperature less than 30° C)
  Decreased myocardial contractility
  Increased ventricular irritability
  Increased SVR
  Cardiac arrest (usually manifests as VF or asystole)
  Electrically silent EEG (if less than 18° C)
  Increased blood viscosity
  Abnormal blood coagulation

SIMILAR EVENTS

Temperature measurement artifact
Local abnormalities in temperature reading (e.g., esophagus cooled by topical pericardial cooling during CPB)

MANAGEMENT

If hypothermia is severe (below 30° C), especially after near-drowning
  Consider CPB for rewarming
  Monitor for and treat myocardial irritability and arrhythmias
  Otherwise apply treatment as for major hypothermia (below)

For major intraoperative hypothermia (below 35° C)
Maintain neuromuscular blockade
Maintain normocarbia by adjusting mechanical ventilation
Warm the patient using
Forced-air warming system
Radiant heaters
Heated and humidified inspired gases
Warm IV fluids
Increased temperature of the OR or ICU room
Warming blanket or hydrogel pad fluid warmers

COMPLICATIONS

Slow metabolism of drugs
Slow awakening from anesthesia
Hypotension from rapid vasodilation during rewarming
Severe shivering
Can increase O_2 consumption by up to 800%
Coagulation abnormalities
Dermal injury due to temperature gradients between tissues and warming devices
Myocardial ischemia secondary to CO increases to meet tissue demands
Arrhythmias

SUGGESTED READING

1. Díaz M, Becker DE. Thermoregulation: physiological and clinical considerations during sedation and general anesthesia. Anesth Prog 2010;57:25-33.
2. Sessler DI. Temperature monitoring. In: Miller RD, editor. Miller's anesthesia. 6th ed. Philadelphia: Churchill Livingstone; 2005. p. 1571-97.

45 Malignant Hyperthermia

DEFINITION

Malignant hyperthermia (MH) is a lethal disorder of skeletal muscle metabolism triggered by volatile anesthetics or succinylcholine.

ETIOLOGY

MH is usually an inherited disorder (autosomal dominant with partial penetrance and variable expressivity), but spontaneous mutations can occur
Certain drugs can trigger MH in susceptible patients
Succinylcholine
Volatile anesthetic agents
Exercise or stress (including the stress of surgery) alone can trigger MH in susceptible individuals

TYPICAL SITUATIONS

In patients with a history (or a family history) of a prior episode of MH
In patients with masseter spasm following administration of succinylcholine
MH is more common in pediatric patients
In association with certain congenital abnormalities (strabismus, musculoskeletal deformities, central core disease, hypokalemic periodic paralysis)

PREVENTION

Obtain an anesthetic history for the patient and the patient's family
Use a nontriggering anesthetic for known susceptible individuals or if the history is suggestive of MH susceptibility
    Includes patients with a history of exercise-induced or heat-induced rhabdomyolysis

MANIFESTATIONS

MH may occur in the OR, in the PACU, or after discharge from the PACU. Approximately 50% of MH events occur in patients previously exposed to general anesthesia.
Initial sign of MH may be masseter muscle rigidity (MMR) after succinylcholine
    Observe such patients carefully for further signs of MH
Unexplained tachycardia, hypertension, cardiovascular instability, and arrhythmias
Increased CO_2 production resulting in
    Increased ET CO_2 and $PaCO_2$
        Tachypnea in spontaneously ventilating patient, overbreathing of ventilator in nonparalyzed patient being mechanically ventilated
        Rapid exhaustion of CO_2 absorbent, increased heat production in soda lime container
Muscle rigidity
Hyperthermia
    A late manifestation
    Core temperature may increase by up to $1°$ C every 5 minutes, and reach a value as high as $45°$ C
Hypoxemia
Abnormal laboratory values
    Lactic acidosis
    Hyperkalemia
    Markedly elevated serum CK
    Myoglobinuria secondary to rhabdomyolysis
Sweating

SIMILAR EVENTS

Monitor artifact (temperature, ET CO_2)
Light anesthesia
Fever secondary to
    Infection (see Event 13, The Septic Patient)
    Hyperthyroidism

Pheochromocytoma

Infected IV fluids or blood products

Inadvertent overheating of the patient by warming devices

Drug reactions causing tachycardia or hyperthermia (neuroleptic malignant syndrome, MAO inhibitors, cocaine, methamphetamines, atropine, scopolamine)

Elevated ET CO_2 for other reasons (see Event 32, Hypercarbia)

Injury to the hypothalamic thermoregulatory center

Muscle rigidity (see Event 98, Masseter Muscle Rigidity)

MANAGEMENT

If MH is suspected (tachycardia, hypercarbia, muscle rigidity, hyperthermia)

Confirm the diagnosis of MH

Check the ECG (HR arrhythmias)

Check O_2 saturation

Check ET CO_2 and its response to hyperventilation

Check temperature, place a temperature probe if necessary, feel temperature of skin and CO_2 absorber

Draw an ABG sample to look for combined respiratory and metabolic acidosis

If uncertain of diagnosis, err on the side of caution by treating MH

Once the diagnosis of MH is made

Declare an MH emergency

Notify the surgeons and nurses, and terminate the surgical procedure as soon as feasible

Call for additional help

Call for the MH kit

Turn off volatile anesthetic agents and N_2O, administer 100% O_2

Intubate the trachea if not already established

Hyperventilate patient with **HIGH** fresh gas flow (10 to 15 L/min)

Do not replace anesthesia workstation as it distracts from primary treatment

Assign one or more individuals to mix dantrolene; it is lifesaving and takes precedence over other supportive measures

Dantrolene comes as a lyophilized powder; each vial contains 20 mg dantrolene and 3 g mannitol (pH 9)

Each vial must be reconstituted with **60 mL sterile water**

Multiple vials will be needed for an older child or an adult

Administer dantrolene IV bolus, 2.5 mg/kg

Administer further doses of dantrolene as necessary, titrated to the HR muscle rigidity, and temperature, to a maximum of 10 mg/kg

Initiate cooling if temperature is elevated

Place core temperature probes (esophageal, nasal, bladder)

Surface cooling with ice packs to axillae and/or groin

Administer cold IV solutions

Gastric or rectal lavage with cold solution

Consider cold peritoneal lavage, especially with access to the peritoneum

Consider cooling via CPB

STOP COOLING WHEN CORE TEMPERATURE REACHES 38° C

Administer $NaHCO_3$ IV, 1 to 2 mEq/kg initially, then as indicated by ABG results

Correct hyperkalemia (see Event 40, Hyperkalemia)

   $CaCl_2$ 10% IV, 500-1000 mg

   $NaHCO_3$ IV, 50-100 mEq

   Furosemide IV, 5 to 20 mg

   IV glucose and insulin

      Dextrose IV 50%, 25 g

      Regular insulin IV, 10 units

Treat myocardial arrhythmias

   Correcting metabolic abnormalities will usually correct the arrhythmias

   Lidocaine IV, 1 to 1.5 mg/kg, is safe to use

   DO NOT USE CALCIUM CHANNEL BLOCKERS (may cause hyperkalemia or cardiac arrest in presence of dantrolene)

Place a urinary catheter

   If there is decreased urine output or if there is evidence of myoglobinuria, force a diuresis (goal is urine output of at least 2 mL/kg/hr to minimize risk of renal tubular injury from rhabdomyolysis)

      Mannitol IV, 0.5 to 1 g/kg (include the 3 g mannitol per vial of dantrolene in calculation)

      Furosemide IV, 5 to 20 mg

      Increase IV fluid infusion rate

Send blood samples to clinical laboratory for

   CK

   Serum K^+

   PT, aPTT, platelet count

Measure mixed venous blood gases if CVP catheter is in place

   MH will be associated with

      Decreased mixed venous O_2 (normal 70% to 80%)

      Increased mixed venous CO_2 (normal 46 mm Hg)

If uncertain at any time of how to proceed

   Consult the **MH Hotline (1-800-644-9737)**, outside the United States (001-303-389-1647)

Transfer patient to ICU when stable

   Watch carefully for signs of recurrent MH (occurs in 25% in the first 24 hours)

   Repeat dantrolene, 4 mg/kg/day, in divided doses for 48 hours, discontinue if no recurrence of symptoms

   Convert to oral dantrolene when patient is extubated and stable

   Refer patient for a medical emergency bracelet and counseling (in the United States contact the Malignant Hyperthermia Association of the United States at 800-986-4287 or 607-674-7901)

COMPLICATIONS

Hypothermia from excessive cooling

Side effects of dantrolene therapy

   Muscle weakness

   Double vision

   Dizziness

   Nausea

   Diarrhea

DIC
Renal failure from myoglobinuria
Interactions between dantrolene and other drugs
Death

SUGGESTED READING

1. Rosenbaum H, Brandom BW, Sambuughin N. Fluids, malignant hyperthermia and other inherited disorders. In: Barash PG, Cullen BF, Stoelting RK, Calahan M, Stock MC, editors. Clinical anesthesia. 6th ed. Philadelphia: Lippincott Williams & Wilkins; 2009. p. 598-613.
2. Larach MG, Gronert GA, Allen GC, . Clinical presentation, treatment, and complications of malignant hyperthermia in North America from 1987 to 2006. Anesth Analg 2010;110:498-507.
3. Hopkins PM. Malignant hyperthermia: pharmacology of triggering. Br J of Anaesth 2011;107:48-56.
4. Malignant Hyperthermia Association of the United States. Emergency therapy for malignant hyperthermia. 2008. http://medical.mhaus.org (last accessed August 2013).

46   Metabolic Acidosis

DEFINITION

Metabolic acidosis is an abnormally high level of circulating acid in the blood, producing a blood pH of <7.35 and an HCO_3^- concentration <21 mEq/L.

ETIOLOGY

Elevated blood levels of metabolic acids (increased anion gap)
    Anion gap = $[Na^+] - ([Cl^-] + [HCO_3^-])$
    Normal range is 9 to 13
Abnormally low blood levels of HCO_3^- (normal anion gap)

TYPICAL SITUATIONS

Lactic acidosis secondary to inadequate perfusion of peripheral tissues
    Increased lactic acid production by ischemic tissues accompanied by normal or decreased
        hepatic utilization of lactic acid
    Shock or profound hypotension
        Hypovolemic
        Cardiogenic
        Distributive (e.g., septic shock, anaphylaxis)
        Neurogenic
        Obstructive (e.g., PE, cardiac tamponade)
    Severe hypoxemia
    Cardiac arrest
    Release of arterial tourniquet or cross-clamp (transient acidosis)
Increased production of metabolic acids
    DKA
    Ingestion of medications

Aspirin (produces organic acids)
Methanol or ethylene glycol (produce formic acid and glycolic acid/oxalic acid, respectively)
Cyanide from IV administration of sodium nitroprusside (produces lactic acid)
Chronic renal failure (accumulation of urea and other byproducts of protein metabolism)
MH
Loss of circulating HCO_3^-
Diarrhea
Pancreatic fistula
Renal tubular acidosis
Early stages of acute renal failure
Large volume fluid resuscitation with NS
Hyperchloremia, low blood level of HCO_3^-

PREVENTION

Maintain CO and tissue perfusion
Maintain urine output
Avoid excessive use of NS for fluid resuscitation
Monitor electrolyte levels frequently during cases with large fluid shifts

MANIFESTATIONS

Hyperventilation
In spontaneously ventilating patient
Overbreathing of ventilator in nonparalyzed ventilated patient
Decreased pH on ABG
Decreased HCO_3^-
Arrhythmias
Decreased myocardial contractility and CO
Vasodilation and hypotension
Decreased response to endogenous catecholamines and IV vasopressors

SIMILAR EVENTS

Hyperventilation due to other causes
Laboratory artifact
Respiratory acidosis (see Event 32, Hypercarbia)

MANAGEMENT

Confirm acidosis
Obtain an ABG (pH < 7.35 or HCO_3^- < 21 mEq/L)
Ensure adequate oxygenation and ventilation
Hyperventilate to a $PaCO_2$ of 28 to 30 mm Hg to compensate for metabolic acidosis
$PaCO_2$ less than 25 mm Hg will produce marked cerebral vasoconstriction
Increase FiO_2 to 100% if acidosis is severe

Administer NaHCO$_3$ only to patients who have severe metabolic acidosis (pH less than 7.1) not associated with tissue hypoxia

Administer NaHCO$_3$ as needed to maintain the pH above 7.1 to 7.2

Administration of large amounts of NaHCO$_3$ during cardiac arrest can result in severe hypernatremia, hyperosmolality, increased lactic acidosis, and decreased survival

Administration of NaHCO$_3$ does not increase the pH of the blood when CO$_2$ excretion is impaired

Ensure adequate CO, perfusion pressure, and tissue O$_2$ delivery

Evaluate cardiac function with TEE, TTE, or with a PA catheter

Optimize CO with IV fluid and vasopressor administration

Administer vasopressors as necessary to maintain an adequate BP; goal is MAP at or above 65 mm Hg (see Event 9, Hypotension)

Optimize O$_2$ delivery

Treat anemia

Maximize PaO$_2$ (100% O$_2$, PEEP, optimize ventilation)

Consider monitoring mixed venous O$_2$ saturation

Establish the cause of the acidosis

Review the clinical course and management to date

Identify possible causes of shock

Draw blood and other cultures as indicated (e.g., urine, sputum)

Check serum electrolyte and glucose levels

Calculate the anion gap

Monitor K$^+$ carefully

Send blood to clinical laboratory to measure blood levels of lactic acid and/or ketoacids

Send blood or urine for a toxicology screen

Institute appropriate therapy for toxic ingestion

If the patient has received sodium nitroprusside and there is no other cause for metabolic acidosis, treat for possible cyanide toxicity

Send blood to laboratory to measure cyanide levels

Administer sodium nitrite IV, 4 to 6 mg/kg, over 3 minutes, followed by sodium thiosulfate IV, 150 to 200 mg/kg, over 10 minutes

COMPLICATIONS

Tetany due to too rapid alkalization of blood
Hypernatremia, hypertension, fluid overload due to fluid resuscitation
Cardiac arrest

SUGGESTED READING

1. Prough DS, Funston JS, Svensen CH, Wolf SW. Fluids, electrolytes and acid–base physiology. In: Barash PG, Cullen BF, Stoelting RK, Calahan M, Stock MC, editors. Clinical anesthesia. 6th ed. Philadelphia: Lippincott Williams & Wilkins; 2009. p. 292-3.
2. Waters JH, Miller LR, Clack S, Kim JV. Cause of metabolic acidosis in prolonged surgery. Crit Care Med 1999;27:2142-6.
3. Park CM, Chun HK, Jeon K, et al. Factors related to post-operative metabolic acidosis following major abdominal surgery. ANZ J Surg 2012; http://dx.doi.org/10.1111/j.1445-2197.2012.06235.x [Epub ahead of print] [accessed July 24, 2013].
4. Neligan PJ, Deutschman CS. Perioperative acid–base balance. In: Miller RD, editor. Miller's anesthesia. 7th ed. Philadelphia: Churchill Livingstone; 2010. p. 1557-72.

47 Methemoglobinemia

DEFINITION

Methemoglobinemia is an abnormally high blood level of oxidized hemoglobin (methemoglobin, metHgb) (in which the iron is in the ferric [Fe^{3+}] form).

ETIOLOGY

Normal metHgb levels are <1% of total Hgb

Acquired methemoglobinemia
    Exposure to oxidizing agents
        Local anesthetics (benzocaine, prilocaine, lidocaine)
        Antibiotics (trimethoprim, dapsone, sulfonamides)
        Other drugs (nitrates, metoclopramide, phenytoin, aniline dyes, bromates, chlorates)
Congenital methemoglobinemia
    NADH metHgb reductase deficiency
    Abnormal Hgb (e.g., Hgb M, Hgb H)
    Glucose-6-phosphate dehydrogenase (G6PD) deficiency

TYPICAL SITUATIONS

Excessive local anesthetic administration
    Topicalization of mucous membranes with benzocaine
Antibiotic administration
Environmental exposure to dyes

PREVENTION

Keep local anesthetic dose within recommended guidelines
Avoid excess administration of topical local anesthetics (especially benzocaine spray, EMLA cream)

MANIFESTATIONS

Pulse oximetry displays saturation around 85%
Arterial blood has a characteristic chocolate-brown color
Healthy patients may be asymptomatic with metHgb levels <15%
Patients with comorbidities may have symptoms with metHgb >5%
    Dyspnea, cyanosis, mental status changes, headache, dizziness, and loss of consciousness
Severe symptoms seen with metHgb levels >50%
    Chest pain, arrhythmias, seizures, coma, and death

SIMILAR EVENTS

Hypoxemia (see Event 10, Hypoxemia)
Congenital heart disease
CHF

Shock (see Event 13, The Septic Patient)
Hypothermia (see Event 44, Hypothermia)
Carbon monoxide poisoning

MANAGEMENT

Ensure adequate oxygenation and ventilation
Stop administration of oxidizing agent, if known
    Wash or wipe off topical local anesthetic
Send blood sample to lab for ABGs and cooximetry
    Specifically request measurement of metHgb
Administer methylene blue IV, 1% solution 1 to 2 mg/kg over 5 minutes
    Do not use in patients with G6PD deficiency
    Alternatives for patients with G6PD deficiency or when methylene blue is ineffective are
        exchange transfusion and hyperbaric O_2 treatment
Obtain a baseline 12-lead ECG
Check troponin levels
In severe cases, admit to ICU for cardiac monitoring for 24 hours
Watch for recurrence, which can occur up to 24 hours from exposure, especially if caus-
ative agent is in depot or slow-release formulation

COMPLICATIONS

Hypoxemic organ dysfunction
Encephalopathy
Seizures
Myocardial ischemia/infarction

SUGGESTED READING

1. Dahshan A, Donovan GK. Severe methemoglobinemia complicating topical benzocaine use during endoscopy in a toddler: a case report and review of the literature. Pediatrics 2006;117:e806-9.
2. Groeper K, Katcher K, Tobias JD. Anesthetic management of a patient with methemoglobinemia. South Med J 2003;96:504-9.
3. Skold A, Cosco DL, Klein R. Methemoglobinemia: pathogenesis, diagnosis, and management. South Med J 2011;104:757-61.

48 Oliguria

DEFINITION

Oliguria is urine production below 0.5 mL/kg/hr for more than 2 hours.

ETIOLOGY

Decreased renal perfusion
Primary renal failure
Increased secretion of vasopressin
Obstruction or diversion of urine outflow

TYPICAL SITUATIONS

During surgical procedures involving large amounts of blood loss or fluid shifts
    Inadequate fluid replacement
    Hypotension
During laparoscopic surgery
When vasopressin production is stimulated by anesthesia or surgery
    Surgical stress
    Administration of opioids or other drugs
    Positive pressure ventilation or application of PEEP
When aortic or renal artery flow is impaired
    Cross-clamping of the aorta (above or below the renal arteries)
    Renal artery stenosis
Patients with CHF or myocardial dysfunction
Patients with renal failure
Surgery on or near the bladder or ureters
Patients who are hypovolemic following bowel preparation
Patients with trauma or shock

PREVENTION

Identify patients with diseases that make them at high risk of oliguria
    Postpone elective surgery until the underlying diseases can be treated appropriately
    Monitor urine output and the cardiovascular system carefully if surgery is necessary
Maintain normal circulating fluid volume and CO during anesthesia and surgery
    Insensible losses and fluid shifts to the "third space" are often underestimated

MANIFESTATIONS

Urine output below 0.5 mL/kg/hr
Empty bladder (if visible or palpable)

SIMILAR EVENTS

Failure to drain urine from the bladder
    Obstructed urinary catheter or collecting tubing
    Urine pooling at dome of bladder (e.g., Trendelenburg position)
    Disconnection of some part of the urine collecting system from the urinary catheter to the urimeter
Obstruction or laceration of one or both ureters

MANAGEMENT

If urine output stops acutely
    Look for acute surgical events such as pressure on the bladder or ureters from surgical
        retraction
    Rule out a mechanical obstruction to urine drainage
        Ensure that the urinary catheter is still in place and patent
            Track the course of the urine collecting system from the patient to the urimeter
            Check for a kink or a disconnection of the tubing

48

Irrigate the urinary catheter

Ask the surgeon to feel the fullness of the bladder and to check for ureteric obstruction if these are in the surgical field

Evaluate the patient for evidence of hypovolemia or decreased CO (see Event 9, Hypotension)

Check for

Hypotension or tachycardia

Low CVP or PA pressure

Increased stroke volume variability or pulse pressure variation

Review blood loss and fluid administration

Consider covert blood loss, insensible losses, and third spacing of fluid

Consider a trial of volume expansion

Administer crystalloid (NS or LR) in 250 to 500 mL increments

Administer 5% albumin in 100 to 250 mL increments

Perform TEE or TTE examination to evaluate myocardial filling and function

If a PA catheter is present, expand fluid volume to achieve a PCWP of 15 to 20 mm Hg

If CO is low after fluid volume is optimized, administer inotropic support

Dopamine, 3 to 10 µg/kg/min

Dobutamine, 3 to 10 µg/kg/min

Epinephrine, 3 to 100 ng/kg/min

If CO is normal or elevated

Consider low-dose dopamine, 2 to 3 µg/kg/min

After optimizing CO, consider diuretic therapy to increase urine output

Furosemide IV, 5 to 10 mg bolus; 10 to 50 mg if the patient is already receiving diuretic therapy

Mannitol IV, 25 g bolus

Check Hgb and hematocrit; transfuse PRBCs if there is significant anemia

In cases in which risk factors for acute renal failure are present

Review the patient's history to evaluate for acute precipitants of renal failure

Shock or hypotension

Crush syndrome (myoglobinuria)

Transfusion reaction (hemoglobinuria)

If the case is otherwise routine, the patient is previously healthy, and there have been no episodes of hypotension, sepsis, or other predisposing factors of acute renal failure

Consider observing the urine output over a longer period of time

Consider administering furosemide IV, 5 to 10 mg bolus

If oliguria persists, obtain laboratory data

Send urine sample for specific gravity

If urine output and specific gravity are both low, this may be due to the kidney's inability to concentrate and excrete electrolytes

Send samples of urine and plasma for concurrent measurement of osmolality and calculate the urine/plasma osmolality ratio

Less than 1:1 suggests intrinsic renal failure

1:1 to 2:1 suggests prerenal cause

More than 2:1 suggests physiologic cause

Progressive rises in BUN and creatinine are indicative of acute renal failure

Until acute renal failure has been ruled out

Restrict K^+ intake unless the patient is symptomatic from hypokalemia

Use caution in administering drugs that are nephrotoxic or that depend on renal excretion
  Pancuronium
  Aminoglycoside antibiotics
  NSAIDs
  Iodinated radio contrast agents

COMPLICATIONS

Pulmonary edema from overhydration
Excessive reduction in preload from diuretic therapy
Acute renal failure

SUGGESTED READING

1. Stafford-Smith M, Shaw A, George R, Muir H. The renal system and anesthesia for urologic surgery. In: Barash PG, Cullen BF, Stoelting RK, Calahan M, Stock MC, editors. Clinical anesthesia. 6th ed. Philadelphia: Lippincott Williams & Wilkins; 2009. p. 1346-73.
2. Tang IY, Murray PT. Prevention of perioperative acute renal failure: what works? Best Practice Res Clin Anaesthesiol 2004;18:91-111.
3. Wilson WC, Aronson S. Oliguria: a sign of renal success or impending renal failure? Anesthesiol Clin North Am 2001;19:841-83.
4. Joseph SA, Thakar CV. Perioperative risk assessment, prevention, and treatment of acute kidney injury. Int Anesthesiol Clin 2009;47:89-105.

---

49 Thyroid Storm

DEFINITION

Thyroid storm is a hypermetabolic state caused by an acute exacerbation of hyperthyroidism characterized by high levels of circulating catecholamines.

ETIOLOGY

Excessive thyroid hormone activity with end-organ system dysfunction
Incidence is 10% in hospitalized hyperthyroid patients and mortality rates approach 20%

TYPICAL SITUATIONS

Hyperthyroid patients with exaggerated symptoms (e.g., exophthalmos, widened pulse pressure, tachycardia or AF, thyromegaly)
Common triggers include
  Discontinuing treatment for hyperthyroidism
  Overreplacement of thyroid hormone
  Surgical stress
  Severe infection or illness in a patient with hyperthyroidism
  Trauma
  Preeclampsia
  Recent radioactive iodine treatment
  Surgical manipulation of hypertrophic thyroid gland

PREVENTION

Continue antihyperthyroid and β-blocker medications up to the day of surgery
Avoid sympathomimetic medications (e.g., ketamine, atropine, pancuronium, ephedrine)
Achieve and maintain adequate anesthetic depth before any stimulus (e.g., laryngoscopy)

MANIFESTATIONS

In the awake patient
    Alteration in consciousness
In any patient
    Fever
    Cardiac symptoms including tachycardia, hypertension, widened pulse pressure, arrhythmias, myocardial ischemia, CHF
    Diarrhea
    Seizures

SIMILAR EVENTS

Pheochromocytoma
Cocaine/methamphetamine intoxication
Delirium tremens
MH (see Event 45, Malignant Hyperthermia)
Neuroleptic malignant syndrome

MANAGEMENT

Thyroid storm requires emergent treatment. Nonemergent procedures should be postponed until hyperthyroid state is controlled.

Decrease sympathetic nervous system activity
    β-blockade
        Esmolol IV, 250 to 500 μg/kg load, then 50 to 100 μg/kg/min infusion
        Metoprolol IV, 1 to 5 mg, to effect
        Propranolol PO, 10 to 40 mg q4-6h
    Administer IV fluids—hyperthyroid patients may be chronically hypovolemic
    Treat hypotension with a direct-acting vasoconstrictor
        Phenylephrine IV, 50 to 100 μg bolus, or infusion to maintain BP
    Reduce T4 to T3 conversion and promote vasomotor stability
        Steroids
            Hydrocortisone IV, 100 mg q8h
            Dexamethasone IV, 4 mg q6h
    Reduce thyroid hormone synthesis
        Propylthiouracil (PTU)
            Load PO or PR with 1000 mg, then 200 to 250 mg q4h
        Methimazole
            Give 30 mg PO or PR q6h

Reduce thyroid hormone release
    Administer one of the following:
        Sodium iodide PO or IV, 250 mg q6h
        Lugol solution PO, 8 drops
        Saturated solution of potassium iodide PO, 6 drops q6h
Inhibit peripheral T4 to T3 conversion
    Sodium ipodate or iopanoic acid PO, 1 g daily
Consider treating patient with dantrolene IV if diagnosis is in question (see Event 45, Malignant Hyperthermia)
    Administer acetaminophen or NSAIDs to decrease fever
    Obtain labs
        Electrolytes
        Thyroid function studies (thyroid-stimulating hormone [TSH], free and total T4, free and total T3)
    Treat arrhythmias (see Event 23, Supraventricular Arrhythmias)

COMPLICATIONS

Hypovolemia
Arrhythmias
Myocardial ischemia
CHF
Seizures
Renal failure
Hepatic failure

SUGGESTED READING

1. Schwartz JJ, Akhtar S, Rosenbaum SH. Endocrine function. In: Barash PG, Cullen BF, Stoelting RK, Calahan M, Stock MC, editors. Clinical anesthesia. 6th ed. Philadelphia: Lippincott Williams & Wilkins; 2009. p. 1282.
2. Klubo-Gwiezdzinska J, Wartofsky L. Thyroid emergencies. Med Clin N Am 2012;96:385-403.
3. Langley RW, Burch HB. Perioperative management of the thyrotoxic patient. Endocrinol Metab Clin North Am 2003;32:519-34.
4. Ebert RJ. Dantrolene and thyroid crisis. Anaesthesia 1994;49:924.

50   Transfusion Reaction

DEFINITION

A transfusion reaction is an immunologic reaction directed against RBCs or WBCs, platelets, or at least one of the immunoglobulins that have been transfused into a patient.

ETIOLOGY

Incompatibility between donor and recipient ABO Rh systems
Incompatibility between donor and recipient minor antibody systems
Allergic reaction to transfused neutrophils, platelets, or other blood component

TYPICAL SITUATIONS

When blood products are transfused
> Physician, nurse, or clerical error in transfusing the unit of blood product to the patient
> In emergency situations requiring rapid transfusion of multiple blood products
>> There may be time for a group-specific crossmatch only
>>> In more urgent situations, uncrossmatched type-specific or O-negative blood may be transfused

Patients who have previously been exposed to ABO or other antigens

PREVENTION

Avoid transfusion of blood products when possible by using blood conservation techniques
> Autologous blood donation prior to surgery (clerical errors may still lead to mismatched transfusion)
> Use of an intraoperative blood salvage device during surgery in which substantial loss of uncontaminated blood is likely
> Isovolemic withdrawal of blood from the patient at the beginning of surgery for later transfusion back to the patient

Ensure positive patient identification and appropriate patient serum sample labeling before sending it to the blood bank for crossmatching

Request crossmatched blood in advance of surgery when there is a significant likelihood of a blood transfusion, allowing time for a full crossmatch to be performed

Use an appropriate protocol to cross-check and verify all blood products (donor and autologous products) prior to transfusion
> More than one individual should check the patient's name and identification number and the identification number of the blood product against the crossmatch report from the blood bank

Monitor the patient for signs of a transfusion reaction when starting a transfusion

MANIFESTATIONS

The onset of a major ABO transfusion reaction is usually rapid and frequently severe. Reactions due to reexposure to a minor antigen are frequently mild and may be delayed.

In the awake patient, the signs and symptoms may include
> Restlessness or anxiety
> Chest, flank, or lumbar pain
> Tachypnea, tightness of the chest
> Flushing and fever
> Development of a rash or hives

Signs may be concealed during anesthesia but may include
> Hypotension
> Tachycardia
> TRALI
>> Bronchospasm or reduced pulmonary compliance
>> Hypoxemia
> Hemoglobinuria
> Bleeding from mucosal membranes or the operative site secondary to the development of DIC
> Hives or edema of the mucosal membranes
>> May be hidden by the surgical drapes

50

SIMILAR EVENTS

Allergic reaction or anaphylaxis (see Event 16, Anaphylactic and Anaphylactoid Reactions)

Bronchospasm from other causes (see Event 29, Bronchospasm)

Transfusion of blood or IV fluids contaminated with bacteria

Septic shock (see Event 13, The Septic Patient)

Coagulopathy or other causes of DIC

ARDS

Pulmonary edema secondary to overtransfusion (see Event 20, Pulmonary Edema)

MANAGEMENT

Stop blood product transfusion immediately if a transfusion reaction is suspected

Double check the identity of the recipient and the blood product against the crossmatch report from the blood bank

Save any blood product containers for further compatibility testing by the blood bank

Notify the surgeon that a transfusion reaction may be occurring

Call for help if symptoms are severe

Management of complications may require more than one person

Contact blood bank and transfusion hematologist for advice on management and to alert them to possible error in blood preparation processes

It may be necessary to abort the surgical procedure

Support the BP with fluids and with vasopressors as needed (see Event 16, Anaphylactic and Anaphylactoid Reactions, and Event 9, Hypotension)

Treat bronchospasm (see Event 29, Bronchospasm)

Administer corticosteroids for severe reactions

Methylprednisolone IV, 1 mg/kg

If oliguria or frank hemoglobinuria develops (see Event 48, Oliguria)

Insert a urinary catheter, if not already in place

Administer 25% mannitol IV, 0.5 g/kg

Administer low-dose dopamine infusion, 2 to 3 μg/kg/min, to promote diuresis

Administer furosemide IV, 5 to 20 mg

Treat DIC as necessary. Send sample to the lab for coagulation studies

Platelet count

PT/aPTT

Fibrinogen

Fibrin split products

Avoid further transfusion unless absolutely necessary

Obtain samples of blood and urine and send to the laboratory to establish the diagnosis of a major transfusion reaction

Demonstration of intravascular hemolysis of RBCs

Free Hgb in the plasma or urine

Repeat determination of donor and recipient blood types (on pretransfusion specimen if possible)

Coombs test may assist in diagnosis of delayed antibody-mediated hemolytic reactions but will not help in the acute phase

COMPLICATIONS

The risk of a fatal hemolytic reaction is less than 1:100,000 units of blood product transfused
DIC
Hypotension
Acute renal failure
Cardiac arrest

SUGGESTED READING

1. Miller RD. Transfusion therapy. In: Ronald D, Miller MD, editors. Miller's anesthesia. 7th ed. Philadelphia: Churchill Livingstone; 2009. p. 1739-66.
2. American Society of Anesthesiologists Task Force on Perioperative Blood Transfusion and Adjuvant Therapies: Practice guidelines for perioperative blood transfusion and adjuvant therapies: an updated report by the American Society of Anesthesiologists Task Force on Perioperative Blood Transfusion and Adjuvant Therapies. Anesthesiology 2006;105:198-208. http://www.ncbi.nlm.nih.gov/pubmed/16810012
3. Sazama K, DeChristopher PJ, Dodd R, et al. Practice parameter for the recognition, management, and prevention of adverse consequences of blood transfusion. College of American Pathologists. Arch Pathol Lab Med 2000;124:61-70.
4. Squires JE. Risks of transfusion. South Med J 2011;104:762-9.
5. Strobel E. Hemolytic transfusion reactions. Transfus Med Hemother 2008;35:346-53.

50

Chapter 9

Neurologic Events

JEREMY S. DORITY

51 Central Nervous System Injury

DEFINITION

A central nervous system (CNS) injury is any new neurologic deficit presenting after anesthesia that can be localized anatomically to the brain or spinal cord.

ETIOLOGY

Cerebral ischemia
    Global
    Focal
Cerebral hemorrhage
Cerebral embolism
Increased ICP
Hypoglycemia
Direct trauma or surgical injury to CNS
Injection of neurolytic solutions into the cerebrospinal fluid or into CNS
Epidural or subdural hematoma

TYPICAL SITUATIONS

In patients with diseases predisposing to cerebral ischemia or embolism
    AF
    Endocardial mural thrombus following a MI
    Known cerebrovascular disease
        Previous stroke or transient ischemic attacks (TIAs)
        Hypertension
        Smoking history
        Diabetes mellitus
        Dyslipidemia
        Obesity
    Pregnancy-induced hypertension
Following surgery that carries a high risk of CNS injury
    Carotid endarterectomy or carotid stenting
    Procedures requiring CPB
        Cardiac surgery
        Repair of descending thoracic aneurysm or dissection (impaired blood flow to the spinal cord)
    Craniotomy or procedures on or near the spinal cord
Following an intraoperative catastrophe with hypotension or cardiac arrest
In patients with raised ICP
In patients positioned with traction on or compromise of blood flow to the spinal cord

51

Procedures in the sitting position
In patients with anatomic abnormalities of the bony covering of the CNS
    Congenital (Down syndrome, Klippel-Feil syndrome)
    Acquired (rheumatoid arthritis with cervical instability)
    Spinal stenosis
Following neuraxial anesthesia (especially in patients taking anticoagulants and antiplatelet agents)

PREVENTION

Identify patients with conditions that predispose to CNS injury
    Optimize treatment of medical conditions (hypertension, diabetes mellitus)
    Monitor neurologic function in patients at risk
      EEG
      Evoked potentials
Position patients carefully and reassess during long cases
    Avoid extreme rotation, flexion, or extension of the cervical spine
    In the sitting position, support patients adequately to prevent traction on the spinal cord or cervical spine
Maintain an adequate cerebral perfusion pressure
    Measure BP at the level of the brain
Maintain adequate perfusion pressure of the spinal cord
    Consider placement of a lumbar drain during thoracic aortic surgery
In patients with raised ICP
    Avoid obstruction to cerebral venous outflow
    Maintain the head in an elevated position
    Ventilate the patient to maintain $PaCO_2$ of 30 to 35 mm Hg
Avoid neuraxial regional anesthesia in patients with a bleeding diathesis

MANIFESTATIONS

Cerebral injuries may be manifested by
    Delayed recovery from anesthesia
    A new focal motor or sensory deficit
    Seizures
    Subarachnoid hemorrhage
      Severe headache, stiff neck, or neurologic deficit
SCI may be manifested by
    Failure of the sensory or motor level to recede after neuraxial block
    Motor and/or sensory deficits
    Cauda equina syndrome
      Loss of bowel and/or bladder function, saddle anesthesia, lower extremity pain and/or weakness

SIMILAR EVENTS

Inadequate reversal of neuromuscular blockade (see Event 56, Postoperative Failure to Breathe)
Slow resolution of spinal or epidural block

Drug administration errors (see Event 63, Drug Administration Error)

Delayed recovery from general anesthesia (see Event 55, Postoperative Alteration in Mental Status)

Transient neurologic deficits secondary to metabolic disorders (see Event 55, Postoperative Alteration in Mental Status, and Event 54, Peripheral Nerve Injury)

Seizure (see Event 57, Seizure)

In patients with prior stroke, there may be a temporary exacerbation of previously compensated stroke symptoms in the recovery period after general anesthesia

Psychosomatic neurologic deficit

MANAGEMENT

Ensure adequate oxygenation and ventilation (see Event 10, Hypoxemia, and Event 32, Hypercarbia)

Mild hypoxemia can cause obtundation but more often causes restlessness, which may be mistakenly treated with further sedation and result in respiratory depression

Severe hypoxemia can cause coma

Hypercarbia generally causes obtundation

Check that all volatile and IV anesthetics have been discontinued

Administer 100% O_2 with high flows into the breathing circuit to enhance elimination of inhalation anesthetics

Check expired anesthetic gas concentrations

Stimulate the obtunded patient

Use verbal or tactile stimuli and gentle suctioning of the upper airway

Perform a neurologic examination

Check pupillary diameter and reaction to light

Anesthetic or ophthalmic drugs may affect pupillary size or response to light

CNS injury may alter pupillary size or might manifest as a blown pupil

Check for the presence of corneal and gag reflexes

Test the response to physical stimulation or deep pain

Check the limb reflexes and plantar responses (Babinski reflex)

If abnormalities on neurologic examination are evident, inform the surgeon

Assume cerebral ischemia, infarction, embolism, or hemorrhage has occurred

Obtain an immediate neurology or neurosurgery consultation

Obtain a CT scan of the head or spinal cord if the patient can be moved safely

Hypertension and hypotension should be managed cautiously in consultation with the neurologist

Other imaging studies may be needed to determine cause of abnormality

Further therapy depends on the diagnosis but may include

Thrombolytics or anticoagulation for cerebral thromboembolism

Surgical decompression of intracranial hemorrhage

External ventricular drain placement for ICP management

For acute, nonpenetrating SCI, consider administering high-dose corticosteroids

Methylprednisolone IV, 30 mg/kg, followed by 5.4 mg/kg/day for 24 or 48 hours

Use of steroids in acute SCI remains controversial

Rule out a metabolic etiology

Send blood and urine samples to the laboratory

Treat hypoglycemia with 50% dextrose IV, 1 mL/kg, or rapid infusion of D5W (see Event 41, Hypoglycemia)

Treat hyperglycemia, DKA, and hyperosmolar nonketotic coma with insulin therapy IV and volume resuscitation (see Event 39, Diabetic Ketoacidosis)

Treat hyponatremia (see Event 43, Hyponatremia and Hypo-osmolality)

Treat metabolic acidosis (see Event 46, Metabolic Acidosis)

Send urine or blood for toxicology screens

Check for drug administration errors (see Event 63, Drug Administration Error)

COMPLICATIONS

Hypoxemia, hypercarbia

Cardiovascular instability

Inability to maintain or protect the airway

Aspiration of gastric contents

Extension of neurologic injury

Permanent CNS injury

Metabolic abnormalities (e.g., hyperglycemia)

Seizures

Death

SUGGESTED READING

1. Stahel PF, VanderHeiden T, Finn MA. Management strategies for acute spinal cord injury: current options and future perspectives. Curr Opin Crit Care 2012;18:651-60.
2. Mashour GA, Shanks AM, Kheterpal S. Perioperative stroke and associated mortality after noncardiac, nonneurologic surgery. Anesthesiology 2011;114:1289-96.
3. Davis MJ, Menon BK, Baghirzada LB, et al. Anesthetic management and outcome in patients during endovascular therapy for acute stroke. Anesthesiology 2012;116:396-405.

52 Local Anesthetic Systemic Toxicity

DEFINITION

Local anesthetic systemic toxicity (LAST) is an adverse systemic effect of high blood concentrations of local anesthetics.

ETIOLOGY

Direct intravascular injection of local anesthetic solution

Excessive amount of local anesthetic absorbed into the circulation over a short period

TYPICAL SITUATIONS

During regional anesthesia in which large volumes of local anesthetic are administered or when there is significant potential for intravascular injection

Epidural anesthesia

Intercostal nerve blocks

Paravertebral block

Lumbar plexus block

Brachial plexus block
Femoral nerve block
Paracervical block for gynecologic procedures
IV regional anesthesia (Bier block)
Pain-related blocks (e.g., stellate ganglion block, lumbar sympathetic block, etc.)
During IV lidocaine infusion
During topicalization of the nasopharynx with local anesthetic

PREVENTION

Create "LAST Treatment Kit" and notify personnel as to its contents and location
Post a LAST treatment cognitive aid at locations where high volumes and concentrations
  of local anesthetics are used (e.g., block areas, ORs, PACUs, labor and delivery)
Pretreating the patient with a benzodiazepine will increase the seizure threshold but may mask
  early LAST neurologic symptoms
Where large volumes of local anesthetic are administered, use standard American Society of
  Anesthesiologists (ASA) monitoring during and after the block for 30 minutes
Use the following techniques during regional blockade to minimize risk of intravascular injection:
    Ultrasound guidance
    Assess the patient's response to a test dose of local anesthetic; consider using epinephrine
      ($5\,\mu g/mL$) as a marker for intravascular injection
    Use an incremental aspiration and injection technique, looking for blood prior to inject-
      ing local anesthetic
    Continuously assess patient's mental, neurologic, and cardiovascular status during and
      after block
    Any abnormality in patient status should be considered LAST until proven otherwise
    Use the least amount of local anesthetic for desired effect
    Do not administer more than the maximum recommended dose
Monitor the surgeon's use of local anesthetic for infiltration and in surgical packing
Use appropriate bolus doses and infusion rates for IV lidocaine therapy
    Check blood lidocaine levels during prolonged infusions

MANIFESTATIONS

CNS abnormalities
    Tinnitus
    Circumoral numbness, heavy tongue, metallic taste
    Nystagmus, diplopia, difficulty in focusing
    Mental status change: agitation, confusion, obtundation, coma
    Preseizure motor irritability (twitching), followed by overt seizure
Airway and respiratory abnormalities
    Airway obstruction
    Loss of airway reflexes
    Respiratory depression followed by apnea
Cardiovascular abnormalities
    Initially may be hyperdynamic (hypertension, tachycardia, ventricular arrhythmias)
    Conduction abnormalities (e.g., increased PR interval, T wave changes, bradycardia,
      asystole)
    Progressive hypotension

Ventricular arrhythmias (VT, VF, torsades de pointes)
Cardiovascular collapse—cardiac arrest
>> Bupivacaine is the local anesthetic most likely to produce cardiovascular collapse, as the cardiovascular collapse:convulsion dosage ratio is lower for bupivacaine than for other local anesthetics
>> Patients with low cardiac ejection fraction are more susceptible to the cardiotoxic effects of local anesthetics
>> Acidosis and hypoxemia markedly potentiate the cardiotoxicity of bupivacaine

SIMILAR EVENTS

Hyponatremia (see Event 43, Hyponatremia and Hypo-osmolality)
IV injection of epinephrine
Hypoxemia (see Event 10, Hypoxemia)
Inadvertent neuromuscular blockade (see Event 63, Drug Medication Error)
High spinal/epidural block (see Event 89, Total Spinal Anesthesia)
Primary seizure disorder (see Event 57, Seizures)
Anaphylaxis (see Event 16, Anaphylactic and Anaphylactoid Reactions)
AFE (see Event 81, Amniotic Fluid Embolism)
Panic reaction

MANAGEMENT

Intra-arterial injection into the carotid or vertebral arteries will result in immediate CNS toxicity, even with small volumes of local anesthetic.

Stop injection of local anesthetic at the first indication of toxicity
Call for help, get LAST Treatment Kit, and use the cognitive aid
> Severe cases of LAST may require prolonged treatment
> Patients who are healthy at the initiation of the event usually can be resuscitated
If respiratory distress, apnea, or loss of consciousness occurs
> Establish bag valve mask airway
> Deliver 100% O_2, assist ventilation as necessary
> Do not hyperventilate the patient, as this decreases the seizure threshold, but ensure adequate ventilation, as hypercapnia and hypoxemia exacerbate toxicity
Ensure adequate IV access
If there is preseizure motor irritability or seizure activity
> Administer
>> Midazolam IV, 0.5 to 1 mg increments
>> Propofol IV, 10 to 20 mg (higher doses can further depress cardiac function)
>>> Seizures are often exquisitely sensitive to these drugs
If seizures occur, cardiovascular collapse may be imminent
> **Immediately administer lipid emulsion (20%)**
>> Bolus 1.5 mL/kg over 1 minute (approximately 100 mL)
>> Continuous infusion 0.25-0.5 mL/kg/min until stable
>> Can repeat bolus dose if symptoms persist or if progresses to cardiac arrest
>> Recommended upper limit: 10 mL/kg in first 30 minutes
>> Continue infusion for at least 10 minutes after attaining circulatory stability

If seizures do not resolve rapidly
    Intubate the patient's trachea using a short-acting muscle relaxant
    Administer higher doses of midazolam
    Administer other anticonvulsant drugs (see Event 57, Seizures)
        Phenytoin IV, loading dose, 10 mg/kg, administered slowly (may cause hypotension)
        Levetiracetam IV, 1000 mg
    Administer muscle relaxant after the airway is protected to minimize peripheral O_2 consumption and resultant acidosis during seizures
        Assess ongoing seizure activity using an EEG monitoring device
Management of Cardiac Instability
  If patient arrests
    Prolonged resuscitation efforts may be necessary
    CPR as per BLS/ACLS with these modifications (see Event 94, Cardiac Arrest, and Event 82, Cardiac Arrest in the Parturient)
    Medications:
        Reduce epinephrine doses to <1 µg/kg initially; high-dose epinephrine (1 mg) might impair resuscitation and efficacy of lipid rescue
        Administer lipid emulsion (20%) as stated previously
        AVOID vasopressin, calcium channel blockers, beta blockers, local anesthetics, and higher doses of propofol
        Consider CPB for refractory cardiac arrest
            Notify the necessary personnel (cardiac surgeon, perfusionist)
            Transferring any patient in cardiac arrest within a hospital is VERY difficult; consider initiation of CPB at the location where the cardiac arrest occurred
            If CPB is not available, alert the nearest facility with CPB capability and arrange transfer of the patient
Monitor patient in the ICU for at least 12 hours, as LAST can persist or recur after initial treatment
Obtain a consultation from a neurologist if seizures do not resolve

COMPLICATIONS

Cardiovascular collapse
Hypoxic brain injury
Status epilepticus
Recurrence of systemic toxicity
Aspiration
Death

NOTE: Infusion of lipid emulsion has proved useful in the treatment of overdose of other lipid-soluble medications (tricyclic antidepressants and sodium channel blockers). Consider the use of lipid emulsion where overdose is a possibility.

SUGGESTED READING
1. Neal JM, Bernards CM, Butterworth 4th JF, et al. ASRA practice advisory on local anesthetic systemic toxicity. Reg Anesth Pain Med 2010;35:152-61.
2. Neal JM, Mulroy MF, Weinberg GL. American Society of Regional Anesthesia and Pain medicine checklist for managing local anesthetic systemic toxicity: 2012 version. Reg Anesth Pain Med 2012;37:16-8.

3. Neal JM, Hsiung RL, Mulroy MF, et al. ASRA checklist improves trainee performance during a simulated episode of local anesthetic systemic toxicity. Reg Anesth Pain Med 2012;37:8-15.
4. Wolfe JW, Butterworth 4th JF. Local anesthetic systemic toxicity: update on mechanisms and treatment. Curr Opin Anesth 2011;24:561-6.
5. Mercado P, Weinberg GL. Local anesthetic systemic toxicity: prevention and treatment. Anesthesiol Clin 2011;29:233-42.

53   Perioperative Visual Loss

DEFINITION

Perioperative visual loss (POVL) is permanent, partial, or total loss of vision during or after general anesthesia.

ETIOLOGY

Ischemic optic neuropathy (ION)
  Anterior ION
  Posterior ION
Central retinal artery occlusion (CRAO)
Direct mechanical trauma to optic nerve or compression from retrobulbar hematoma (e.g., during sinus surgery)
Retinal arterial or venous hemorrhages involving the macula or leading to optic nerve atrophy
Acute closed-angle glaucoma
Cortical blindness
Photic injury from laser techniques
Direct ocular trauma

TYPICAL SITUATIONS

Prolonged spine or other surgery in the prone position
Procedures with substantial blood loss or hypotension
Procedures performed in the steep Trendelenburg position (e.g., robotic prostatectomy or robotic gynecology cases)
Perioperative globe compression
Procedures requiring CPB
Retrobulbar or peribulbar block administration
Male gender
Obesity

PREVENTION

Not all of the causative factors in POVL are known, the following are based on current recommendations.

Consider "staging" long, complex spine procedures as two or more separate operations
Maintain head in neutral position

Avoid head below heart position
Avoid use of Wilson positioning frame
Maintain BP within 20% of baseline
Avoid deliberate hypotension
Avoid hemodilution
  Balance crystalloid administration with colloid
  Monitor hematocrit at frequent intervals
    Discuss transfusion threshold with patient and surgeon
Avoid direct pressure on globe and reassess at frequent intervals
  Consider using mirrored headrest in prone cases
Avoid prolonged CPB times
Avoid N_2O during and after intraocular sulfur hexafluoride (e.g., surgery for detached retina)
Cover patient's eyes with appropriate goggles during nonocular laser surgery
Monitor visual-evoked potentials in procedures that affect the ophthalmic artery or optic nerve

MANIFESTATIONS

Loss of vision evident after recovery from anesthesia
  Bilateral or unilateral
  Partial or total
Periorbital edema and chemosis
Decreased ocular movements
Nystagmus
Ocular pain
Abnormal fundoscopic examination
Loss of or abnormal pupillary reflexes
CRAO
  Unilateral vision loss or changes in light perception, decreased extraocular movements
  Periorbital edema and chemosis
  Cherry-red spot and pale, edematous retina on fundoscopic examination
  Afferent pupillary defect
Anterior ION
  Painless visual loss
  MRI evidence of enlarged optic nerve
  Afferent pupillary defect
Posterior ION
  Bilateral visual loss or changes
  Onset may be delayed a few days
  Afferent pupillary defect or nonreactive pupil
Cortical blindness
  Normal pupillary response and fundoscopic examination results
  Occipital infarction on MRI
Acute closed-angle glaucoma
  Presents as ocular pain and blurred vision with a red eye
  Raised intraocular pressure (IOP)
  Fixed, dilated pupil

SIMILAR EVENTS

Residual petroleum-based ophthalmic ointment
Corneal abrasion
Photophobia
Residual anticholinergic medication effects
Glycine toxicity during TURP

MANAGEMENT

Examine the patient and evaluate the severity of visual impairment or ocular trauma
    Check visual fields
    Check pupillary responses to light
If examination is abnormal, obtain urgent ophthalmologic consultation
Obtain MRI examination
Manage patient with ophthalmology
    In the absence of a treatable cause, visual loss is likely to be permanent
        The ASA Task Force on Perioperative Blindness found that there is no role for antiplatelet agents, steroids, or IOP-lowering agents in the treatment of ION
The following therapies have been attempted, but efficacy has not been proved.
    Head-up position
    Hyperbaric O_2
    Augmenting O_2 delivery (optimization of BP, hematocrit, and arterial oxygenation)
    Acetazolamide to lower IOP
    Diuretics
    Steroids
    Anterior chamber paracentesis
    Ocular massage to lower IOP and possibly dislodge emboli
    Inhaled CO_2 in O_2 to enhance retinal artery dilation
    Endovascular fibrinolysis of the ophthalmic artery for retinal artery occlusion
    Optic nerve sheath decompression

COMPLICATIONS

Partial or total permanent visual loss

SUGGESTED READING

1. Roth S. Perioperative visual loss: what do we know, what can we do? Br J Anaesth 2009;103(Suppl. 1):i31-40.
2. Practice advisory for perioperative visual loss associated with spine surgery: an updated report by the American Society of Anesthesiologists Task Force on Perioperative Visual Loss. Anesthesiology 2012;116:274-85.
3. Lee LA, Roth S, Posner KL, et al. The American Society of Anesthesiologists Postoperative Visual Loss Registry: analysis of 93 spine surgery cases with postoperative visual loss. Anesthesiology 2006;105:652.

54 Peripheral Nerve Injury

DEFINITION

A peripheral nerve injury is a new neurologic deficit localized anatomically to a site distal to the CNS, which presents after anesthesia.

ETIOLOGY

Peripheral nerve or nerve plexus injury secondary to
> Direct trauma (e.g., direct injection into a nerve during regional anesthesia)
> Ischemia
> Compression
> Stretch
> Metabolic derangements
> Idiopathic causes

TYPICAL SITUATIONS

Following surgery in which a support frame, stirrups, straps, or other mechanical device has
> placed pressure on a peripheral nerve

Surgical trauma to peripheral nerves

Direct injection into a nerve during regional anesthesia

Patients with preexisting dysfunction of peripheral nerves

Following cardiac surgery (thoracic inlet and first rib injury to the brachial plexus from sternal
> retraction)

Following surgery where the patient is immobilized for prolonged procedures

Following the use of a limb tourniquet (time and/or pressure related)

After encountering a sustained paresthesia during regional blockade

Surgical procedures requiring anticoagulation

Administration of excessive amounts of vasoconstrictor
> During local infiltration around a nerve
> During direct application of a vasoconstrictor to a nerve root

Surgical procedures involving prolonged hypotension

PREVENTION

Ensure proper positioning of the patient
> The anesthesiologist is responsible for checking the positioning of the patient by other
> > OR personnel
> Avoid pressure on the ulnar nerve at the elbow or abduction of the arm of more than 90
> > degrees
> Avoid pressure on the common peroneal and saphenous nerves by leg holders in the
> > lithotomy position
> Use axillary rolls for patients in the lateral position
> When the patient is in the steep Trendelenburg position
> > Place, protect, and secure the arms at the patient's side or on armboards
> > Place, protect, and secure the legs
> > Position shoulder pads over the acromioclavicular joint
> Carefully pad all areas between the patient and support structures

Surgical use of nerve stimulation during procedures where peripheral nerves are at risk (e.g.,
> facial nerve during ear, nose, and throat surgery)
> Do not use neuromuscular blocking agents if nerve stimulators are used

Periodically relieve pressure on the extremities or the head during anesthesia

Use the minimum limb tourniquet pressure required to achieve adequate hemostasis
> Communicate tourniquet time to the surgeon every 30 minutes for 1 hour, and document
> > this in the record

Release the tourniquet for at least 15 minutes after 2 hours

If further tourniquet time is required by the surgeon, discuss the limits prior to inflating the tourniquet, and document this discussion in the chart

MANIFESTATIONS

Loss of motor or change in sensory function in the distribution of a peripheral nerve or nerve plexus evident after emergence from general or regional anesthesia

Symptoms are sometimes delayed and rarely progress over time

SIMILAR EVENTS

Excessive spread of local anesthetic following regional or local blockade

Delayed recovery from regional anesthesia

CNS injury (see Event 51, Central Nervous System Injury)

MANAGEMENT

Perform a neurologic examination and treat any factors that might cause further nerve injury

Prevent further injury to affected nerves (e.g., pressure from cast due to secondary swelling)

Inform the surgeon of the problem

Obtain a consultation from a neurologist or neurosurgeon about management options

Discuss the situation with the patient

Review the patient's history

Identify any predisposing factors in the patient's history

Diabetes

Preexisting neurologic disorders

Hypertension

Smoking

Check for possible intraoperative factors

Tourniquet time(s) during surgery

Patient positioning and positioning aids

Intraoperative hypotension

Impound and inspect any equipment that might have been involved in the injury

Tourniquets

Positioning aids

Operating table

Peripheral nerve injuries can be classified into one of three categories

Neurapraxia is a temporary injury, frequently caused by compression. Full and rapid recovery is likely without specific treatment.

Axonotmesis is a destructive injury of the axons but not the supporting matrix. Proximal degeneration of the nerve occurs, with regeneration beginning in 3 weeks.

Neurotmesis is a severe crush injury, avulsion, or severing of the nerve. Prognosis is poor without surgical intervention.

COMPLICATIONS

Temporary or permanent loss of function of the distal musculature

Temporary or permanent sensory changes

Contractures

SUGGESTED READING

1. Welch MB, Brummett CM, Welch TD, et al. Perioperative peripheral nerve injuries: a retrospective study of 380,680 cases during a 10-year period at a single institution. Anesthesiology 2009;111:490-7.
2. American Society of Anesthesiologists Task Force on Prevention of Perioperative Peripheral Neuropathies. Practice advisory for the prevention of perioperative peripheral neuropathies: an updated report by the American Society of Anesthesiologists Task Force on prevention of perioperative peripheral neuropathies. Anesthesiology 2011;114:741-54.
3. Barrington MJ, Snyder GL. Neurologic complications of regional anesthesia. Curr Opin Anaesthesiol 2011;24:554-60.
4. Cheney FW, Domino KB, Caplan RA, Posner KL. Nerve injury associated with anesthesia: a closed claims analysis. Anesthesiology 1999;90:1062-9.

55   Postoperative Alteration in Mental Status

DEFINITION

Postoperative changes in mental status include failure to recover consciousness, responsiveness, or baseline mental status within the expected time frame following general anesthesia.

ETIOLOGY

Absolute or relative overdose of drugs that impair mental status
    Volatile anesthetics
    Benzodiazepines
    Other anesthetic adjuvants (ketamine, dexmedetomidine)
    Opioids
    Nonanesthetic CNS-active medications
        Psychiatric medications
        Antihypertensive medications (clonidine)
Severe pain
Urinary retention
Metabolic abnormalities affecting the level of consciousness
    Hypoxemia or hypercarbia
    Endocrinopathies (thyroid disorders, adrenal disorders, diabetes)
    Electrolyte disorders (Na^+, K^+, Ca^{++}, Mg^{++})
    Endogenous toxins (uremia, porphyria, hepatic encephalopathy)
Neurologic abnormalities affecting the level of consciousness
    Cerebral injury due to ischemia, hemorrhage, embolism, tumor, or edema
    Ictal and postictal states
    CNS infection
Hypothermia
Recent use of or withdrawal from drugs (alcohol, prescribed or illicit drugs)
Overwhelming systemic infection/sepsis
Psychiatric disorders (e.g., posttraumatic stress disorder)
Carbon monoxide in the anesthesia circuit

TYPICAL SITUATIONS

Following shorter than anticipated surgical procedure
Following cardiac, TURP, and major vascular surgery

In patients with compromised renal or hepatic function
Following major trauma, massive fluid resuscitation, or metabolic acidosis
In neonates and the elderly
In patients with preexisting CNS disorders
    Diminished cognitive reserve, such as dementia or Parkinson disease
    Psychiatric conditions
    Substance abuse problems including alcoholism
    Seizure disorders

PREVENTION

Identify and treat patients with metabolic or neurologic abnormalities that might contribute to impaired level of consciousness
Avoid excessive preoperative sedation, especially benzodiazepines in elderly or compromised patients
Titrate anesthetics, opioids, hypnotics, and anticholinergics to clinical effect or a processed EEG-guided anesthetic
Monitor blood sugar during anesthesia when clinically indicated
Prevent buildup of carbon monoxide in the anesthesia circuit (e.g., turn off fresh gas flow if the anesthesia workstation will not be used for a long period of time)

MANIFESTATIONS

Failure to recover consciousness, alertness, or appropriate responses to stimuli following general anesthesia
Confusion
    Agitation, restlessness, incoherence
    Disorientation
    Inability to follow commands or unintentional, uncooperative behavior
    PTSD symptoms (e.g., flashbacks)
Focal neurologic signs

SIMILAR EVENTS

Residual neuromuscular blockade (see Event 56, Postoperative Failure to Breathe)
Drug withdrawal syndromes
Drug administration errors (see Event 63, Drug Administration Error)
Stroke
Psychiatric disorders
Nonconvulsive status epilepticus
Carbon monoxide in the anesthesia circuit (see Event 58, Carbon Monoxide in the Anesthesia Circuit)

MANAGEMENT

Ensure adequate oxygenation and ventilation (see Event 10, Hypoxemia and Event 32, Hypercarbia)
    Mild hypoxemia can cause obtundation or restlessness, which can be mistakenly treated with further sedation
    Severe hypoxemia can cause coma
    Hypercarbia generally causes obtundation

Check that all volatile and IV anesthetics have been discontinued

Administer 100% O_2 with high flows into the breathing circuit to enhance elimination of inhalation anesthetics

Check expired anesthetic gas concentrations

Stimulate the obtunded patient

Use verbal or tactile stimuli and gentle suctioning of the upper airway

Restrain the combative patient to prevent injury to the patient and staff

Call for help to safely restrain the patient

Mechanical or chemical restraints should only be used to protect the patient or the staff while determining a definitive diagnosis

Reassure the patient

Carefully place physical restraints

Administer a small dose of opioid if severe pain suspected

Consider using benzodiazepines, haloperidol, or dexmedetomidine as pharmacologic restraint

Rule out a metabolic etiology

Check glucose, electrolytes, and ABG

Treat hypoglycemia with 50% dextrose IV, 1 mL/kg or rapid infusion of D5W (see Event 41, Hypoglycemia)

Treat hyperglycemia, DKA, and hyperosmolar nonketotic coma with insulin therapy IV and volume resuscitation (see Event 39, Diabetic Ketoacidosis)

Treat hyponatremia (see Event 43, Hyponatremia and Hypo-osmolality)

Treat metabolic acidosis (see Event 46, Metabolic Acidosis)

Order urine or blood toxicology screen

Check for medication administration errors (see Event 63, Drug Administration Error)

Consider reversing the effects of specific drugs

Opioids

Naloxone IV, 20 to 40 μg increments, titrated to effect

Benzodiazepines

Flumazenil IV, 0.2 mg over 15 seconds, repeat q1min until effective (maximum dose is 1 mg in 5 minutes, 3 mg in 1 hour)

Perform a neurologic examination

Check pupillary diameter and reaction to light

Anesthetic or ophthalmic drugs may affect pupillary size or response to light

CNS injury may alter pupillary size or might manifest as a blown pupil (see Event 51, Central Nervous System Injury)

Check for the presence of corneal and gag reflexes

Test the response to physical stimulation or deep pain

Check the limb reflexes and plantar responses (Babinski reflex)

If the neurologic examination suggests a focal abnormality, obtain urgent neurology or neurosurgery consultation and CT scan (see Event 51, Central Nervous System Injury)

Inform the surgeon of the concern

If the confused or agitated patient does not recover baseline mental status

Keep the environment as quiet as possible

Reassure the patient with verbal contact

Repeatedly orient the patient to time, place, and person

Keep the patient warm and comfortable

Obtain neurology and/or psychiatry consultation for continuing care

COMPLICATIONS

Prolonged endotracheal intubation
Self-inflicted injury
Prolonged hospital stay

SUGGESTED READING

1. Bryson GL, Wyand A. Evidence-based clinical update: general anesthesia and the risk of delirium and postoperative cognitive dysfunction. Can J Anaesth 2006;53:669-77.
2. Radtke FM, Franck M, Hagemann L, et al. Risk factors for inadequate emergence after anesthesia: emergence delirium and hypoactive emergence. Minerva Anestesiol 2010;76:394-403.
3. Lepousé C, Lautner CA, Liu L, Gomis P, Leon A. Emergence delirium in adults in the post-anaesthesia care unit. Br J Anaesth 2006;96:747-53.
4. Sato M, Shirakami G, Tazuke-Nishimura M, et al. Effect of single-dose dexmedetomidine on emergence agitation and recovery profiles after sevoflurane anesthesia in pediatric ambulatory surgery. J Anesth 2010;24:675-82.
5. Rudolph JL, Marcantonio ER. Review articles: postoperative delirium: acute change with long-term implications. Anesth Analg 2011;112:1202-11.

56 Postoperative Failure to Breathe

DEFINITION

Postoperative failure to breathe is inadequate ventilation or apnea following anesthesia.

ETIOLOGY

Decreased ventilatory drive
    Opioids
    Benzodiazepines
    Residual sedative hypnotic agents
    Volatile anesthetics
Residual neuromuscular blockade
    Overdosage
    Impaired metabolism/clearance of drug
    Administration of drugs that potentiate neuromuscular blockade
    Inadequate pharmacologic reversal
CNS impairment or injury
    Hypoxemia
    Metabolic abnormality
    Structural abnormality
Neuromuscular disorders

TYPICAL SITUATIONS

Altered respiratory drive
    Patients receiving opioids, benzodiazepines
    Hyperventilated patients

56

Patients with sleep apnea or COPD
Patients status post carotid endarterectomy
Neonates and elderly patients
Normal respiratory drive with impaired ventilatory ability
    Inadequate reversal of neuromuscular blocking agent
        Shorter than anticipated surgical procedure
        Recent dosing of neuromuscular blocking agent
        Compromised drug metabolism/clearance
        Patients receiving aminoglycoside antibiotics
        Parturients receiving $MgSO_4$
        Metabolic acidosis
    Upper airway obstruction, edema, or hematoma
Hypothermia
Syringe or ampule swap
Following major trauma or massive fluid resuscitation

PREVENTION

Identify patients with metabolic or neurologic abnormalities that might contribute to postoperative failure to breathe
Preoperative optimization of respiratory status of patients with chronic lung disease
Identify patients with undiagnosed OSA (using STOP-BANG screening questionnaire)
Avoid profound hypocarbia
Carefully administer supplemental O_2 and opioids in patients status post carotid endarterectomy
Titrate the dose of opioids to the patient's RR and ET CO_2 levels near the end of general anesthesia
Strict attention to labeling and identification of medications
Use the minimum necessary dose of neuromuscular blocking agents as determined by peripheral nerve stimulation
Avoid hypothermia

MANIFESTATIONS

Inadequate or absent efforts to breathe
Apparent decreased level of consciousness
    Level of consciousness may be normal if there is residual neuromuscular blockade
    Signs of residual neuromuscular blockade
        Nonsustained tetanus or fade in the train-of-four (nondepolarizing relaxants)
        Inability to sustain headlift
        Lack of muscle strength or coordination
        Maximum inspiratory force less than 25 to 30 cm H_2O
        Hypertension and tachycardia (awake but paralyzed)
Low RR and miosis after opioid administration
Signs of hypercarbia or hypoxemia are late manifestations
    Tachycardia
    Hypertension

Bradycardia
Ventricular ectopy

SIMILAR EVENTS

Failure to awaken (see Event 55, Postoperative Alteration in Mental Status)

MANAGEMENT

At the end of anesthesia, if you are concerned about the patient's ability to ventilate and to protect their airway, do not extubate the trachea.

Ensure adequate oxygenation and ventilation
    Maintain normocarbia or mild hypercarbia
    Ensure that oxygenation is maintained and that significant tachycardia or hypertension does not develop
Check that all anesthetics, both volatile and IV, have been discontinued
    Increase fresh gas flow into the anesthesia breathing circuit to enhance elimination of inhalation anesthetics
    Check expired anesthetic gas concentrations
Stimulate the patient
    Use verbal or gentle tactile stimuli
Check neuromuscular function
    If residual neuromuscular blockade is present
        Administer additional neostigmine to a maximum dose of 70 µg/kg (max dose is 5 mg)
        Consider use of sugammadex if available
    If neuromuscular blockade persists after a full dose of reversal agents have been administered
        Reassure the patient that weakness is temporary
        Sedate the patient until there is recovery of neuromuscular function
        Extubate the trachea only when there is full recovery of neuromuscular function
        Consider any synergistic effects of neuromuscular blocking agents and other drugs, including calcium channel blockers, aminoglycoside antibiotics, or bacitracin (often included in irrigation solutions)
Review the doses of medications administered and check for syringe or ampule swap (see Event 63, Drug Administration Error)
    Opioids
    Neuromuscular blocking agents
    Hypnotics
    Anticholinergics
    Epidural or intrathecal administration of local anesthetics and opioids
Consider reversing the effects of specific drugs if neuromuscular blockade is not present
    Opioids
        Naloxone IV, 20 to 40 µg increments, titrated to effect
            Monitor for excessive sympathetic response and pulmonary edema
    Benzodiazepines
        Flumazenil IV, 0.2 mg over 15 seconds, repeat q1min until effective (maximum dose is 1 mg in 5 minutes, 3 mg in 1 hour)
Inform the surgeon of the problem

56

Send blood samples to the laboratory for
    ABG analysis
    Serum electrolyte and Mg^{2+} levels
    Toxicology screen
Conduct a neurologic examination to exclude CNS injury as the cause of failure to breathe
    (see Event 55, Postoperative Alteration in Mental Status, and Event 51, Central Nervous
    System Injury)
If failure to breathe persists
    Arrange to transfer the patient to PACU or ICU for mechanical ventilation and further evaluation
    Obtain a consultation from a neurologist
    Follow the patient postoperatively for underlying abnormalities
        Plasma cholinesterase deficiency
        Myasthenia gravis or myasthenic syndrome
        Abnormalities of metabolism

COMPLICATIONS

Hypercarbia
Hypoxemia
Inability to reintubate the trachea
Postoperative pain on reversal of opioids
Hypertension and tachycardia on reversal of opioids

SUGGESTED READING

1. American Society of Anesthesiologists Task Force on Neuraxial Opioids, Horlocker TT, Burton AW, et al. Practice guidelines for the prevention, detection, and management of respiratory depression associated with neuraxial opioid administration. Anesthesiology 2009;110:218-30.
2. Chung F, Yegneswaran B, Liao P, et al. STOP questionnaire: a tool to screen patients for obstructive sleep apnea. Anesthesiology 2008;108:812-21.
3. Thilen SR, Hansen BE, Ramaiah R, et al. Intraoperative neuromuscular monitoring site and residual paralysis. Anesthesiology 2012;117:964-72.

57   Seizures

DEFINITION

Seizures are paroxysmal discharges from abnormally excited neuronal foci, which can be classi-
    fied as convulsive, nonconvulsive, or refractory status epilepticus. Specific subtypes include:
    Tonic-clonic, generalized seizures (grand mal)
    Partial focal motor seizures (Jacksonian)
    Temporal lobe seizures (complex partial)
    Absence seizures (petit mal)

ETIOLOGY

CNS injury
Hypoxemia
Drugs, including local anesthetics and alcohol
Metabolic abnormality

Infection
Pyrexia (especially in children)
Noncompliance with antiepileptic drug treatment
Idiopathic causes

TYPICAL SITUATIONS

Patients with local anesthetic toxicity
Patients with preexisting seizure disorders
Parturients with eclampsia
Patients with acute head trauma or raised ICP
Patients with brain tumors
Patients who are hypoxemic
Patients undergoing TURP surgery
Hypoglycemia in patients who receive insulin
Patients who are taking illicit drugs
Acute alcohol toxicity or withdrawal
Patients who are post hemodialysis
Patients with metabolic disorders
Children with fevers

PREVENTION

Identify patients with preexisting seizure disorders
        Question patients about drug and alcohol use
        Continue preoperative antiepileptic drugs and confirm therapeutic blood levels
        Avoid hyperventilation/hypocapnia
        Discuss prophylactic antiepileptic drug with neurosurgeons
        Administer benzodiazepines as a preoperative medication or in patients at risk of drug
            withdrawal
                Adhere to institutional acute withdrawal protocols
        Serially monitor glucose levels
Avoid local anesthetic toxicity
Treat preeclamptic patients with $MgSO_4$
Monitor for and treat hyponatremia during TURP surgery

MANIFESTATIONS

Awake patients may report an aura prior to a seizure
Generalized seizures
        Uncontrolled tonic-clonic motor activity involving most or all extremities
        Loss of consciousness
        Loss of bowel or bladder control
        Forced gaze preference
        Airway obstruction
Partial focal motor seizures
        Tonic-clonic motor activity restricted to all or part of an isolated limb
        May progress to full generalized seizures
Temporal lobe seizures
        Bizarre behavior, motions, or utterances

Absence seizures
    Blank stare, unresponsiveness
Following seizures there is often a postictal state of deep "sleep" or depressed responsiveness
    The patient may be slow to awaken from general anesthesia

SIMILAR EVENTS

Cardiac arrest may present as "seizure" or seizure-like activity
Nonepileptic myoclonus (etomidate administration)
Muscle fasciculations secondary to succinylcholine
Opioid-induced chest wall rigidity
Partial neuromuscular blockade in the awake patient
    Incomplete reversal of neuromuscular blockade
Syringe or ampule swap (see Event 63, Drug Administration Error)
Light anesthesia
Loss of consciousness for other reasons
Panic reaction or psychogenic nonepileptic seizures
Shivering

MANAGEMENT

Primary goal is the cessation of both clinical and electroencephalographic seizure activity.

Prevent traumatic injury to the patient
If respiratory distress, apnea, or loss of consciousness occurs
    Establish mask airway
    Administer 100% O_2, assist ventilation as necessary
        Do not hyperventilate the patient; hypocarbia decreases the seizure threshold
Ensure adequate IV access
Administer an antiepileptic drug
    Propofol IV, 10 to 20 mg
    Midazolam IV, 0.5 to 2 mg increments, intranasal 0.2 mg/kg
    Lorazepam IV, 1 to 4 mg increments
    Avoid overdoses of antiepileptic drugs as they may cause hypotension and contribute to depressed mental status in the postictal state
        Seizures caused by intrinsic disease of the CNS may not respond to small doses of these drugs, but seizures due to other etiologies are often exquisitely sensitive to them
If there is difficulty ventilating the patient
    Administer a short-acting muscle relaxant and intubate the trachea
    Assess ongoing seizure activity using EEG
    May require long-acting muscle relaxation to allow adequate ventilation and avoid or control complications of excessive muscular activity
If seizures do not resolve rapidly, administer additional antiepileptic drugs
    Levetiracetam IV, 1000 to 2000 mg
    Phenytoin IV, loading dose 10 mg/kg administered slowly (may cause hypotension)
    Phenobarbital IV, 1 to 2 mg/kg
    Propofol IV infusion, 30 to 200 µg/kg/min
    Volatile anesthetic agents
Treat cardiovascular complications following ACLS protocols

Obtain consultation from a neurologist
Administer $MgSO_4$ to parturients with eclampsia (see Event 88, Preeclampsia and Eclampsia)
Investigate underlying etiologies if not already established
  Check blood glucose
  Send samples to laboratory for serum Na^+ and osmolality (particularly during or after TURP surgery), toxicology screen, serum antiepileptic drug levels
  Examine the patient for signs of infection, occult head trauma, drug reaction, or new intracranial disaster
If seizures are secondary to an acute head injury or increased ICP
  Hyperventilate to reduce the arterial $PaCO_2$ to 30 to 35 mm Hg
  Administer mannitol IV, 1 g/kg rapidly
  Administer dexamethasone IV, 10 to 20 mg bolus
  Elevate the head of the patient's bed 30 degrees if possible to ensure adequate venous drainage

COMPLICATIONS

Hypoxemia
Aspiration of gastric contents
Cardiac arrhythmias
Electrolyte and glucose abnormalities
Rhabdomyolysis
Pulmonary edema
Neurologic injury from
  Refractory status epilepticus
  Prolonged hypoxemia during an uncontrolled seizure
  Too rapid reversal of hyponatremia with hypertonic saline
  Impaired cerebral autoregulation
Hypotension and respiratory depression from anticonvulsant therapy
Side effects of $MgSO_4$ therapy, including neuromuscular and CNS depression

SUGGESTED READING

1. Brophy GM, Bell R, Claassen J, et al. Guidelines for the evaluation and management of status epilepticus. Neurocrit Care 2012;17:3-23.
2. Rossetti AO, Lowenstein DH. Management of refractory status epilepticus in adults: still more questions than answers. Lancet Neurol 2011;10:922-30.
3. Turner C. The management of tonic-clonic status epilepticus (TCSE). Curr Anaesth Crit Care 2007;18:86-93.

Chapter 10
Equipment Events
JAN EHRENWERTH and JAMES B. EISENKRAFT

58 Carbon Monoxide in the Anesthesia Circuit

DEFINITION

Carbon monoxide present in the anesthesia breathing circuit

ETIOLOGY

Carbon monoxide is produced by degradation of volatile anesthetic agents in the presence of desiccated CO_2 absorbents

The amount of carbon monoxide produced depends upon the degree of desiccation, temperature in the breathing circuit, volatile anesthetic concentration, and fresh gas flow

   Production is greatest with absorbents containing strong bases (e.g., KOH > NaOH)

   Production is greatest with desflurane and isoflurane but has also been reported with sevoflurane

CO_2 absorbent desiccation is typically caused by fresh gas flow into circle system of anesthesia workstation allowing CO_2 absorbent drying (e.g., fresh gas flow left on overnight)

TYPICAL SITUATIONS

After period of anesthesia workstation nonuse (e.g., over a weekend)

PREVENTION

Use CO_2 absorbents whose composition does not facilitate significant volatile anesthetic degradation

Awareness of the potential for carbon monoxide production if a machine has not been used for some time

Develop institutional, hospital, and/or departmental policies regarding steps to prevent desiccation of the CO_2 absorbent, such as

   Turn off all gas flow when the workstation is not in use

   Change the absorbent regularly

   Change absorbent whenever the color change indicates exhaustion

   Change all absorbent (both cartridges in a two cartridge system)

   Change absorbent when uncertain of the state of hydration

   If compact canisters are used, consider changing them more frequently

   Place a date on the canister when it is changed

   If available, monitor patient using a multiwavelength pulse oximeter capable of continuously measuring carboxyhemoglobin

MANIFESTATIONS

Moderate decrease in O_2 saturation

Unexpectedly rapid change of absorbent indicator color after anesthesia induction

Unusually high temperature of absorbent canister

On emergence from anesthesia, unexplained confusion, nausea, dyspnea, headaches, blurred vision, and dizziness

SIMILAR EVENTS

Emergence delirium after general anesthesia (see Event 55, Postoperative Alteration in Mental Status)
Hypoxemia (see Event 10, Hypoxemia)
Hypercarbia (see Event 32, Hypercarbia)
MH (see Event 45, Malignant Hyperthermia)

MANAGEMENT

Use high fresh gas flow to purge carbon monoxide from breathing circuit
Confirm diagnosis
    Draw an arterial blood sample for co-oximetry analysis, looking for elevated carboxyhemoglobin (COHb)
Ventilate lungs with 100% O_2 to decrease the half-life of COHb
    Patient may require mechanical ventilation until COHb has fallen to safe levels
Replace absorbent with fresh absorbent

COMPLICATIONS

Hypoxemia
Nausea, vomiting, severe headache, syncope
Coma, convulsions
Myocardial ischemia
Neuropsychologic abnormalities
Cardiac arrest

SUGGESTED READING

1. Olympio MA. Carbon dioxide absorbent desiccation safety conference convened by APSF. APSF Newsletter 2005;20:25-9.
2. Berry PD, Sessler DI, Larson MD. Severe carbon monoxide poisoning during desflurane anesthesia. Anesthesiology 1999;90:613-6.
3. Woehlck HJ, Dunning M, Connolly LA. Reduction in the incidence of carbon monoxide exposures in humans undergoing general anesthesia. Anesthesiology 1997;87:228-34.
4. Feiner JR, Rollins MD, Sall JW, et al. Accuracy of carboxyhemoglobin detection by pulse co-oximetry during hypoxemia. Anesth Analg 2013;117:847-58.

59 Circle System Expiratory Valve Stuck Closed

DEFINITION

The expiratory valve of a circle system is "stuck closed" when the valve does not open properly during expiration, thus preventing exhalation of gas from the lungs

ETIOLOGY

Valve components are misassembled
Extra parts or foreign bodies are present in the valve assembly
Dirt, blood, moisture, or secretions contaminating the valve assembly

TYPICAL SITUATIONS

After cleaning or reassembly of the valve

PREVENTION

Ensure that only trained individuals assemble and maintain the valve systems
Conduct a thorough preuse check of the circle system and the unidirectional valves
    Check for normal appearance of the valve assembly
    Check that the valve disk moves appropriately when breathing from the circuit or when
        ventilating a "test lung" (reservoir bag)
        Check breathing circuit pressure at end-expiration during mechanical ventilation of
           the test lung
                With a standing bellows ventilator, the pressure should be 2 to 3 cm H_2O
                With a piston or hanging bellows ventilator, the pressure should be zero
                An automated machine check would probably **not** detect this problem

MANIFESTATIONS

Progressive increase in PIP and PEEP
    The increase in PIP may plateau at a high value owing to the performance envelope of the
        ventilator and to gas escaping through a high-pressure relief valve during inspiration
    The continuing pressure alarm will sound after 15 seconds if pressure limit is set appropriately
Hypotension secondary to increased intrathoracic pressure and impaired venous return
    Delayed or diminished response to injected vasoactive medications and fluids
        They may not reach the arterial circulation because of impeded venous return
Increasing difficulty in ventilating the patient's lungs due to apparent low total thoracic compliance (i.e., "stiff lungs")
Decreased or absent ET CO_2
Decreased O_2 saturation
Pulmonary barotrauma
    Pneumothorax
    Pneumomediastinum
    SC emphysema

SIMILAR EVENTS

Kinked or obstructed ETT or breathing circuit hose (see Event 7, High Peak Inspiratory Pressure)
Obstruction of the WAGD system (see Event 73, Waste Anesthesia Gas Disposal System Malfunction)
Bronchospasm (see Event 29, Bronchospasm)
Pneumothorax from other causes (see Event 35, Pneumothorax)

MANAGEMENT

Disconnect the patient from the anesthesia breathing circuit to relieve high intrathoracic pressure

Use an alternative system to ventilate the lungs (e.g., self-inflating bag or a nonrebreathing system)

> If total thoracic compliance is still low (e.g., "stiff lungs" or tension pneumothorax), the problem is in the patient, not the breathing circuit (see Event 7, High Peak Inspiratory Pressure)

If the circle system must be used

> Reduce the fresh gas flow into the circuit
>
> Ventilate the lungs manually, disconnecting the patient from the breathing circuit as often as necessary to relieve the excess pressure
>
> Attempt to relieve the obstruction
>
>> Tap the valve dome
>>
>> Remove the expiratory valve disk
>>
>>> Increase the fresh gas flow to minimize rebreathing of CO_2
>>
>> Ventilate the lungs
>
> Repair or replace the expiratory valve or valve-CO_2 absorber assembly

COMPLICATIONS

Hypotension

Pneumothorax

Following relief of the high intrathoracic pressure

> Hypertension and tachycardia due to relief of the venous obstruction and accumulated doses of vasoactive drugs reaching the arterial circulation

SUGGESTED READING

1. Eisenkraft JB. Hazards of the anesthesia delivery system. In: Ehrenwerth J, Eisenkraft JB, Berry JM, editors. Anesthesia equipment: principles and applications. 2nd ed. Philadelphia: Saunders; 2013. p. 591-620.
2. American Society of Anesthesiologists. ASA recommendations for pre-anesthesia checkout procedures. Park Ridge, Ill: American Society of Anesthesiologists; 2008. Available at http://www.asahq.org/For-Members/Clinical-Information/2008-ASA-Recommendations-for-PreAnesthesia-Checkout.aspx.

---

60 Circle System Inspiratory Valve Stuck Closed

DEFINITION

The inspiratory valve of a circle system is "stuck closed" when it does not open properly during inspiration, thus preventing ventilation of the lungs.

ETIOLOGY

Valve components are misassembled

Extra parts or foreign bodies are present in the valve assembly

Dirt, blood, moisture, or secretions contaminating the valve assembly

TYPICAL SITUATIONS

After cleaning or reassembly of the valve

PREVENTION

Ensure that only trained individuals assemble and maintain the valve systems
Conduct a thorough preuse check of the circle system and the unidirectional valves
>   Automated check of the newer anesthesia workstations should detect this fault
>   Check for normal appearance of the valve assembly
>   Check that the valve disk moves appropriately when breathing from the circuit or when
>   ventilating a "test lung" (reservoir bag)
>   Check that PIP is normal during ventilation of the test lung and that there is appropriate
>   flow of gas into the test lung during inspiration

MANIFESTATIONS

Markedly increased PIP
>   The high-pressure alarm may sound
>   Most anesthesia workstations have a default setting of 40 cm H_2O
Apparent low total thoracic/pulmonary compliance
>   The reservoir bag feels "stiff" during manual ventilation
Diminished or absent breath sounds
Decreased expired minute volume
Absent or decreased ET CO_2
>   Increased arterial $PaCO_2$
Hypoxemia

60

SIMILAR EVENTS

Kinked or obstructed ETT or breathing circuit hose (see Event 7, High Peak Inspiratory Pressure)
Obstruction of the WAGD system (see Event 73, Waste Anesthesia Gas Disposal System
>   Malfunction)
Bronchospasm (see Event 29, Bronchospasm)
Pneumothorax (see Event 35, Pneumothorax)
Endobronchial intubation (see Event 30, Endobronchial Intubation)

MANAGEMENT

**Use an alternative system to ventilate the lungs (e.g., self-inflating bag or a nonrebreath-
ing system)**
>   Maintain oxygenation and ventilation
>   Convert to an IV anesthetic if necessary
To diagnose the obstruction in the inspiratory limb of the circle system
>   Disconnect the patient from the anesthesia breathing circuit at the Y piece and activate
>   the O_2 flush
>   If the breathing circuit pressure rises dramatically but there is no gas flow from the
>   circuit, the inspiratory limb is obstructed
>   Inspect the valve assembly

If the circle system must be used
> Remove the disk from the inspiratory valve, effectively leaving the valve stuck open
> Maximize the fresh gas flow to minimize rebreathing
> Ventilate the patient's lungs

COMPLICATIONS

Hypoventilation
Hypoxemia
Hypercarbia

SUGGESTED READING

1. Eisenkraft JB. Hazards of the anesthesia delivery system. In: Ehrenwerth J, Eisenkraft JB, Berry JM, editors. Anesthesia equipment: principles and applications. 2nd ed. Philadelphia: Saunders; 2013. p. 591-620.
2. Walker SG, Smith TC, Sheplock G, Acquaviva MA, Horn N. Breathing circuits. In: Ehrenwerth J, Eisenkraft JB, Berry JM, editors. Anesthesia equipment: principles and applications. 2nd ed. Philadelphia: Saunders; 2013. p. 95-124.

61   Circle System Valve Stuck Open

DEFINITION

A valve in the circle system is "stuck open" when it does not fully occlude the inspiratory or expiratory limb, thereby permitting rebreathing of exhaled gases containing CO_2.

ETIOLOGY

The valve disk or valve ring is broken or deformed
Valve components are misassembled or missing
Extra parts or foreign bodies are present in the valve assembly
Dirt, blood, moisture, or secretions contaminating the valve assembly

TYPICAL SITUATIONS

After cleaning or reassembly of the valve
Long-duration cases with humidification

PREVENTION

Ensure that only trained individuals assemble and maintain the valve systems
Conduct an appropriate preuse check of the circle system and the one-way valves
> Check for normal appearance of the valve assembly
> Check that the valve disks move appropriately when breathing from the circuit or when ventilating a "test lung" (reservoir bag)
> Check for agreement between the tidal volume set on the ventilator and the volumes delivered and exhaled from the test lung
> An automated machine check would most likely not detect this problem

MANIFESTATIONS

Increased inspiratory CO_2
    This is pathognomonic for rebreathing or for exogenous administration of CO_2
    Observe both the digital readout of $FiCO_2$ and the capnogram
        $FiCO_2 > 0$ to 1 mm Hg
        Elevated baseline of capnogram
Increased ET CO_2 and $PaCO_2$
    Hypertension, tachycardia, and vasodilation secondary to hypercarbia
Hyperventilation in patients who are breathing spontaneously
Reverse flow alarm may be activated by a spirometer that can sense the direction of flow and is located in the limb of the incompetent valve
If the incompetent valve is in the inspiratory limb, there may be a disparity between the inspiratory movement of the ventilator bellows and the expired volumes measured by a spirometer in the expiratory limb

SIMILAR SITUATIONS

Failure or exhaustion of the CO_2 absorbent
CO_2 absorber bypass valve accidentally left in the bypass position
CO_2 absorber out of circuit
CO_2 infused into the circuit from a pipeline supply or tank

MANAGEMENT

Check for CO_2 absorbent exhaustion and replace if necessary
Check that CO_2 absorber bypass valve (if present) is correctly positioned
Check that the CO_2 absorber (disposable cartridge) is in the circuit
Use an alternative system to ventilate the lungs (e.g., self-inflating bag or a nonrebreathing system) if the ET CO_2 or $PaCO_2$ is significantly increased or if there are systemic signs of hypercarbia
    Repair or replace the valve assembly or anesthesia workstation as soon as feasible
Maintain anesthesia with IV agents
If the circle system must be used
    Maximize fresh gas flow into the breathing circuit
    Ventilate the patient's lungs

COMPLICATIONS

Hypercarbia
    Tachycardia
    Hypertension
Arrhythmias

SUGGESTED READING

1. Walker SG, Smith TC, Sheplock G, Acquaviva MA, Horn N. Breathing circuits. In: Ehrenwerth J, Eisenkraft JB, Berry JM, editors. Anesthesia equipment: principles and applications. 2nd ed. Philadelphia: Saunders; 2013. p. 95-124.
2. Eisenkraft JB, Jaffe MB. Respiratory gas monitoring. In: Ehrenwerth J, Eisenkraft JB, Berry JM, editors. Anesthesia equipment: principles and applications. 2nd ed. Philadelphia: Saunders; 2013. p. 191-222.
3. Giordano CR, Gravenstein N. Capnography. In: Ehrenwerth J, Eisenkraft JB, Berry JM, editors. Anesthesia equipment: principles and applications. 2nd ed. Philadelphia: Saunders; 2013. p. 245-55.

62 Common Gas Outlet Failure

DEFINITION

Common (fresh) gas outlet failure is the disconnection or obstruction of the fresh gas supply between the common gas outlet of the anesthesia workstation and the anesthesia breathing circuit (many contemporary anesthesia workstations do not have a user-accessible common gas outlet).

ETIOLOGY

Disconnection of the connecting hose from the common gas outlet or the CO_2 absorber housing
Obstruction of the common gas outlet or connecting hose
Failure of the auxiliary common gas outlet present on some anesthesia workstations (e.g., GE/ Datex-Ohmeda Aestiva and the GE Aisys Carestation)

TYPICAL SITUATIONS

After the connecting hose has been disconnected from the common gas outlet so that the common gas outlet can be used as a source of O_2 or an O_2-air mixture for delivery to a face mask or nasal cannulae
After cleaning or maintenance of the anesthesia workstation

PREVENTION

Use an antidisconnect device at each end of the connecting hose between the common gas outlet and the anesthesia breathing circuit
Do not connect O_2 nasal cannulae or face masks to the common gas outlet or connecting hose
    Connect to a separate O_2 source
    Connect to auxiliary O_2 flowmeter
    Connect to the Y piece of the breathing circuit
    Connect to auxiliary common gas outlet if an air/O_2 mixture is desired to avoid an O_2 enriched atmosphere
Conduct a thorough preuse check of the anesthesia workstation
Discourage nonessential activity in the vicinity of the anesthesia workstation and the anesthesia breathing circuit

MANIFESTATIONS

The reservoir bag or ventilator bellows will progressively empty
    In ventilators in which the bellows falls during exhalation ("hanging bellows"), the loss of gas from the circuit may not be apparent
When the O_2 flush is activated, there will be a loud sound of rushing gas but the reservoir bag or ventilator bellows will not fill
The breathing circuit low airway pressure alarm will sound
The low minute ventilation alarm may sound
Decrease in the O_2 concentration of the inspired gas
The signs of hypoventilation, hypoxemia, and hypercarbia will appear later

SIMILAR EVENTS

Major leak in the anesthesia circuit from other causes (see Event 69, Major Leak in the Anesthesia Breathing Circuit)

MANAGEMENT

Increase the fresh gas flow into the anesthesia breathing circuit
> This will not compensate for the leak from a disconnection of the common gas outlet or connecting hose

Switch to the reservoir bag, close the pop-off valve, and attempt to fill the anesthesia breathing circuit by activating the O_2 flush
> Activating the O_2 flush will not fill the anesthesia circuit
>> If the common gas outlet is obstructed, there will be no flow of gas
>> If the connecting hoses are disconnected, there will be a loud sound of escaping gas but the reservoir bag will not fill

Scan for an obvious disconnection or interruption of the hose between the common gas outlet and the anesthesia breathing circuit
> Reconnect the hose

Check whether the auxiliary common gas outlet (present on some anesthesia workstations) has been selected

If problem persists, use an alternative system to ventilate the lungs (e.g., self-inflating bag or a nonrebreathing system)
> Call for help to identify and correct the problem
> If necessary, replace the anesthesia workstation if this is feasible

Maintain anesthesia with IV agents until the common gas outlet is restored

Inform biomedical engineering of the failure and have the equipment inspected

COMPLICATIONS

Hypoventilation
> Hypercarbia
> Hypoxemia

Awareness

SUGGESTED READING

1. Raphael DT, Weller RS, Doran DJ. A response algorithm for the low pressure alarm condition. Anesth Analg 1988;67:876.
2. Eisenkraft JB. The anesthesia machine and workstation. In: Ehrenwerth J, Eisenkraft JB, Berry JM, editors. Anesthesia equipment: principles and applications. 2nd ed. Philadelphia: Saunders; 2013. p. 25-63.

---

63 Drug Administration Error

DEFINITION

A drug administration error involving a syringe, ampule, or infusion pump may occur in the following ways:
> *Ampule swap:* The incorrect drug is drawn up into a labeled syringe or infusion pump

Syringe swap: Medication from the wrong syringe is administered to the patient
Infusion pump error: Incorrect drug or drug dosage administration from an infusion pump

ETIOLOGY

Failure to label syringes or infusion pump
Incorrect labeling of syringes or infusions
Failure to read the label on the ampule, syringe, or infusion pump
  Mix-up of drugs with similar names (e.g., epinephrine and ephedrine)
  Mix-up of drugs with similar packaging (drugs from different vendors may look similar)
  Wrong drug in storage bin
Failure to properly dilute a concentrated preparation of a drug (e.g., regular insulin)

TYPICAL SITUATIONS

When the anesthesia professional is working in unfamiliar settings or with unfamiliar devices
When drug packaging or ampules are changed (e.g., new vendor)
When drugs are restocked
When there is time pressure or in the presence of distractions
When ampules have a similar appearance, especially if they are located close to each other in
  a drug cart
When syringe and infusion pump labels are written by hand
When syringes are prepared by other personnel
When it is dark in the OR or procedure room

PREVENTION

Check the drug name and concentration on each drug ampule carefully (ASTM standard D 6398-08)
Use drug ampules whose labels conform to ASTM standard D 5022-07
Label syringes carefully
  Use preprinted, color-coded adhesive syringe labels (ASTM D 4774-11e1)
  For emergency drugs, use "ready to use" syringes (ASTM D 4775-88/D 4775M-09)
  Discard unlabeled syringes
  Discard syringes if there is any doubt about their actual contents
Use commercially premade syringes (especially with high-potency medications requiring dilution)
Arrange drug trays to separate similar appearing or named medications
Pharmacy should notify anesthesia professionals when changing drug vendors
Use "high risk" labels for high-risk drugs (e.g., neuromuscular blockers)

MANIFESTATIONS

Unusual response or lack of response to drug administration
  Unusual increase or decrease in BP or HR
  The awake patient may complain of an unusual sensation
    Pounding heart or palpitations
    Lightheadedness
    Unexpected change in level of consciousness
    Visual disturbance
    Unexpected muscle weakness

The anesthetized patient may exhibit
>> Hypertension, tachycardia, hypotension, bradycardia
>> Unexpected occurrence or persistence of muscle relaxation
>> Unexpected change, or lack of change, in level of consciousness
Incorrect ampule or vial found to be open in the anesthesia professional's work area

SIMILAR EVENTS

Seizures (see Event 57, Seizures)
Airway obstruction
Hypertension (see Event 8, Hypertension)
Hypotension from other causes (see Event 9, Hypotension)
Failure to awaken or breathe from other causes (see Event 56, Postoperative Failure to Breathe, and Event 55, Postoperative Alteration in Mental Status)
Anaphylaxis (see Event 16, Anaphylactic and Anaphylactoid Reactions)
Failure of the IV infusion (see Event 67, Intravenous Line Failure)

MANAGEMENT

If the error in drug administration is recognized immediately after injection
Stop the IV line carrying the drug
Disconnect IV tubing from IV catheter and drain IV line
If there is a BP cuff on the same arm as the IV catheter, inflate it to slow down the entry of the drug into the central circulation
Maintain the patient's airway and ensure adequate oxygenation and ventilation
If the medication error involved administration of a muscle relaxant to an awake patient
>> Reassure the patient, provide sedation with a short-acting IV agent, and assess the need to place an ETT for ventilation and anesthesia
>> Assess neuromuscular function with a nerve stimulator and reverse neuromuscular blockade when sufficient recovery has occurred
If the medication error involved administration of a muscle relaxant to an anesthetized patient
>> Assess neuromuscular function with a nerve stimulator and reverse neuromuscular blockade when sufficient recovery has occurred
>> Maintain anesthesia until adequately reversed
If the patient is hypotensive (see Event 9, Hypotension)
Expand the circulating fluid volume rapidly
Administer a vasopressor (e.g., phenylephrine IV, 50 to 100 µg bolus)
Treat any associated bradycardia with atropine IV, 0.6 mg bolus; or glycopyrrolate IV, 0.2 to 0.4 mg bolus, repeated as necessary
If the patient is hypertensive (see Event 8, Hypertension)
Depending on the drug and dose, the hypertensive episode may resolve quickly. In particular, it is often better to wait for the effects of epinephrine (especially tachycardia) to resolve spontaneously than to treat it aggressively with β-blockade, which can lead to unopposed adrenergic effects
Administer a short-acting vasodilator (NTG IV 0.2 to 1 µg/kg/min; sodium nitroprusside IV 0.2 to 2 µg/kg/min)
Consider treating prolonged tachycardia
>> Esmolol IV, 0.5 mg/kg loading dose, followed by an infusion as necessary to control the HR
>> Labetolol IV, 5 to 20 mg, repeat as needed

Attempt to determine what drug was administered
> Check infusion pumps
>> Check to see whether infusions are running
>> Check drug infusion settings and labeling
>> Check tubing from source to patient
> Check the syringes and ampules used during the case
>> Check the label on the syringe just used to determine whether it was the desired one
>> Check to see whether one syringe has an unexpectedly low volume of drug remaining
> Inspect opened ampules and vials to determine whether an incorrect medication was opened
> Have the trash and "sharps" containers impounded to allow inspection of ampules, vials, and syringes at a later time

Treat any additional side effects of the medications that were administered

COMPLICATIONS

Awareness
Residual or prolonged neuromuscular blockade
Hypoventilation, hypoxemia, or hypercarbia
Myocardial ischemia or infarction
Cerebral ischemia
Arrhythmias
Cardiac arrest

SUGGESTED READING

1. Eichhorn JH. APSF hosts medication safety conference consensus group defines challenges. APSF Newsletter 2010;25:1-9.
2. Stratman RC, Wall MH. Implementation of a comprehensive drug safety program in the perioperative setting. Int Anesthesiol Clin 2013;51:13-30.
3. Cooper L, Nossaman B. Medication errors in anesthesia: a review. Int Anesthesiol Clin 2013;51:1-12.
4. Orser BA, Hyland S, U D, Sheppard I, Wilson CR. Review article: improving drug safety for patients undergoing anesthesia and surgery. Can J Anaesth 2013;60:127-35.

64   Electrical Power Failure

DEFINITION

Electrical power failure is loss of all or part of the electrical power supply, including the possible loss of the emergency power generation system.

ETIOLOGY

Power failure external to the hospital
Power failure internal to all or part of the hospital
Failure of an electrical circuit within the OR
Failure of the emergency power generation system or battery backup system

TYPICAL SITUATIONS

During severe weather
During or after a fire in the hospital
Following a natural disaster (e.g., earthquake)
During or after construction within or outside the hospital

PREVENTION

Ensure that backup batteries in anesthesia equipment are charged and that the batteries continue to hold charge
   Nickel-cadmium batteries may need to be fully discharged occasionally to maintain their ability to hold a full charge
Plug critical electrical equipment into circuits connected to the emergency power generation system (typically red colored outlets)
Test the emergency power generation system on a regular basis, and correct any faults that might prevent a rapid switchover to emergency power
Use an uninterruptible power supply (UPS) for critical pieces of equipment
   Check the operating manual of each anesthesia workstation and ventilator for the need of a UPS
      Some newer anesthesia workstations have a battery backup that can power the ventilator for a short time
Conduct periodic power failure drills with OR staff

MANIFESTATIONS

Failure of primary and emergency electrical power
   Room lights go off
   All electrical equipment without a battery backup goes off
   Electronically controlled or powered anesthesia workstations without battery backup will stop working
      Some anesthesia ventilators are both pneumatically powered and pneumatically controlled and will continue to function
      Most contemporary anesthesia ventilators are electronically controlled or electrically powered and will stop working
      Delivery of anesthetic gases to the circuit may also stop
Failure of primary power only; emergency power is on
   Lights and equipment go off transiently
      There will be a variable time interval while emergency generators are activating and power is restored to the emergency power outlets
   When switching to emergency power, microprocessor-based equipment may reset to factory defaults or lock up owing to power surge
   Equipment that is not connected to an emergency power outlet will not operate

SIMILAR EVENTS

Localized failure of a single outlet or circuit
Failure of an individual monitor, device, or light
Tripping of a ground fault circuit interrupter (GFCI) outlet

MANAGEMENT

Find an emergency flashlight

    A flashlight should be stored in the anesthesia cart

    Many ORs have battery-powered emergency lights

    Use the laryngoscope light to assist in finding other lights

    Use a smartphone flashlight

    Open the OR door to let in light from the corridor

If emergency power is on, ensure that all critical devices are connected to emergency power outlets

Ensure that the O_2 supply is still intact

    If not, disconnect wall O_2 hose, open backup O_2 cylinders on the anesthesia workstation, and manually ventilate the patient's lungs

If both the primary and emergency power systems have failed

    The internal backup battery may power the anesthesia workstation for a short time, usually 30 to 60 minutes

    Prolong battery life in workstations by reducing screen brightness to a minimum

    Check the anesthesia workstation to determine what systems are functional. If there is any doubt about ability to oxygenate and ventilate the patient using the anesthesia workstation, ventilate with a self-inflating bag and a separate O_2 source

        Check gas flow

            If there is no gas flow, activate the manual emergency O_2 flowmeter if available and ventilate with self-inflating bag. Send help to obtain additional O_2 tanks and regulator

        Check the ventilator to ensure the patient's lungs are being mechanically ventilated

            If the ventilator is not operating, initiate manual ventilation using the anesthesia workstation and breathing circuit or self-inflating bag

            Consider manual ventilation to prolong battery life of the anesthesia workstation

        Check that monitors are functioning

            Send for battery-operated transport monitor

Confer with the surgeon

    Consider the status of the surgical procedure and its urgency

    If the surgery is at a critical point, the highest priority for lighting should go to the surgical field

Establish monitoring of the patient

    Place esophageal or precordial stethoscope

    Place manual BP cuff and check periodically

    Palpate peripheral pulses or have the surgeon palpate arterial pulses in the operative field

    Check that routine monitors with battery backups are still operating

        Allocate available battery-operated transport monitors (high-acuity cases have priority)

Consider the need for additional IV anesthesia drugs

Ensure that OR staff and engineers are informed of the power failure and have activated the hospital disaster plan if appropriate

Allocate personnel and equipment where needed most

    Patients undergoing CPB

        Some pump oxygenators have battery backups but all have hand cranks

    Complex or urgent surgical cases

    ICU (all ventilators may be inoperative if there has been a large-scale power loss)

    Reassess allocation of personnel and resources as the situation evolves

Determine time until power will be restored, if possible

> If power supply is likely to take more than a few minutes to restore, terminate all non-emergent cases as soon as possible
>
> Do not start non-emergent cases until a reliable electrical power supply is ensured

COMPLICATIONS

Hypoxemia
Surgical mishap
Hemodynamic instability
Intraoperative awareness

SUGGESTED READING

1. Ehrenwerth J, Seifert HA. Electrical and fire safety. In: Ehrenwerth J, Eisenkraft JB, Berry JM, editors. Anesthesia equipment: principles and applications. 2nd ed. Philadelphia: Saunders; 2013. p. 621-52.
2. Ehrenwerth J, Seifert HA. Electrical and fire safety. In: Barash PB, Cullen BF, Stoelting RK, et al, editors. Clinical anesthesia. 7th ed. Philadelphia: Lippincott Williams and Wilkins; 2013, chapter 8.
3. NFPA-99. Health care facilities code. 2012 ed. Quincy, Mass: National Fire Protection Association; 2012.
4. Eichhorn JH, Hessel EA. Electrical power failure in the operating room: a neglected topic in patient safety. Anesth Analg 2010;110:1519-21.
5. Carpenter T, Robinson ST. Response to a partial power failure in the operating room. Anesth Analg 2010;110:1644-6.

65   Faulty Oxygen Supply

DEFINITION

Faulty O_2 supply is when the O_2 supply to the anesthesia workstation does not contain 100% O_2

ETIOLOGY

Crossing of pipelines with other medical gases (central air, N_2O, or N_2) during construction or repair of the central O_2 delivery system
Incorrect connector on the O_2 hose to the wall O_2 outlet
Connection of the O_2 hose and connector to the wrong gas outlet

> Failure or misuse of the Diameter Index Safety System (DISS) or proprietary "quick connect" systems

Substitution of a non-O_2 cylinder at the O_2 yoke

> Failure or misuse of the Pin Index Safety System (PISS)

Central O_2 supply contaminated with another gas (i.e., N_2O or N_2)
Supply lines to the anesthesia workstation have been reversed
O_2 cylinders contain another gas

TYPICAL SITUATIONS

Following construction, modification, or repair of the piped gas delivery system
Construction of an OR room or remodeling of an existing OR
Following initial installation or maintenance of the anesthesia workstation
Following disconnection of the O_2 supply hose from the O_2 outlet in the OR
Following delivery of bulk O_2 or N_2O to the central supply system

PREVENTION

Ensure all work on medical gas pipelines is performed by properly trained and certified
  individuals
Analyze all medical gases at all outlets following any construction or repair of the piped gas
  supply
Use a redundant O_2 analyzer with a low O_2 alarm (set to >21%) in the anesthesia breathing
  circuit along with respiratory gas analyzer
Ensure O_2 analyzer reads 100%, with pure O_2 flowing
Calibrate the O_2 analyzer as part of a thorough machine check
Use DISS connectors on high-pressure medical gas supply hoses
Use PISS on all gas cylinders and cylinder yokes
    Do not force a cylinder onto the hanger yoke
    Do not attempt to bypass the PISS
Use appropriately color-coded gas cylinders, but always check the label on the tank for content
    Color codes differ in different countries

MANIFESTATIONS

If the O_2 supply is contaminated with CO_2, N_2O, N_2, or air
    The anesthesia breathing circuit O_2 analyzer indicates an abnormally low O_2 concentra-
    tion for the setting of the flowmeters
    Manifestations will depend on the gas and its concentration that is contaminating the supply
        The low O_2 concentration alarm may sound
        O_2 saturation may fall
    The O_2 concentration in the anesthesia breathing circuit might not be increased by in-
    creasing the O_2 flow
If the O_2 supply is crossed with N_2O, N_2 or CO_2
    Rapid decrease in FiO_2 and O_2 saturation during preoxygenation, and it is worsened by
    increasing the flow of "O_2"
If N_2O is crossed with O_2:
    Rapid decrease in FiO_2 and O_2 saturation during preoxygenation or when N_2O is discon-
    tinued at the end of the case
        Gas analyzer will read high N_2O
    Crossover may not be immediately apparent if equal flows of N_2O and O_2 are used dur-
    ing the case
    Arrhythmias
    Bradycardia
    Cardiac arrest
If CO_2 and N_2O supplies are crossed
    Very high levels of ET CO_2 and no N_2O on the gas analyzer
    Tachycardia, hypertension, or arrhythmias
    Could be mistaken for MH

SIMILAR EVENTS

Hypoxemia secondary to other causes (see Event 10, Hypoxemia)
Artifact or malfunction of O_2 analyzer or pulse oximeter
Anaphylaxis (see Event 16, Anaphylactic and Anaphylactoid Reactions)

65

PE (see Event 21, Pulmonary Embolism)
Loss of pipeline O_2 (see Event 68, Loss of Pipeline Oxygen)
MH (see Event 45, Malignant Hyperthermia)

MANAGEMENT

Ventilation with a non-O_2 containing gas causes hypoxemia more rapidly than does apnea or airway obstruction secondary to replacement of O_2 with the other gas.

Verify that the O_2 concentration is abnormally low
　　Check the O_2 analyzer and respiratory gas analyzer
　　Check the settings of flowmeters on the anesthesia machine
Do NOT use the anesthesia machine auxiliary O_2 flowmeter, as this will also deliver the crossed gas
Open an O_2 cylinder on the anesthesia machine AND disconnect the O_2 and other gases from the pipeline supply
　　The anesthesia machine will preferentially draw O_2 from the pipeline even if the O_2 cylinders on the anesthesia machine are opened
　　　　Pipeline supply pressure is 50 psig, whereas the cylinder pressure is reduced to 45 psig
Activate the O_2 flush valve and fill the anesthesia breathing circuit with O_2 from the cylinder
Verify that the circuit O_2 concentration rises appropriately
　　Check the O_2 analyzer and the respiratory gas analyzer
　　Maintain ventilation with 100% O_2 until the patient's oxygenation is normal
If the O_2 concentration in the anesthesia breathing circuit does not rise appropriately
　　Ventilate the patient with an alternate ventilation system (e.g., self-inflating bag or non-rebreathing circuit), using a fresh O_2 cylinder as the O_2 source
　　If no other O_2 cylinder is available, ventilate with a self-inflating bag using room air, or perform mouth-to-ETT ventilation
Immediately alert personnel in other ORs, critical care areas, hospital engineering, and other parts of the hospital
Terminate all cases as soon as possible

COMPLICATIONS

Hypoxemia
Hypoxic injury to the heart or brain
Cardiac arrest

SUGGESTED READING

1. Malayaman SN, Mychaskiw G, Ehrenwerth J. Medical gases: storage and supply. In: Ehrenwerth J, Eisenkraft J, Berry J, editors. Anesthesia equipment: principles and applications. 2nd ed. Philadelphia: Saunders; 2013. p. 3-24.
2. It could happen to you! Construction contaminates oxygen pipeline. APSF Newsletter 2012;27:35.
3. Weller J, Merry A, Warman G, Robinson B. Anaesthetists' management of oxygen pipeline failure: room for improvement. Anaesthesia 2007;62:122-6.
4. Mudumbai SC, Fanning R, Howard SK, et al. Use of medical simulation to explore equipment failures and human-machine interactions in anesthesia machine pipeline crossover. Anesth Analg 2010;110:1292-6.
5. Rose G, Durbin K, Eichhorn JH. Gas cylinder colors ARE NOT an FDA standard! Anesthesia Patient Safety Foundation Newsletter 2010;25:16.

65

66   Gas Flow Control Malfunction

DEFINITION

Gas flow control malfunction is failure of the gas flow control system

ETIOLOGY

Leak
>   Broken or cracked flowmeter
>   Leaking seal between the flowmeter and the anesthesia workstation
>   Leaking flow control valve (no gas flow)
>   Failure of the electronic gas mixer module

Obstruction
>   Foreign body or dirt in the flowmeter tube
>   Bobbin stuck at the top of the flowmeter tube

Misleading reading
>   Bobbin stuck at the bottom, top, or inside of the flowmeter without obstructing flow
>   Worn, distorted, or damaged bobbins
>   Wrong gas for the flowmeter in use
>   Interchange of parts during repair
>   Improper alignment of the flowmeter
>   Gas leak between electronic flow sensors and the total gas outflow (backup) flowmeter
>   Artifact created by high pressure in the breathing circuit

TYPICAL SITUATIONS

After installation or repair of the anesthesia workstation
Mechanical damage to the anesthesia workstation
When initially turning on the gas supply to the anesthesia workstation or flowmeter
Failure of the O_2/N_2O proportioning systems
Failure of gas mixer

PREVENTION

Provide appropriate routine maintenance of anesthesia workstation
>   Some flowmeters are sealed units and require no preventive maintenance

Turn off gas flows at flowmeters before turning off the gas supply to the anesthesia workstation
Check that gas flows are turned off at the flowmeters before connecting pipeline hoses to the
>   machine or before opening cylinders on the anesthesia workstation

Conduct appropriate preuse check of the anesthesia workstation
Monitor FiO_2 throughout each case
Ensure backup flowmeters are functioning on anesthesia workstations with electronic flow sensors

MANIFESTATIONS

Hypoxemia (if O_2 flowmeter leaks)
Abnormal readings on respiratory gas analyzer

Different concentrations than those set at flowmeters

Presence of an unexpected gas in the inspired gases (e.g., CO_2, N_2, helium)

Light anesthesia (if N_2O flowmeter is obstructed or leaks)

Discrepancy between gas flows measured by electronic flowmeters and total gas flow measured by backup flowmeter upstream of machine common gas outlet

SIMILAR EVENTS

Incorrect calibration of the respiratory gas analyzer

Operator error in adjusting the gas flow controls

O_2/N_2O pipeline crossover (see Event 65, Faulty Oxygen Supply)

MANAGEMENT

Check FiO$_2$ and O$_2$ saturation

If FiO_2 is abnormally low, check for O_2 flowmeter leak or inappropriate flow through another flowmeter

Check that the appropriate O_2 concentration can be maintained with mechanical ventilation

If unable to ventilate manually or if O$_2$ saturation is low, switch to backup ventilation system (e.g., self-inflating bag with a separate source of O$_2$)

Call for help to assist in identifying and correcting the problem

If the FiO$_2$ is appropriate and the patient's lungs can be mechanically ventilated, arrange to replace the anesthesia workstation

Have an alternative ventilation system ready

Monitor the FiO_2, O_2 saturation, anesthetic gas concentrations, and airway pressures carefully

Check for a leak in the machine's low-pressure circuit

Visually check each flowmeter bobbin for free rotation and for appropriate rise and fall with changes in gas flow

If there is any question about the anesthesia workstation and its operating condition, withdraw it from service immediately and have it tested and repaired by a qualified technician

COMPLICATIONS

Hypoxemia

SUGGESTED READING

1. Eisenkraft JB. The anesthesia machine and workstation. In: Ehrenwerth J, Eisenkraft JB, Berry JM, editors. Anesthesia equipment: principles and applications. 2nd ed. Philadelphia: Saunders; 2013. p. 25-63.
2. Eng TS, Durieux ME. Case report: automated machine checkout leaves an internal gas leak undetected: the need for complete checkout procedures. Anesth Analg 2012;114:144-6.

67 Intravenous Line Failure

DEFINITION

An intravenous line failure is a previously functioning IV line that fails for any reason

ETIOLOGY

Obstruction of the IV catheter or tubing
    Stopcock turned in the wrong direction
    Roller clamp on the IV tubing closed
    IV tubing taped so that it can kink
    Precipitation of incompatible drugs in the IV tubing
    Tip of the IV catheter up against a valve in the vein
    Thrombus in IV catheter or IV tubing and filters
Disconnection of, or leak from, the IV catheter or tubing
Migration of the IV catheter outside the vein
External compression of the vein at a site between the IV insertion and the heart
    Because of limb position
    Because of surgical compression on the arm
    BP cuff left in venous stasis mode
    Tourniquet left in place on the limb

TYPICAL SITUATIONS

IV catheter was inserted prior to coming to OR
After repositioning the patient
    From one bed or table to another (e.g., turning to the prone position)
    On the operating table
    Rotating the operating table relative to the anesthesia workstation
During induction of anesthesia
    Failure to turn stopcocks after administering drugs
When large amounts of fluid are infused through a small vein
After a difficult IV placement
When using an unfamiliar IV administration set

PREVENTION

Carefully assess IV catheters placed by other personnel
    Determine how well the IV runs
    Look for signs of erythema or infiltration
    Observe for pain if IV is forcibly flushed or on injection of a test dose of induction agent
Check all IV lines after placement and after repositioning the patient
Use Luer Lock IV connectors
Ensure that all IV connections are tight
Secure the IV catheter to the patient

MANIFESTATIONS

Obstruction to flow or external compression of the vein
    IV infusion stops running
    High resistance to injection or forcible flush
    No blood return when the tubing is open to the atmosphere below the level of the heart
Disconnection
    IV infusion runs excessively fast

Unusually low resistance to injection
A pool of fluid or blood accumulates on the mattress cover or on the floor
SC migration of the IV catheter
Hematoma, swelling, or pain at the IV site or on injection through the IV
Lack of patient response to drug or fluid administration

SIMILAR EVENTS

Irrigation fluid or blood from the wound on the surgical drapes or pooling on the floor
Excessively small-gauge IV catheter or connecting tubing

MANAGEMENT

If the IV infusion stops
Check for a high resistance to the injection of IV fluid
Trace the IV from the solution bag to the catheter hub
Check that all stopcocks and roller clamps are open
Check for kinks in the IV catheter and IV tubing
Look for surgical clamps or surgical retractors that may be obstructing the IV tubing
Inspect the IV catheter insertion site for signs of extravasation
Check for external compression of extremity
Check for a BP cuff that may not have fully deflated
Check for compression of the arm by a surgical team member or a surgical retractor
attached to the side of the OR table
Check for tourniquet left in place
If using TIVA and the IV fails, ensure anesthesia and amnesia with inhaled agents until
IV problem is solved
If the cause cannot be found or cannot be alleviated, insert a new IV line
If access is limited and the need is urgent, ask the surgeons whether they have direct
access to a vein in the surgical field
If there is suspicion of a disconnection of the IV line
Trace the IV tubing to exclude disconnection
Check that stopcocks are in the correct position
Check that all connections are tight
Check that the IV catheter is still in the patient
If a disconnection has occurred, reconnect or replace the appropriate components
Decontaminate connectors as thoroughly as possible with alcohol or other disinfectant
**If no disconnection is found and there is pooling of blood on the drapes or floor, rule out
the surgical site as the source**

67

COMPLICATIONS

Hypovolemia
Venous air embolism
Local tissue necrosis, ulceration, or compartment syndrome due to extravasation of vasoactive
medications or large volumes of fluid
Failure to respond to IV drug's anticipated effects
Light anesthesia
Patient movement; inadequate relaxation during infusion of neuromuscular-blocking drug
Awareness

68   Loss of Pipeline Oxygen

DEFINITION

Loss of pipeline O_2 occurs when pipeline O_2 pressure drops to zero or below the operating threshold pressure of the anesthesia workstation

ETIOLOGY

Exhaustion of the hospital's central O_2 storage supply
Rupture or obstruction of O_2 piping connecting the central O_2 storage to the OR
O_2 shutoff valve to the OR or zone turned off
Obstruction, disconnection, or rupture of the O_2 hose connecting the wall or ceiling outlet to the anesthesia workstation within the OR
Failure of O_2 regulator in anesthesia workstation

TYPICAL SITUATIONS

When pipeline system or central O_2 storage is under repair
During or following natural disasters that damage the central O_2 storage or delivery system or prevent refilling of the central supply
    Electrical power, water, and vacuum may fail simultaneously
    The building may suffer structural damage
After disconnecting the pipeline hose to the machine to check "fail-safe" system
When quick-connect hose couplers are used
During delivery of O_2 to the central storage supply tank

PREVENTION

Before beginning each case, conduct a thorough preuse check of the anesthesia workstation and O_2 supply system
    Verify a normal pipeline pressure
    Check that O_2 couplers and hoses are tightly connected
    Check that backup O_2 tank(s) have >1000 psig, and then close tank valve
Arrange for hospital engineering department to notify the anesthesia department and the OR when the O_2 delivery system requires service or modification

MANIFESTATIONS

Manifestations will vary depending on how quickly pressure is lost and the type of anesthesia machine in use.

Pipeline O_2 pressure gauge indicates a fall in line pressure
Low O_2 supply pressure alarm will sound when the threshold is reached
O_2 flow in flowmeter falls to zero (bobbin drops)
O_2 flow in "virtual" electronic flow sensor shows zero flow
Flow of N_2O falls to zero as long as the anesthesia workstation fail-safe system is operational
O_2 flush becomes inoperative
Bag or ventilator fails to fill completely

Loss of ventilator pneumatic drive
Hiss from leak or partial disconnection in O_2 couplers or hoses
Late signs
    Apnea alarms on spirometer and capnograph
    Decrease in FiO_2 as remaining O_2 in circuit is consumed
    Signs of hypoxemia and hypercarbia

SIMILAR EVENTS

Major leak from the anesthesia breathing circuit (see Event 69, Major Leak in the Anesthesia
    Breathing Circuit)
Isolated N_2O failure
Failure of the O_2 flush valve
Failure of the O_2 flowmeter or gauge (see Event 66, Gas Flow Control Malfunction)

MANAGEMENT

Verify loss of O_2 supply
    Check pipeline pressure gauge
    Check function of O_2 flush
    Check O_2 flowmeter
    Check O_2 analyzer for hypoxic gas mixture
Open O_2 tank on the anesthesia machine
If O_2 tank is empty
    Obtain a replacement O_2 tank and additional O_2 tanks for backup
    Close the breathing circuit pop-off valve (converts to closed circuit)
    Ventilate manually using reservoir bag with gas contained in circle system
        Refill the volume of reservoir bag as necessary with your own breath
Switch to self-inflating bag or nonrebreathing circuit if a separate O_2 tank is available
Use self-inflating bag with room air, or mouth-to-ETT ventilation only if absolutely necessary
Switch to IV agents to maintain anesthesia if anesthesia workstation cannot be used
Notify surgeon of problem
Notify OR personnel and have them check other ORs for O_2 failure
If O_2 tank is full
    Use manual ventilation to conserve O_2, because O_2 is used to drive the bellows in pneu-
        matic ventilators
        On some workstations (e.g., GE Aisys) that have a supply of compressed air (pipe-
            line or tank), if O_2 supply fails, ventilator drive gas source automatically switches
            to air and workstation will deliver air via its flowmeter to the common gas outlet
            and breathing circuit
    Call for additional O_2 tanks as backups
Check hoses, couplers, anesthesia workstation, and in-room shutoff valve
    Hoses may be kinked by the wheels of the anesthesia workstation or other equipment
    Couplers may be partially disconnected
    Notify biomedical engineering or machine service technician if there is a failure in an
        anesthesia workstation, hose, coupler, or in-room shutoff valve
If the failure is not isolated to a single anesthesia workstation hose, or coupler
    Notify hospital engineering
    Do not start elective cases until the problem has been resolved

68

COMPLICATIONS

Hypoxemia
Hypercarbia
Light anesthesia, patient recall of intraoperative events

SUGGESTED READING

1. Schumacher SD, Brockwell RC, Andrews JJ, Ogles D. Bulk liquid oxygen supply failure. Anesthesiology 2004;100:186-9.
2. Malayaman SN, Mychaskiw G, Ehrenwerth J. Medical gases: storage and supply. In: Ehrenwerth J, Eisenkraft JB, Berry JM, editors. Anesthesia equipment: principles and applications. 2nd ed. Philadelphia: Saunders; 2013. p. 3-24.
3. Lorraway PG, Salvoldelli GL, Joo HS, et al. Management of simulated oxygen supply failure: is there a gap in the curriculum? Anesth Analg 2006;102:865-7.
4. Eisenkraft JB. The anesthesia machine and workstation. In: Ehrenwerth J, Eisenkraft JB, Berry JM, editors. Anesthesia equipment: principles and applications. 2nd ed. Philadelphia: Saunders; 2013. p. 25-63.

69   Major Leak in the Anesthesia Breathing Circuit

DEFINITION

A major leak has occurred when there is a significant loss of gas from the anesthesia workstation or breathing circuit

ETIOLOGY

Ventilator/bag selector switch or pop-off valve in the wrong position for positive pressure ventilation
Leak in the anesthesia breathing circuit
    Disconnection of any component of the breathing circuit (e.g., ETT disconnect, gas sampling line open)
    Structural failure of, or defect in, an anesthesia breathing circuit
Leak in or around the ETT
    ETT not in the trachea
    ETT cuff does not seal the trachea
    Hole or laceration in the ETT itself or in the ETT cuff
    Placement of a NGT into the trachea
Leak in the low-pressure system of the anesthesia workstation
    Component failure
    Disconnection
Leak from the lungs
    Pneumothorax
    Bronchopleural-cutaneous fistula

TYPICAL SITUATIONS

When the patient's position is changed
    Moving the operating table relative to the anesthesia workstation

Moving the patient from one bed or table to another
During manipulation of the head and neck
When the airway is shared with the surgeon
After changing components of the anesthesia breathing circuit
When first initiating positive pressure ventilation
After a difficult endotracheal intubation or the use of Magill forceps to guide the ETT
After the common gas outlet has been disconnected to provide a source of O_2 for a face mask
or nasal cannula, or use of an auxiliary common gas outlet
After service of the anesthesia workstation
After the CO_2 absorbent has been changed

PREVENTION

Perform a thorough preuse check of the anesthesia workstation and breathing circuit
    Perform a positive-pressure leak test of the anesthesia breathing circuit
        Repeat the test after any component of the breathing circuit has been changed
    Perform a low-pressure system leak test on the anesthesia workstation and ventilator
        Turn on any vaporizer and flowmeter that may be used during anesthesia
    Test the integrity of the ETT cuff for leaks
Following endotracheal intubation, inflate the ETT cuff to minimal occlusion volume and
check carefully for leaks around the cuff
Check again for leaks around the cuff and for changes in the position of the ETT after any
movement of the patient or the ETT
Check the position of the ventilator/bag selector switch and pop-off valve before initiating
mechanical ventilation
Have an appropriate range of ETT sizes available

MANIFESTATIONS

During spontaneous ventilation
    An abnormally high fresh gas flow is required to fill the reservoir bag between each
breath
    Signs of light anesthesia
        Tachycardia
        Hypertension
        Movement
    Strong odor of volatile anesthetic agent
    Capnograph may appear abnormal
During positive pressure ventilation
    Leaking gas may be heard
    No breath sounds or abnormal breath sounds heard through the esophageal or precordial
stethoscope
    Decreased or zero PIP
    Decreased or zero expiratory gas flow measured by a spirometer in the expiratory limb of
the anesthesia breathing circuit
        Expired volume will be significantly less than inspired volume
    Little or no ET CO_2
    Patient's chest does not rise with inspiration
    Ventilator bellows either does not refill at an appropriate rate during exhalation or col-
lapses (only for a bellows that normally ascends during exhalation)

69

Abnormally high fresh gas flow required to prevent bellows from collapsing

Alteration of tone of the ventilator if the bellows empties completely and is compressed against the bottom of the housing

ETT may be visualized outside the trachea

SIMILAR EVENTS

Low fresh gas flow in the presence of a small leak from the anesthesia breathing circuit

Unplanned extubation (see Event 37, Unplanned Extubation)

Failure of the ventilator or bellows to operate correctly (see Event 71, Ventilator Failure)

Tracheobronchial gas leak during thoracic surgery (see Event 35, Pneumothorax)

MANAGEMENT

Maintain adequate ventilation and oxygenation of the patient at all times

Switch to an alternative system for ventilation (e.g., self-inflating bag or nonrebreathing circuit) and call for help early if the leak cannot be found and resolved quickly

During Spontaneous Ventilation

Close the pop-off valve

Increase the fresh gas flow into the circuit

The reservoir bag should fill

If the reservoir bag does not fill

Activate the O_2 flush

A major leak should become apparent

Check for and tighten loose connections

Switch to an alternative circuit (e.g., nonrebreathing circuit) if the leak cannot be identified or corrected quickly

During Positive Pressure Ventilation

Increase the fresh gas flow into the anesthesia breathing circuit

If the leak can be compensated for, continue positive pressure ventilation while determining the cause of the leak

Switch to the reservoir bag, close the pop-off valve, and attempt to fill the anesthesia breathing circuit by activating the O_2 flush

If the reservoir bag fills, ventilate the patient's lungs

Check the compliance of the reservoir bag and look for the rise of the chest on inspiration

Listen for breath sounds and look for a CO_2 waveform on the capnograph

If manual ventilation is possible

Continue manual ventilation

Call for help to identify the leak, which is probably in the ventilator circuit

If the reservoir bag fills but there is still a leak with positive pressure ventilation

Ventilate with a self-inflating bag

Call for help

Listen for a leak around the ETT during inspiration

If there is a leak, add air to the ETT cuff to determine whether the leak can be stopped

If there is still a leak

Assess the position and integrity of the ETT (see Event 37, Unplanned Extubation)

Perform direct or videolaryngoscopy

Consider removing the ETT, ventilating the patient's lungs by mask with the alternative ventilation system, and replacing the ETT

Perform high pressure leak test of the anesthesia breathing circuit by occluding the Y piece and activating the O_2 flush

If the breathing circuit can be pressurized and maintain pressure, the problem is either in the ETT, in the ETT cuff, or in the patient

If the leak persists after all mechanical components have been checked, evaluate the patient for a possible pneumothorax or bronchopleural-cutaneous fistula

A bronchopleural fistula may only be apparent after chest tubes are connected to suction

If the reservoir bag does not fill when the O_2 flush is activated

Scan for an obvious disconnection

The connection of the anesthesia breathing circuit to the ETT

The connection of the anesthesia breathing circuit to the common gas outlet

Sites at which external devices such as spirometers and respiratory gas analyzers are connected to the anesthesia breathing circuit

Use a self-inflating bag to ventilate the patient's lungs

Call for help to identify the leak

Check the O_2 pipeline pressure and the function of the O_2 flowmeter

If the pipeline pressure is low, open the O_2 cylinder on the anesthesia workstation

Check for a vaporizer leak

Feel for a gas leak around the vaporizer mountings

Turn off the vaporizer and check for a persistent leak

If all the previous are normal, consider an internal malfunction in the anesthesia workstation

Continue to ventilate the patient using the self-inflating bag

Replace the anesthesia workstation

Maintain anesthesia with IV agents

Inform biomedical engineering of the failure and have the equipment inspected by a biomedical engineer

COMPLICATIONS

Hypoventilation
Hypoxemia
Hypercarbia
Accidental extubation

SUGGESTED READING

1. Raphael DT, Weller RS, Doran DJ. A response algorithm for the low pressure alarm condition. Anesth Analg 1988;67:876-83.
2. Seif DM, Olympio MA. Expiratory limb ventilation during unique failure of the anesthesia machine breathing circuit. Anesthesiology 2013;118:751-3.
3. Gravenstein D, Wikhu H, Liem EB, Tilman S, Lampotang S. Aestiva ventilation mode selector switch failures. Anesth Analg 2007;104:860-2.

70   Pop-Off Valve Failure

DEFINITION

A pop-off (adjustable pressure limiting [APL]) valve failure in the anesthesia breathing circuit

ETIOLOGY

Pop-off valve inappropriately left open or closed by the user
Failure of the pop-off valve control knob
Internal failure in the pop-off valve mechanism
Failure of the ventilator pressure relief valve (internal "pop-off" valve of the ventilator)

TYPICAL SITUATIONS

After switching from manual ventilation to mechanical ventilation or vice versa (user error)
Mechanical failure of the pop-off valve
After service of breathing circuit components or the ventilator

PREVENTION

Conduct a thorough preuse check of the anesthesia breathing circuit
  Set the ventilator/bag selector switch to BAG and occlude the breathing circuit at the Y piece
  Close the circuit pop-off valve, and pressurize the anesthesia circuit. Ensure that pressure builds up in the circuit (this discloses a pop-off valve that is stuck open)
  Open the circuit pop-off valve fully and ensure that there is a decrease in circuit pressure to 1 to 2 cm H_2O (this checks for a circuit pop-off valve that is stuck closed or a failure of the control knob)
  Increase the fresh gas flow rate to 10 L/min and check for any increase in circuit pressure (an increase in pressure would indicate either a faulty pressure gauge or a partially closed circuit pop-off valve)
  Set the ventilator/bag selector switch to VENTILATOR, maintain the fresh gas flow at 10 L/min, and ventilate a test lung (reservoir bag). Check for any increase in circuit pressure during the expiratory phase (an increase in pressure indicates either a faulty pressure gauge or a closed ventilator pressure relief valve)
Open the pop-off valve and observe the anesthesia circuit while preoxygenating the patient and maintaining a tight seal between the mask and the patient's face
  Ensure that inspiratory and expiratory unidirectional valves move appropriately and that circuit pressure does not rise to more than 1 to 2 cm H_2O

MANIFESTATIONS

Circuit Pop-Off Valve Stuck Closed or Inappropriately Set to CLOSED
If the ventilator/bag selector switch is on BAG (the relevant pop-off valve is in the breathing circuit)
  Progressive increase in PIP and PEEP
    The increase in PIP may plateau at a high value owing to gas escaping through a high-pressure relief mechanism in the pop-off valve. This occurs at 70 to 80 cm H_2O

The sustained pressure alarm will sound if set appropriately

Increasing distention of the reservoir bag

The awake patient will complain of difficulty breathing

Hypotension secondary to increased intrathoracic pressure and impaired venous return

Lack of response to injected vasoactive medications because drugs may be slow to reach the arterial circulation secondary to decreased venous return

Progressive difficulty in ventilating the patient's lungs due to apparent low total thoracic compliance (i.e., "stiff lungs")

Decreased or absent ET CO_2

Decreased O_2 saturation

Pulmonary barotrauma

Pneumothorax

Pneumomediastinum

SC emphysema

If the ventilator/bag selector switch is on VENTILATOR (the relevant pressure relief valve is internal to the ventilator)

The same manifestations listed previously, PLUS

Unusual sound of the pneumatic ventilator as it struggles to work against the increased circuit pressure

Decreased tidal volume (the performance of most ventilators degrades as the circuit pressure increases)

Circuit or Ventilator Pop-Off Valve Stuck Open or Inappropriately Set to OPEN

If the patient is breathing spontaneously, the reservoir bag may fail to fill adequately

If the patient's lungs are being mechanically ventilated

There will be a major leak during inspiration

The ventilator standing bellows will fall or the reservoir bag will collapse, making ventilation impossible

Tidal volume and minute ventilation will decrease

SIMILAR EVENTS

Closed Pop-Off Valve

Expiratory valve stuck in the closed position (see Event 59, Circle System Expiratory Valve Stuck Closed)

WAGD system malfunction (see Event 73, Waste Anesthesia Gas Disposal System Malfunction)

Obstruction of the expiratory limb of the anesthesia circuit

Pneumothorax (see Event 35, Pneumothorax)

Bronchospasm (see Event 29, Bronchospasm)

Open Pop-Off Valve

Major leak from other circuit component (see Event 69, Major Leak in the Anesthesia Breathing Circuit)

MANAGEMENT

If Pop-Off Valve Stuck Closed or Inappropriately Set to CLOSED

Check that the pop-off valve and selector switch are set appropriately for the desired mode of ventilation

If the circuit pressure remains high, change the selector switch to its alternative setting (from BAG to VENTILATOR or vice versa). This may decrease pressure within the breathing circuit and assist in diagnosing the problem

> Ventilate the patient's lungs with an alternative ventilation system (e.g., self-inflating bag or nonrebreather system) as soon as possible

> Call for help to repair or replace defective components in the circuit or ventilator

>> This may require replacement of the anesthesia workstation

If Pop-Off Valve Stuck Open or Inappropriately Set to OPEN

Check that the pop-off and selector switch are set appropriately for the desired mode of ventilation

Ensure adequate oxygenation and ventilation

> Use an alternative ventilation system if controlled ventilation is in use and there is a large, uncorrectable leak through the circuit pop-off valve

> Call for help to repair or replace defective components in circuit or ventilator

>> This may require replacement of the anesthesia workstation

Maintain anesthesia with IV medications

COMPLICATIONS

Hypotension
Hypoxemia
Hypercarbia
Pulmonary barotrauma
> Pneumothorax
> Gas embolism
Cardiac arrest

SUGGESTED READING

1. Walker SG, Smith TC, Sheplock G, Acquaviva MA, Horn N. Breathing circuits. In: Ehrenwerth J, Eisenkraft JB, Berry JM, editors. Anesthesia equipment: principles and applications. 2nd ed. Philadelphia: Saunders; 2013. p. 95-124.
2. Oprea AD, Ehrenwerth J, Barash PG. A case of adjustable pressure-limiting (APL) valve failure. J Clin Anesth 2011;23:58-60.
3. Eisenkraft JB. Potential for barotrauma or hypoventilation with the Drager AV-E ventilator. J Clin Anesth 1989;1:452-6.
4. Vijayakumar A, Saxena DK, Sivan Pillay A, Darsow R. Massive leak during manual ventilation: adjustable pressure limiting valve malfunction not detected by pre-anesthetic checkout. Anesth Analg 2010;111:579-80.
5. Hennenfent S, Suslowicz B. Circuit leak from capnograph sampling line lodged under adjustable pressure limiting valve. Anesth Analg 2010;111:578.

71   Ventilator Failure

DEFINITION

A ventilator failure is the inability of the ventilator to deliver the required inspired gas volume to the patient

ETIOLOGY

Circuit disconnect or misconnect
Stuck bellows

Improper seal between ventilator housing and bellows
Improper assembly of ventilator or connecting hoses
Failure of fresh gas flow to the anesthesia circuit and ventilator
Electrical power failure of an electrically controlled ventilator
Ventilator pressure relief valve stuck open or missing
Lung compliance outside the performance envelope of the ventilator
Failure of fresh gas decoupling valve

TYPICAL SITUATIONS

When the patient's position is changed, causing a disconnect
Bag/ventilator selector switch incorrectly set
After changing components of the anesthesia breathing circuit
After service of the anesthesia workstation
When the user is unfamiliar with the anesthesia workstation or ventilator controls
In patients with severe lung disease and low lung compliance
During interruptions of electrical power or O_2 supply
> Severe weather
> Earthquake

PREVENTION

Change patient position carefully
Provide appropriate routine maintenance for the anesthesia workstation and ventilator
Train personnel in correct assembly and use of ventilator
Conduct a thorough preoperative check of the anesthesia workstation and ventilator
> Place a breathing bag on the end of the Y piece and use it as a "test lung" for the ventilator
Ensure that the ventilator power is turned on and that the bag/ventilator selector valve is set properly

MANIFESTATIONS

Ventilator bellows moves inadequately or sticks in a tilted position
Ventilator fails to cycle, bellows does not move at all
Abnormal sound of the ventilator during inspiration
Ventilator alarm sounds (e.g., "unable to drive bellows" alarm)
If a piston ventilator, piston moves normally but lungs are not ventilated
Signs of hypoventilation of the patient
> Decreased or absent chest movement on inspiration
> Little or no ET CO_2 present on capnograph waveform
> Low or zero tidal volume measured by spirometry
> Apnea alarm may sound
> Low pressure alarm may sound
> As $PaCO_2$ rises, the patient may make respiratory efforts if not fully paralyzed
> Hypoxemia
> Reduced or absent breath sounds
If there has been a loss of electrical power, other devices may lose power or OR lights may go out
> Ventilator may work if battery backup is functional
If the main O_2 supply to the OR fails, the bobbins will fall to the bottom of the flowmeters and a low O_2 pressure alarm will sound

SIMILAR EVENTS

Ventilator never turned on
Breathing circuit bag/ventilator selector switch set incorrectly
Pop-off valve failure (see Event 70, Pop-Off Valve Failure)
Major leak from the anesthesia circuit (see Event 69, Major Leak in the Anesthesia Breathing Circuit)
WAGD system malfunction (see Event 73, Waste Anesthesia Gas Disposal System Malfunction)
Inspiratory valve stuck closed (see Event 60, Circle System Inspiratory Valve Stuck Closed)
Obstruction of the inspiratory tubing of the anesthesia circuit or the ETT

MANAGEMENT

Attempt to manually ventilate the patient using the bag on the anesthesia breathing circuit
Switch to manual ventilation using the reservoir bag on the anesthesia workstation
Activate the O_2 flush device to fill the reservoir bag
If able to ventilate, continue manual ventilation
Call for help to identify the problem in the ventilator and to assist you in caring for the patient
Prepare to use alternative ventilation system (e.g., self-inflating bag or nonrebreathing circuit)
If unable to fill the anesthesia breathing circuit using the O_2 flush
Visually check for a major circuit disconnection, checking the ETT, Y piece, hoses, and reservoir bag
Ensure that the bag/ventilator selector switch is set to BAG for manual ventilation
If there is no disconnect and bag/selector switch is in BAG position
Ventilate the patient using a self-inflating bag, nonrebreathing circuit, or mouth-to-ETT
Check the flowmeters and pipeline O_2 pressure gauge
Switch to O_2 cylinders if the external O_2 supply has failed (see Event 68, Loss of Pipeline Oxygen)
If the anesthesia breathing circuit and bag fill but the patient cannot be ventilated manually
Check again that bag/ventilator selector switch is in BAG position
Ventilate the patient using an alternative ventilation system (self-inflating bag, nonrebreathing circuit, or mouth-to-ETT)
Check the inspiratory limb of the anesthesia breathing circuit for obstruction
If unable to ventilate with alternative ventilation system
Check for kinked ETT, bronchospasm, endobronchial intubation, pneumothorax (see Event 29, Bronchospasm, Event 30, Endobronchial Intubation, and Event 35, Pneumothorax)
Once you have established adequate ventilation
Maintain anesthesia with IV agents, if necessary
Assign your help to diagnose and correct the problem
Check the circuit hoses, bag/ventilator selector switch, and the ventilator ON switch again
Find and correct the fault in the ventilator
Problem may require replacing the anesthesia workstation
In the event of an electrical power failure, the emergency power system should automatically activate
The emergency power generator may fail or may itself be damaged by an event that cuts the main power supply (see Event 64, Electrical Power Failure)
Make sure that the ventilator is plugged into an emergency power outlet
Battery backup function is limited in time, so plan for alternative means of ventilation
If electrical power cannot be restored quickly, obtain a pneumatically controlled ventilator

COMPLICATIONS

Hypoxemia
Hypercarbia
Cardiac arrest

SUGGESTED READING

1. Modak RK, Olympio MA. Anesthesia ventilators. In: Ehrenwerth J, Eisenkraft JB, Berry JM, editors. Anesthesia equipment: principles and applications. 2nd ed. Philadelphia: Saunders; 2013. p. 148-78.
2. Ortega RA, Zambricki ER. Fresh gas decoupling valve failure precludes mechanical ventilation in a Draeger Fabius GS anesthesia machine. Anesth Analg 2007;104:1000-1.
3. Hilton G, Moll V, Zumaran AA, Jaffe RA, Brock-Utne JG. Failure to ventilate with the Dräger Apollo® Anesthesia Workstation. Anesthesiology 2011;114:1238-40.
4. Schulte TE, Tinker JH. Narkomed 6400 anesthesia machine failure. Anesth Analg 2008;106:1018-9.

72   Volatile Anesthetic Overdose

DEFINITION

A volatile anesthetic overdose is either an absolute or a relative excess inspired anesthetic concentration

Absolute overdose: delivered concentration of volatile anesthetic substantially greater than that intended

Relative overdose: intended concentration of volatile anesthetic that causes hemodynamic and/or respiratory compromise

ETIOLOGY

Error in setting the anesthetic vaporizer to desired concentration
Vaporizer accidentally left on after a previous case
Failure to decrease a high concentration of volatile anesthetic used for induction or deepening of anesthesia
Malfunction of the anesthetic vaporizer
Vaporizer filled with the wrong agent
Failure of vaporizer interlock device (allowing two vaporizers to be on at the same time)
Vaporizer has been tilted, causing liquid anesthetic to enter the bypass portion of the vaporizer or the anesthesia workstation piping
Faulty delivery from anesthesia workstation (e.g., electronic failure on new anesthesia workstations)

TYPICAL SITUATIONS

When rapidly changing depth of anesthesia by turning on high concentration of volatile anesthetic
High fresh gas flow and mechanical ventilation will result in rapid equilibration of volatile anesthetic in the anesthesia breathing circuit and the patient
After conducting an inhalation induction with a volatile anesthetic
In patients who have preexisting cardiovascular or pulmonary compromise
When a vaporizer has just been installed on the anesthesia workstation

PREVENTION

Ensure vaporizers are checked regularly during preventive maintenance
Use a respiratory gas analyzer (including volatile anesthetics)
    Set volatile anesthetic high alarm limits appropriately
Use care when administering high concentrations of volatile anesthetic
    Ensure that the concentration is decreased as necessary
Maintain vaporizers in the upright position at all times
Follow manufacturer's recommended filling procedures for vaporizer
Ensure that vaporizer is off during filling
Use agent-specific filling devices to prevent filling with incorrect agent
Do not overfill vaporizer
Use a processed EEG monitor of anesthetic depth and set alarm limits to alert to a possible anesthetic overdose
Never connect a freestanding vaporizer between the machine common gas outlet and the breathing circuit

MANIFESTATIONS

Volatile anesthetic overdose should be included in the differential diagnosis of any unexpected hypotension or bradycardia during anesthesia.

If the vaporizer is accidentally left on from a previous case
    The patient may complain of the odor during preoxygenation
    The patient may become unresponsive during preoxygenation
A high concentration of volatile anesthetic may be detected by a respiratory gas analyzer
Respiratory depression or apnea in the spontaneously ventilating patient
Increased anesthetic depth as measured by processed EEG
Hypotension
Bradycardia
Ventricular arrhythmias
PEA
Failure to breathe or to awaken at the end of the anesthesia

SIMILAR EVENTS

Hypotension and cardiovascular collapse from other causes (see Event 9, Hypotension)
Respiratory depression or apnea from other causes (see Event 56, Postoperative Failure to Breathe)
Overdose of IV medication(s) (see Event 63, Drug Administration Error)
Cardiac Arrest (see Event 2, Cardiac Arrest)

MANAGEMENT

Confirm a volatile anesthetic overdose
    Check the vaporizer and flowmeter settings
    Check the respiratory gas analyzer to determine whether volatile anesthetic concentrations measured in the anesthesia breathing circuit are appropriate
Turn off all volatile anesthetic vaporizers
Ensure adequate oxygenation and ventilation

72

Increase the FiO_2 to 100% with a high flow rate of O_2 into the anesthesia breathing circuit
Purge volatile anesthetic from the breathing circuit into the waste gas scavenging system by activating the O_2 flush between breaths
Confirm that the concentration of volatile anesthetic in the anesthesia breathing circuit has decreased
If the anesthetic concentration does not decrease, ventilate with an alternative ventilation system (e.g., self-inflating bag or nonrebreathing circuit)
There may be an internal fault in the anesthesia workstation or vaporizer
Check vital signs frequently (rule out PEA)
BP
Palpate the peripheral pulses
Pulse oximetry
Auscultate the heart sounds
Support the circulation
Bolus IV fluids
Administer vasopressors (see Event 9, Hypotension)
Administer vagolytic if indicated (see Event 22, Sinus Bradycardia)
Call for help if there is severe hemodynamic compromise
If cardiac arrest occurs, follow ACLS guidelines (see Event 2, Cardiac Arrest)
Arrhythmias may occur when using catecholamines in the setting of a volatile anesthetic overdose
Terminate the surgery as soon as possible if there has been profound hypotension or cardiac arrest
Sequester the anesthesia machine if there is any possibility of misfilling or malfunction of the vaporizer or of a fault in the anesthesia workstation

COMPLICATIONS

Respiratory arrest
Cardiac arrest

SUGGESTED READING

1. Eisenkraft JB. Anesthesia vaporizers. In: Ehrenwerth J, Eisenkraft JB, Berry JM, editors. Anesthesia equipment: principles and applications. 2nd ed. Philadelphia: Saunders; 2013. p. 64-94.
2. Eisenkraft JB. Hazards of the anesthesia delivery system. In: Ehrenwerth J, Eisenkraft JB, Berry J, editors. Anesthesia equipment: principles and applications. 2nd ed. Philadelphia: Saunders; 2013. p. 607-11.
3. Geffroy JC, Gentili ME, Le Pollès R, Triclot P. Massive inhalation of desflurane due to vaporizer dysfunction. Anesthesiology 2005;103:1096-8.
4. Sinclair A, van Bergen J. Vaporizer overfilling. Can J Anaesth 1993;40:77-8.
5. Mehta SP, Eisenkraft JB, Posner KL, Domino KB. Patient injuries from anesthesia gas delivery equipment: a closed claims update. Anesthesiology 2013;119:788-95.
6. Adler AC, Connelly NR, Ankam A, Raghunathan K. Technical communication: inhaled anesthetic agent-vaporizer mismatch: management in settings with limited resources: don't try this at home. Anesth Analg 2013;116:1272-5.

73 Waste Anesthesia Gas Disposal System Malfunction

DEFINITION

The waste anesthesia gas disposal (WAGD) system malfunctions

ETIOLOGY

Internal obstruction or external compression of the WAGD system hose
Mechanical failure of components of the WAGD system
Incorrect assembly or operation of the WAGD system
Lack of adequate vacuum pressure

TYPICAL SITUATIONS

Operator error
When the anesthesia workstation or other equipment is rolled over WAGD system hoses lying
    on the OR floor
Following service of the WAGD system or the anesthesia workstation
Failure to connect the evacuation hose to the WAGD system outlet
Failure to cap unused ports on the WAGD system interface block

PREVENTION

Use of a WAGD system that incorporates safety devices
    Positive and negative pressure relief mechanisms in closed active WAGD interface design
    Ports open to atmosphere in open active WAGD system design
    In-line breathing circuit pressure gauges and alarms to indicate and warn of excessive
        positive or negative pressure
Do not allow untrained users to alter WAGD system settings
Avoid external compression of WAGD system hoses
    Use WAGD system hoses that are constructed to be resistant to kinking or twisting
    Keep WAGD system hoses off the floor
    Move anesthesia workstation and carts carefully to avoid obstructing WAGD system
        hoses
    Visually inspect the WAGD system hoses during the routine preuse machine check and
        after the anesthesia workstation has been moved
Confirm that WAGD system hoses are connected to the correct ports on the WAGD system
During the preuse machine check, occlude the anesthesia breathing circuit at the Y piece
    Activate the O_2 flush and ensure that the gas pressure can be relieved through the pop-off
        valve (tests both the valve and the WAGD system)
    With zero fresh gas flow, occlude the anesthesia breathing circuit and ensure that negative
        pressure does not develop in the circuit (active WAGD system)
    If present, ensure that vacuum pressure monitors are indicating adequate pressure in the
        WAGD system
    If a closed interface WAGD system, ensure that the positive and negative pressure relief
        valves are not obstructed or clogged

MANIFESTATIONS

Abnormal end-expiratory pressure (either positive or negative) in the anesthesia circuit
    When passive WAGD is used, only positive pressure should develop
    When active WAGD (vacuum) is in use, a failure of the WAGD interface can result in
        either excess positive or negative pressure
Inability to ventilate the patient's lungs

Possible difficulty in keeping the circuit filled with gas
Hypotension due to increased intrathoracic pressure
Hypoxemia
Odor of volatile anesthetic gas may be detected by OR personnel
With an active closed interface WAGD system
> Interface reservoir bag should fill at end-exhalation when waste gas enters the interface from the breathing circuit
> Interface reservoir bag should empty during inspiration when no gas enters the interface but gas is being removed by the vacuum

SIMILAR EVENTS

Closed or obstructed pop-off valve (see Event 70, Pop-Off Valve Failure)
Expiratory valve of a circle system stuck in the closed position (see Event 59, Circle System Expiratory Valve Stuck Closed)
Stuck closed ventilator pop-off valve (see Event 71, Ventilator Failure)
Faulty pressure gauge
Pneumothorax (see Event 35, Pneumothorax)
Loss of anesthetic gas from the anesthesia breathing circuit (see Event 69, Major Leak in the Anesthesia Breathing Circuit)

MANAGEMENT

Confirm a fault in the WAGD system
> Observe the pressure in the anesthesia breathing circuit
> If abnormal pressure (either positive or negative) is observed, disconnect the patient from the anesthesia breathing circuit
>> Use an alternative ventilation system
> Adjust amount of vacuum entering an active WAGD system
>> Close relief valve to decrease amount of vacuum
>> Open relief valve to increase amount of vacuum

Check for an obstruction of the WAGD system hoses
> Between the circuit pop-off valve and the WAGD system interface
> Between the ventilator and the WAGD system interface
> Between the WAGD system interface and the OR WAGD system exhaust

If there is an obstruction of the WAGD system hose between the WAGD system interface and either the CO_2 absorber or the ventilator
> Relieve any obvious obstruction
> Consider switching from the ventilator to the reservoir bag or vice versa for positive pressure ventilation
>> Use an alternative ventilation system if there is any doubt
> If the patient is breathing spontaneously, either the reservoir bag or the ventilator bellows can be used as a gas reservoir

If the obstruction of the WAGD system hose is between the WAGD interface and the OR exhaust point
> Relieve any obvious obstruction
> Continue to use the alternative ventilation system if the obstruction cannot be relieved
> Alternatively, disconnect the WAGD system interface from the anesthesia breathing system, venting the waste gases into the OR

Check for other causes of high airway pressure (see Event 7, High Peak Inspiratory Pressure)

Get help to repair and replace the faulty WAGD system components

COMPLICATIONS

Pulmonary barotrauma
  Pneumothorax
  Pneumomediastinum
  SC emphysema
Hypotension
Hypoventilation
Exposure of OR personnel to waste anesthetic gases

SUGGESTED READING

1. Eisenkraft JB, McGregor DG. Waste anesthetic gases and scavenging systems. In: Ehrenwerth J, Eisenkraft JB, Berry JM, editors. Anesthesia equipment: principles and applications. 2nd ed. Philadelphia: Saunders; 2013. p. 125-47.
2. Tavakoli M, Habeeb A. Two hazards of gas scavenging. Anesth Analg 1978;57:286-7.

Chapter 11
Cardiac Anesthesia Events
ANKEET UDANI

74   Cardiac Laceration

DEFINITION

A cardiac laceration is an inadvertent incision into the right atrium, right ventricle, great vessels, or vein graft(s) during sternotomy or resulting from other traumatic injury

ETIOLOGY

Adhesion of scar tissue and/or myocardial tissue to the sternum
CPR
Penetrating chest trauma (e.g., gunshot wound, knife injury, MVA)

TYPICAL SITUATIONS

Patients who have had a previous sternotomy ("redo" sternotomy), especially those with vein
   grafts crossing under the sternum
Inexperienced surgeon
When the lungs are ventilated during sternotomy
Emergency sternotomy
Patients with ascending aortic aneurysms or multivessel aortic arch disease
Patients with an anatomic abnormality of the chest wall (kyphoscoliosis, pectus excavatum)
Patients who have received mediastinal radiation
Patients who have had CPR with rib or sternal fractures
Patients with penetrating injury to the chest
Patients following MVA

PREVENTION

Obtain preoperative lateral CXR and/or CT scan to evaluate the extent of adhesions to the
   heart, great vessels, and sternum
Stop ventilating the lungs prior to primary sternotomy; maintain ventilation at reduced tidal
   volumes during redo sternotomy
Reduce myocardial chamber size during sternotomy
      Place the patient in reverse Trendelenburg position
      Vasodilate the patient with an IV infusion of sodium nitroprusside or NTG
Consider instituting femoral artery–to–femoral vein CPB prior to sternotomy
Suggest that sternotomy be performed following deep hypothermia and complete circulatory
   arrest if an aortic aneurysm is adherent to the underside of the sternum

MANIFESTATIONS

Large volumes of blood welling out of the surgical field or other site of injury

Hypotension
>   May be due to blood loss
>   Acute cardiac failure may occur if a critical vein or internal mammary artery graft to a coronary artery is lacerated

Tachycardia

Obvious signs of chest trauma—knife or bullet holes, seat belt burns

Hemopneumothorax

SIMILAR EVENTS

Bleeding from other intrathoracic structures (see Event 1, Acute Hemorrhage)

Hypotension from other causes (see Event 9, Hypotension)

MANAGEMENT

Cardiac laceration may occur during any sternotomy or chest trauma.

In cardiac surgery, be prepared for major hemorrhage during sternotomy
>   Ensure adequate IV access is in place for redo sternotomy
>   If a blood salvage device is to be used during surgery, have it set up prior to sternotomy
>   Stop ventilating the lungs prior to primary sternotomy; maintain ventilation at reduced tidal volumes during redo sternotomy
>   Ensure at least two units of PRBCs are available in the OR prior to sternotomy
>   Observe the operative field carefully during sternotomy
>   Ensure rapid fluid infuser is available

If major hemorrhage is apparent during sternotomy
>   Stop administering volatile anesthetics and flush the anesthesia breathing circuit with 100% O_2
>   Increase FiO_2 to 100% and resume ventilation
>   Stop administering vasodilators

Maintain the circulating fluid volume
>   Administer IV fluid (crystalloid, colloid, blood)
>   Get help to administer volume rapidly
>   Hook up rapid fluid infuser

Maintain perfusion pressure
>   Administer vasopressors as required (see Event 9, Hypotension)
>>   Administer phenylephrine IV, 50 to 200 µg, and escalate as needed
>>   Administer epinephrine IV, 10 to 50 µg, and escalate as needed

Conserve the patient's blood
>   Ensure that the blood salvage device is used by the surgeons

If surgical repair on CPB is necessary
>   Heparin should be administered (300 to 400 units/kg IV) by the anesthesiologist through a central line
>>   Check ACT as soon as feasible
>>   Administer more heparin if ACT is less than 400 seconds
>   After heparinization, blood can be salvaged by the cardiotomy suction line of the CPB pump ("sucker bypass")
>   The femoral artery may have to be cannulated for the arterial perfusion line
>   A right ventriculotomy and the cardiotomy suction can be used as venous return for CPB

After CPB is initiated, anticipate and plan for problems associated with prolonged CPB time and myocardial injury (see Event 78, Low Cardiac Output State After Cardiopulmonary Bypass; Event 75, Coagulopathy Following Cardiopulmonary Bypass; and Event 15, Acute Coronary Syndrome)

Following penetrating or blunt injury to the chest or in patients who have had CPR, patients may need

Chest tube placement
Fluid resuscitation
Sternotomy/thoracotomy to control bleeding and/or cross-clamping of the descending aorta
Transfer to the OR for definitive surgery

COMPLICATIONS

Failure to wean from CPB
Acute myocardial failure
Myocardial ischemia
Arrhythmias
Cardiac arrest
ARDS
Hypothermia
Systemic air embolism

SUGGESTED READING

1. Mehta AR, Romanoff ME, Licina MG. Anesthetic management in the precardiopulmonary bypass period. In: Hensley FA, Martin DE, Gravlee GP, editors. The practical approach to cardiac anesthesia. Philadelphia: Lippincott Williams & Wilkins; 2008. p. 182-3.
2. Despotis G, Avidan M, Eby C, et al. Prediction and management of bleeding in cardiac surgery. J Thromb Haemost 2009;7(Suppl. 1):111-7.
3. Misao T, Yoshikawa T, Aoe M, et al. Bronchial and cardiac ruptures due to blunt trauma. Gen Thorac Cardiovasc Surg 2011;59:216-9.
4. Nyawo B, Botha P, Pillay T, et al. Clinical experience with assisted venous drainage cardiopulmonary bypass in elective cardiac reoperations. Heart Surg Forum 2008;11:E21-3.
5. Hellevuo H, Sainio M, Nevalainen R, et al. Deeper chest compression: more complications for cardiac arrest patients? Resuscitation 2013;84:760-5.

75 Coagulopathy Following Cardiopulmonary Bypass

DEFINITION

Coagulopathy following CPB as a result of deficiency or dysfunction of platelets or of the coagulation cascade

ETIOLOGY

Circulating anticoagulant
    Inadequate heparin neutralization
    Heparin rebound
    Protamine overdose
Thrombocytopenia
Impaired platelet function

Low plasma concentrations of coagulation factors
DIC
Primary fibrinolysis
Preexisting congenital or acquired coagulopathy

TYPICAL SITUATIONS

Postoperative cardiac surgery patients
Prolonged time on CPB
    Increased platelet activation
    Thrombocytopenia
    Consumption of coagulation factors
Massive hemorrhage or transfusion
Vigorous cardiotomy suction
Patients requiring a circulatory assist device
Patients undergoing deep hypothermia (core temperature below 20° C)
Preexisting coagulopathy
    Drug therapy inhibiting platelet function (aspirin, dipyridamole, clopidogrel)
    Anticoagulant therapy
    Thrombolytic therapy (streptokinase or similar agents)
    Hepatic dysfunction
    Chronic renal failure
    Myeloproliferative disorders

75

PREVENTION

Identify patients with preexisting clinical, subclinical, or pharmacologically induced coagulation disorders
    Obtain preoperative laboratory studies of coagulation function
        PT, PTT
        Platelet count
        Thromboelastogram, if available
Keep CPB time as short as possible
Minimize the negative pressure applied to the cardiotomy suction to reduce platelet trauma
Administer heparin and protamine in appropriate doses
    Monitor coagulation during and immediately after CPB
    Maintain adequate anticoagulation during CPB (ACT >400 seconds)
Consider the use of acute normovolemic hemodilution (remove whole blood pre-CPB for retransfusion post-CPB)
Coordinate the discontinuation of preoperative medications known to cause platelet dysfunction with the surgical team
Consider administering pharmacologic therapy in high-risk cases
    ε-Aminocaproic acid
    Tranexamic acid
Have blood products available at the end of CPB for patients at high risk of a coagulopathy
    Patients who have had previous cardiac surgery
    Duration of CPB longer than 3 hours

MANIFESTATIONS

Bleeding into the surgical field from multiple sites and from wound edges after administration
   of an adequate dose of protamine
Increased mediastinal chest tube output after the chest has been closed
Bleeding from IV insertion sites, wounds, or mucous membranes
Abnormalities in laboratory tests of coagulation function
   Prolonged ACT that does not correct with additional protamine
   Thrombocytopenia
   Prolonged PT and PTT
   Decreased fibrinogen level
   Increased levels of fibrin split products
   Abnormal thromboelastogram
Hypotension, tachycardia
Cardiac tamponade

SIMILAR EVENTS

Surgical bleeding
Acute hemorrhage (see Event 1, Acute Hemorrhage)
Transfusion reaction (see Event 50, Transfusion Reaction)
Cardiac tamponade from other causes (see Event 18, Cardiac Tamponade)

MANAGEMENT

Surgical exploration is indicated if
   The mediastinal chest tube drainage exceeds 300 to 400 mL in 1 hour, drainage is con-
      tinuing, and laboratory tests of coagulation are normal
   Signs of cardiac tamponade are occurring (see Event 18, Cardiac Tamponade)
      Equilibration of filling pressures
      TEE/TTE examination is suggestive of cardiac tamponade
Provide supportive therapy until bleeding is controlled
   Maintain the circulating fluid volume
      Infuse crystalloid, colloid, and blood products as necessary to maintain perfusion
         pressure
   Administer vasopressors as required to maintain perfusion pressure (see Event 9,
      Hypotension)
      Phenylephrine IV, 50 to 100 μg, and escalate as needed
      Epinephrine IV, 10 to 50 μg, and escalate as needed
   Maintain normothermia (see Event 44, Hypothermia)
      Use heating blankets and/or a forced-air warming device
      Warm all IV fluids
   Prevent hypertension
      Maintain adequate sedation
      Administer vasodilator agents as needed
   Consider PEEP to decrease the amount of venous mediastinal bleeding following chest
      closure

Assess laboratory tests of coagulation function

Check the ACT

Administer additional protamine until the ACT returns to control or until there is no further reduction in the ACT

Send samples to the clinical laboratory for

Platelet count

PT

PTT

Fibrinogen

Fibrin split products

Check thromboelastogram

Begin empirical therapy while waiting for laboratory results if bleeding is severe (see Event 1, Acute Hemorrhage)

Restore platelet numbers and function

Reinfuse any fresh whole blood removed from the patient prior to CPB after administration of protamine

Administer platelets (one apheresis unit should increase platelet count by 50,000 to 80,000/μL)

Consider desmopressin (DDAVP) IV by slow infusion, 0.3 μg/kg. Can cause hypotension if given too quickly

Infuse 2 to 4 units of fresh frozen plasma (adults)

Further use of blood products should be guided by laboratory results if practical

Consult a hematologist for further management of a coagulopathy that does not resolve

Consider recombinant factor VIIa IV, 15 to 180 μg/kg (dosage for the treatment of uncontrolled hemorrhage in nonhemophiliac patients vary; consult a hematologist)

If primary fibrinolysis is thought to be the cause of bleeding

Administer ε-aminocaproic acid IV, 5 g bolus infusion followed by 1 g/hr for 6 hours

COMPLICATIONS

Transfusion reaction

Hypovolemia

Hypervolemia

DIC

Hypercoagulable states

Renal failure

Mediastinitis following reexploration

Bloodborne virus infection

Death

SUGGESTED READING

1. Avery EG. Massive bleeding post bypass: rational approach to management. In: ASA refresher course lectures. Park Ridge, Ill: American Society of Anesthesiologists; 2012. p. 214.
2. Mazer CD. Update on strategies for blood conservation and hemostasis in cardiac surgery. In: ASA refresher course lectures. Park Ridge, Ill: American Society of Anesthesiologists; 2012, p. 424.
3. Romanoff ME, Royster RL. The postcardiopulmonary bypass period: weaning to ICU transport. In: Hensley FA, Martin DE, Gravlee GP, editors. The practical approach to cardiac anesthesia. Philadelphia: Lippincott Williams & Wilkins; 2008, p. 233.
4. DiNardo JA. Management of cardiopulmonary bypass. In: DiNardo JA, Zvara DA, editors. Anesthesia for cardiac surgery. Malden, Mass: Blackwell; 2008. p. 369.

5. Speiss BD, Horrow J, Kaplan JA. Transfusion medicine and coagulation disorders. In: Kaplan JA, editor. Kaplan's cardiac anesthesia. 5th ed. Philadelphia: Saunders; 2006. p. 972.
6. Lam MS, Sims-McCallum RP. Recombinant factor VIIa in the treatment of nonhemophiliac bleeding. Ann Pharmacother 2005;39:885-91.

76 Emergent "Crash" onto Cardiopulmonary Bypass

DEFINITION

Emergent initiation of CPB

ETIOLOGY

Cardiac surgery
  Perioperative cardiac arrest, myocardial ischemia, hypotension, or massive hemorrhage
Airway catastrophe
  Inability to establish an airway by routine methods (e.g., anterior mediastinal mass with tracheomalacia)
LAST requiring prolonged CPR

TYPICAL SITUATIONS

Acute coronary graft occlusion
Failure of PCI
Severe valvular dysfunction
  Failure of valve (e.g., ruptured chordae), valve repair or replacement
  Endocarditis with acute severe valvular incompetence
Acute severe myocardial dysfunction
  Severe hypotension
  Severe protamine reaction
Massive perioperative hemorrhage
Massive PE
Obstetrical catastrophes (e.g., LAST, AFE, and cardiac arrest in the parturient)

PREVENTION

Wean from CPB with all necessary inotropic and mechanical myocardial support
Verify protamine reversal and obtain good hemostasis prior to chest closure
Perform a post-CPB TEE examination to evaluate ventricular and valvular function

MANIFESTATIONS

Signs of global or regional myocardial dysfunction
  Visible cardiac distention and poor myocardial contractility
  Systemic hypotension with increased filling pressures
  Wall motion abnormalities on TEE (global or regional)

Abnormalities of ECG morphology or rhythm
> ST elevation, often on the inferior leads II, III, AVF
> Heart block
> Ventricular arrhythmias (VT, VF)
> Asystole

Severe hemorrhage
EEG activity may slow or become quiescent
Cardiac arrest

MANAGEMENT

Alert cardiac surgeon, perfusionist, and nursing team of the situation
> Emergent CPB usually takes some time to organize for heparinization, CPB circuit preparation, and placement of arterial and venous cannulae (not in the context of ongoing cardiac surgery)

Resuscitate the patient
> Check that the patient is being oxygenated (deliver 100% O_2) and ventilated and that infusions of vasopressors are running; adjust ventilation and infusion rates as necessary
> Administer boluses of vasopressors IV as necessary (see Event 9, Hypotension)
>> Phenylephrine IV, 100 to 200 μg, and escalate as necessary
>> Ephedrine IV, 10 to 20 mg
>> Epinephrine IV, 10 to 50 μg, and escalate as necessary
> Administer IV fluids
>> Crystalloid bolus IV, 500 mL, and additional boluses as needed
>> Colloid bolus IV
>>> Hetastarch 500 mL
>>> 5% albumin 250 to 500 mL
>>> RBCs—if massive hemorrhage, inform blood bank of the ongoing need for blood products; initiate your facility's MTP

Once the decision has been made to go on CPB stat, ANTICOAGULATE THE PATIENT
> Administer heparin through a central line *or* surgeons may choose to administer heparin intra-atrially
> Heparin dose will depend on the current level of anticoagulation and whether the patient has received protamine.
>> Aim for ACT >400 seconds
> Initial heparin dose should be at least 300 units/kg

Perfusionist should immediately prime the oxygenator and CPB pump circuit
> If there is any question about the circulation of heparin, have an additional 15,000 units of heparin added to the pump prime
> Volume can be delivered to the patient via arterial cannula once it is in place

Cardiac surgeon should cannulate the arterial system (aorta or femoral artery) first, then the venous system (right atrium or femoral vein)
> If there is massive hemorrhage, the cardiotomy suction cannulae can be used as the source of venous drainage (MUST heparinize before doing this)

Anesthesiologist should consider administering additional anesthetic agents if the case is prolonged once the patient is stable
Check an ABG; correct acidosis if present

COMPLICATIONS

Difficulty in separation from CPB
Myocardial ischemia or infarction
Coagulopathy
Stroke
Arrhythmias
Cardiac arrest
Death

SUGGESTED READING

1. Mora-Mangano CT, Chow JL, Kanevsky M. Cardiopulmonary bypass and the anesthesiologist. In: Kaplan JA, editor. Kaplan's cardiac anesthesia. 5th ed. Philadelphia: Saunders; 2006. p. 908.
2. Birdi I, Chaudhuri N, Lenthall K, Reddy S, Nashef SA. Emergency reinstitution of cardiopulmonary bypass following cardiac surgery: outcome justifies the cost. Eur J Cardiothorac Surg 2000;17:743-6.

77 Hypotension During Cardiopulmonary Bypass

DEFINITION

Hypotension during CPB is a MAP of less than 50 mm Hg

ETIOLOGY

Loss of pulsatility during CPB
Decreased flow from the pump
    Roller pump malocclusion
    Error in calculating the required flow rate for a patient
    Reduced venous return to the oxygenator reservoir
    Hypovolemia
Problem with aortic cannulation
    Aortic dissection by the aortic cannula
    Aortic cannula advanced too far into the aorta
        Carotid artery or innominate artery cannulation
    Clamping of the aortic cannula by the aortic cross-clamp
Decreased SVR
    Vasodilator overdose
    Hyperthermia
Low blood viscosity secondary to hemodilution

TYPICAL SITUATIONS

Acute reduction of viscosity when instituting CPB
Antihypertensive medication use by patient (e.g., ACEIs)
Administration of vasodilator
    Vasodilator infusion pump or IV administration device

Accidentally turned on
Incorrect settings
Malfunction of the pump
Vasodilation during the rewarming phase following hypothermia
Aortic cannula advanced too far into the aorta
More likely to be occluded by the aortic cross-clamp
Cannula may kink
Roller pump malocclusion
Reversal of tubing in the roller pump
Occult hemorrhage in anticoagulated patient
Recent cannulation of a major blood vessel (e.g., femoral artery)
GI bleed

PREVENTION

Control the BP (MAP < 80 mm Hg) at the time of aortic cannulation and when the aortic cross-clamp is applied or removed
Observe the process of cannulation, initiation of CPB, and cross-clamping the aorta; inform the surgeon if abnormalities are seen
Aortic dissection
Aortic cannula advanced too far
Occlusion of the aortic cannula with the aortic cross-clamp
Reversal of flow in the CPB circuit
When using vasodilators, take care in setting infusion pumps and IV administration devices
Maintain a minimum hematocrit of 20% during routine CPB
Monitor temperature from at least two sites during CPB (oropharynx and bladder)

MANIFESTATIONS

Decreased MAP while on CPB
Signs of organ hypoperfusion
Oliguria
Slowing or "flat line" EEG
May be seen normally during CPB secondary to hypothermia or anesthetic administration
If aortic dissection occurs, there may be
Acute dilation and bluish discoloration of the aorta
Low MAP
Increase in the aortic line perfusion pressure
Decrease in venous return
Insertion of the tip of the aortic cannula into the brachiocephalic artery will be manifested by
Increase in the arterial pressure to the right arm and right cerebral hemisphere
Low systemic MAP
Otorrhea, rhinorrhea, conjunctival edema, and facial edema from cerebral hyperperfusion on the right side
Unexpectedly rapid administration of vasodilator manifested by
Rapid flow in the drip chamber (not present in all infusion sets)
Excessive movement of any visible moving parts of the infusion pump mechanism

SIMILAR EVENTS

Artifacts of invasive BP measurement (see Event 20, Hypotension)
Anaphylaxis (see Event 20, Anaphylaxis and Anaphylactoid Reactions)

MANAGEMENT

Confirm hypotension
Flush the arterial line
Check the transducer, tubing, and arterial line for obstruction, kinking, or loose connections
Re-zero the transducer at the correct height
Check the pressure of the arterial side of the CPB pump circuit
If there is pulsatile flow, measure BP using a NIBP device
Inform the surgeon and perfusionist of the hypotension
Have the surgeon palpate the aorta distal to the cross-clamp to assess the intra-aortic pressure
Inspect the aorta using TEE to exclude dissection
If possible, check the position of the tip of the aortic cannula using TEE
Check face for signs of hyperperfusion
Have the perfusionist check for and correct CPB circuit problems
Inspect the CPB tubing for kinks, obstruction, or venous airlock
Check the flow setting on the CPB pump
Inspect the occlusion settings on the CPB roller pump
Discontinue volatile anesthetics being administered into the oxygenator
Inspect all vasoactive infusion pumps
Stop administration of all vasodilators
Effects of IV infusion of nitroprusside or nitroglycerin are short acting: turning them off may be all that is necessary to correct hypotension
If a vasodilator is not being infused
Turn stopcocks to the OFF position to exclude accidental administration of vasodilator
Look for IV crossover (vasodilator for vasopressor)
Ensure that vaporizers are off or turned down
Restore the BP
Have the perfusionist transiently increase the CPB pump flow rate
Administer phenylephrine IV (or directly into the oxygenator reservoir), 50 to 200 µg bolus
If hypotension is persistent, consider instituting a phenylephrine or vasopressin infusion
Give steroids in case of adrenal suppression
Dexamethasone IV, 8 mg
Hydrocortisone IV, 100 mg
Check the hematocrit
If the hematocrit is below 20%, add PRBCs to raise hematocrit and blood viscosity
Check ABGs and mixed venous blood gases
If mixed venous O_2 saturation is low or there is marked metabolic acidosis, tissue hypoperfusion is present
Increase the FiO_2 to 100%
Increase the pump flow rate

Administer $NaHCO_3$ to reverse severe metabolic acidosis

If aortic dissection has occurred
Immediately terminate CPB
Recannulate the true aortic lumen distal to the dissection or cannulate the femoral artery
Surgical repair of the aortic dissection may be required

COMPLICATIONS

Aortic or great vessel dissection
Neurologic injury
Acute renal failure
Myocardial ischemia or infarction
Death

SUGGESTED READING

1. DiNardo JA. Management of cardiopulmonary bypass. In: DiNardo JA, Zvara DA, editors. Anesthesia for cardiac surgery. Malden, Mass: Blackwell; 2008. p. 351.
2. Gibbs NM, Larach DR. Anesthetic management during cardiopulmonary bypass. In: Hensley FA, Martin DE, Gravlee GP, editors. The practical approach to cardiac anesthesia. Philadelphia: Lippincott Williams & Wilkins; 2008. p. 212.

78 Low Cardiac Output State After Cardiopulmonary Bypass

DEFINITION

Inadequate CO that occurs after separation from CPB

ETIOLOGY

Poor left ventricular function before surgery (ejection fraction less than 40%)
Myocardial ischemia or infarction in the preoperative or pre-CPB period
Long aortic cross-clamp time
Inadequate surgical repair or revascularization
Inadequate myocardial protection while on CPB, especially when there has been
    Prolonged VF before or after application of the aortic cross-clamp
    Inadequate myocardial cooling
    Ventricular distention
Arrhythmias

TYPICAL SITUATIONS

Severe CAD
Severe valvular disease of the heart
Coronary embolism during CPB (particulate matter or air)
Redo operations

Acidosis
Hypoxemia
Hypovolemia
Increased SVR (from hypothermia or injudicious use of vasopressor agents)
Inadequate inotropic support
Surgically induced structural changes
    Residual intracardiac shunting
    Residual valvular obstruction or incompetence (in prosthetic or native valve)
    Coronary artery dissection
Following administration of protamine
Acute cardiac tamponade following chest closure

PREVENTION

Discuss with surgeons the adequacy of myocardial preservation and surgical repair
Control the patient's hemodynamic status carefully as guided by TEE, ECG, invasive pressure measurements, and direct observation of the heart
Optimize the patient's condition prior to terminating CPB
    Commence IV infusions of inotropes and/or vasopressors or vasodilators as indicated clinically
    Correct metabolic acidosis, if present
    Ensure that there is sufficient blood volume in the oxygenator reservoir to restore the patient's circulating blood volume as CPB is terminated
Use the checklist **THRIVE** to prepare for weaning from CPB
    T: Temperature—ensure patient is normothermic
    H: Hemodynamics and cardiac function are acceptable
    R: Rhythm is acceptable
    I: Infusions are selected as desired and infusing properly
    V: Ventilation is appropriate for termination of CPB
    E: Electrolytes are acceptable

MANIFESTATIONS

Poor myocardial contractility and cardiac distention as seen on the surgical field and on TEE
Decreased CO
Low ejection fraction on TEE—can be global or regional wall motion abnormality
Valvular dysfunction on TEE—inadequate surgical repair or ischemic papillary muscle dysfunction
Elevated filling pressures
Hypotension
Arrhythmias
Small increases in fluid volume cause disproportionate elevations of CVP and PCWP
Increased SVR
Reduced tissue perfusion
    Decreased mixed venous O_2 saturation
    Oliguria
    Acidosis

SIMILAR EVENTS

Artifact of BP measurement system
>   Faulty BP transducer
>   Transducer height above the patient's heart

Spasm of radial artery or other lack of correlation between radial and central arterial pressure

MANAGEMENT

Optimize the cardiac rate and rhythm
>   Maintain the HR at 70 to 100 bpm
>   Epicardial pacemaker
>> Sequential AV pacing will improve ventricular filling and increase stroke volume, especially if atrial contraction is required for maintenance of adequate CO (e.g., low compliance of left ventricle)
>   Optimize heart rhythm
>> Convert or control AF or junctional rhythms (see Event 23, Supraventricular Arrhythmias)
>> Treat arrhythmias (see Event 19, Nonlethal Ventricular Arrhythmias)
>>> Amiodarone 150 mg IV over 10 minutes, followed by an infusion of 1 mg/min
>>> $MgSO_4$ IV, 2 to 4 g by slow infusion
>>> Lidocaine IV, 1 mg/kg bolus followed by an infusion of 1 to 4 mg/min

Optimize inotropic support
>   Dopamine 2 to 10 μg/kg/min IV
>   Dobutamine 3 to 10 μg/kg/min IV
>   Epinephrine 10 to 100 ng/kg/min IV
>   Milrinone 0.25 to 0.5 μg/kg/min IV, after a loading dose (50 μg/kg over 10 minutes, as indicated)

Perform TEE examination
>   Evaluate for hypovolemia, left ventricular dysfunction, adequacy of valve repair or replacement, presence of new valvular regurgitation or perivalvular leak

Optimize the cardiac filling pressures
>   Use TEE to assess ventricular function and optimize filling pressures
>   If PA catheter in place, administer fluid boluses to optimize PCWP
>   Higher filling pressures may be required in patients with a very low-compliance left ventricle

Ensure adequate oxygenation and ventilation
>   Ventilate the patient with 100% O_2
>   Check ABG—correct abnormalities
>> Respiratory or metabolic acidosis will compromise ventricular function

Give steroids if adrenal suppression is a concern
>   Dexamethasone IV, 8 mg
>   Hydrocortisone IV, 100 mg

Ensure that vasoactive drugs are reaching the circulation
>   Check that infusion pumps are administering vasoactive agents to the patient's circulation
>   Check calculations to ensure that the appropriate dose is set on each infusion pump

Do not allow the heart to become overdistended
  Administer small boluses of epinephrine IV, 5 to 20 µg
  Be prepared to go back on CPB emergently
If low CO state persists, consider placement of a mechanical device to augment CO
  IABP
  Left, right, or biventricular assist device as indicated

COMPLICATIONS

Myocardial ischemia or infarction
Cerebral ischemia
Renal failure
Pulmonary edema
Complications of IABP or ventricular assist device
  Impaired perfusion of lower extremity
  Thrombocytopenia
  Gas embolization
  Renal failure
Death

SUGGESTED READING

1. Romanoff ME, Royster RL. The postcardiopulmonary bypass period: weaning to ICU transport. In: Hensley FA, Martin DE, Gravlee GP, editors. The practical approach to cardiac anesthesia. Philadelphia: Lippincott Williams & Wilkins; 2008. p. 231.
2. DiNardo JA. Management of cardiopulmonary bypass. In: DiNardo JA, Zvara DA, editors. Anesthesia for cardiac surgery. Malden, Mass: Blackwell; 2008. p. 354.

79 Massive Systemic Air Embolism

DEFINITION

Massive systemic air embolism is a large volume of air in the patient's arterial circulation during or after CPB

ETIOLOGY

Air pumped into the aortic cannula from the CPB pump
Air entrained into the heart through a cardioplegic solution cannulation site when active suction has been applied to the left ventricle or PA for venting of the heart

TYPICAL SITUATIONS

Air pumped into the aorta from the CPB pump
  Failure to set, or malfunction of, the oxygenator low-volume alarm during CPB
  When blood is being returned to the patient from the oxygenator following CPB and low-level alarms have been turned off

When the perfusionist is distracted by the operation of other devices
>   Intraoperative RBC salvage equipment
>   IABP
>   Blood gas analyzer
>   Use of "hard shell" oxygenator or cardiotomy suction reservoirs

Urgent/emergent CPB requiring rapid setup of the oxygenator and CPB pump circuit

Reversal of vent or perfusion lines in pump head
>   Flow would occur in the opposite direction to that intended
>   The cardiotomy suction reservoir might become pressurized with air

PREVENTION

Ensure that the perfusionist takes appropriate care in the setup and pre-bypass check of the oxygenator and circuit
>   Prime and remove all air from the oxygenator and lines prior to CPB
>   Set the oxygenator low-volume alarm
>   Incorporate an arterial line filter with a continuous vent to the oxygenator reservoir

Check that there is an adequate blood volume in the oxygenator reservoir during CPB
>   Add volume to the circuit as necessary
>   An air lock in the venous drainage line will cause venous return to the oxygenator to stop abruptly

Use extreme care when returning blood back to the patient following CPB
>   The perfusionist typically disables the oxygenator low-volume alarm at this time
>   If possible, return the blood through the venous line
>   If reinfusing blood through an aortic line, the surgeon should visually monitor the line for bubbles of air
>>   The surgeon should have a clamp available immediately to occlude the aortic line should air become visible in the tubing
>   The perfusionist should clamp the blood return line when not in use in case the CPB pump head becomes activated inadvertently

Avoid the use of N_2O during and after CPB

MANIFESTATIONS

Air may be visible
>   In the aortic cannula from the oxygenator to the patient
>   In the vein grafts
>   In the chambers of the heart on TEE
>   If the tubing in the roller pumps is reversed, air may be visible in other portions of the CPB pump circuit tubing

The oxygenator reservoir may be empty or may have an abnormally low air/blood level
>   Air emboli are more likely to enter the vein grafts if the site of the proximal anastomosis is the anterior portion of the aorta
>   Abnormalities of ECG morphology or rhythm
>>   ST elevation, often on the inferior leads II, III, AVF
>>   Heart block
>>   Ventricular arrhythmias (VT, VF)
>>   Asystole
>   Regional wall motion abnormalities on TEE
>   Low CO state after CPB

EEG activity may slow or "flat line"

The patient may be slow to awaken

> There may be major focal or diffuse cerebral dysfunction, which can be severe or even indicate brain death

SIMILAR EVENTS

Hypotension due to other causes (see Event 9, Hypotension)

Systemic embolization of particulate matter from the operative field

MANAGEMENT

The perfusionist should stop the CPB pump immediately

Place the patient in the steep Trendelenburg position

> This will reduce embolization to the cerebral circulation

> Be prepared to temporarily occlude carotid arteries manually

Remove as much air as possible from the circulation

> The surgeon should immediately make a stab incision into the ascending aorta to allow air to escape

> The surgeon should remove the aortic cannula because

>> This allows more air to escape

>> This makes it easier to reprime the CPB pump

>> If CPB is to be continued, the surgeon must replace the aortic cannula

> The surgeon should massage the heart and great vessels to dislodge trapped air

> The surgeon can vent air from vein grafts using a small (25-gauge) needle and syringe, massaging the vein grafts

Have the perfusionist reprime the oxygenator and CPB pump circuit immediately

> The surgeon may elect to attempt retrograde perfusion of the cerebral circulation through a SVC cannula to backwash air out of the cerebral arteries

>> If retrograde cerebral perfusion is to be attempted, it must be instituted quickly, especially if the patient is normothermic

> The heart can be perfused in a retrograde manner via a coronary sinus catheter

> CPB must be reinstituted emergently if there has been significant coronary air embolization and the patient is unable to maintain an adequate CO

>> Begin CPB gradually, increasing the flow rate up to twice normal

>> Partial aortic clamping distal to the aortic perfusion cannula may help force remaining air through the coronary arteries

Provide 100% O_2 to the patient

> The goal is to denitrogenate the patient

> If CPB is terminated, ventilate the lungs with 100% FiO_2

> When CPB is reinstituted, use only O_2 and CO_2 in the gases supplied to the oxygenator

Increase the arterial pressure and support the heart

> Use vasopressors as necessary (see Event 9, Hypotension)

> Consider the use of a mechanical assist device (IABP or LVAD) to aid separation from CPB

For treatment of cerebral air embolism, consider administering medications that might reduce cerebral injury, although there is no definitive evidence that any medications improve outcome

Dexamethasone IV, 20 mg (or methylprednisone IV, 2 to 4 g); consider neurology consultation to assist in management

Institute systemic hypothermia (32° to 34° C) to increase the solubility of air in the tissues

Compression in a hyperbaric chamber has been reported to reverse the adverse cerebral effects of a major systemic air embolism

This therapy is only available in a few medical centers

Most patients are too sick to be transported to a suitable hyperbaric chamber

COMPLICATIONS

Stroke

Brain death

Myocardial ischemia or infarction

Difficulty in separation from CPB

Arrhythmias

Renal failure

Cardiac arrest

SUGGESTED READING

1. Stammers AH, Brindisi N, Kurusz M, High KM. Cardiopulmonary bypass circuits: design and use. In: Hensley FA, Martin DE, Gravlee GP, editors. The practical approach to cardiac anesthesia. Philadelphia: Lippincott Williams & Wilkins; 2008. p. 553.
2. Kurusz M, Mills NL. Management of unusual problems encountered in initiating and maintaining cardiopulmonary bypass. In: Gravlee GP, Davis RF, Kurusz M, Utley JR, editors. Cardiopulmonary bypass: principles and practice. Philadelphia: Lippincott Williams & Wilkins; 2000. p. 591.

80

80 Protamine Reaction

DEFINITION

Allergic or anaphylactic response to protamine administration

Anaphylactic reaction (immunologic) involves antigen and IgE antibodies; requires previous sensitization to protamine

Anaphylactoid reaction (nonimmunologic) mediated primarily by histamine; may occur with the first exposure to protamine

ETIOLOGY

Administration of protamine to a patient with a protamine allergy

TYPICAL SITUATIONS

Rapid administration of protamine

Sensitization of the patient by prior exposure to protamine, vertebrate fish, or NPH insulin with production of antigen-specific IgE antibodies

Patients with other drug allergies

PREVENTION

Administer protamine slowly
      Consider using an infusion pump
Administer a test dose of 10 to 20 mg
In patients with prior protamine reaction, administer 1 mg diluted in 100 mL over 10 minutes; if no adverse effects, administer full neutralizing dose as described

MANIFESTATIONS

Cardiovascular
      Severe hypotension
      Bradycardia may be initial sign
      Arrythmias
      Cardiac arrest
      Acute pulmonary hypertension secondary to formation of heparin-protamine complexes that cause thromboxane-induced pulmonary vasoconstriction
            RV failure on TTE/TEE
Respiratory
      Hypoxemia
      Decreased lung compliance
      Severe bronchospasm
      Pulmonary edema
Cutaneous—may be obscured by surgical drapes
      Flushing, hives, urticaria, pruritus
Swelling of mucosal membranes, conjunctiva, airway (e.g., lips, tongue, and uvula)

SIMILAR EVENTS

Anesthetic overdose (see Event 72, Volatile Anesthetic Overdose)
Pulmonary edema (see Event 20, Pulmonary Edema)
Cardiac tamponade (see Event 18, Cardiac Tamponade)
Venous air embolism (see Event 24, Venous Air or Gas Embolism)
PE (see Event 21, Pulmonary Embolism)
Pneumothorax (see Event 35, Pneumothorax)
Bronchospasm (see Event 29, Bronchospasm)
Skin manifestations of drug reactions not associated with anaphylaxis
Hypotension from other causes (see Event 9, Hypotension)
Allergic reaction to other drugs (See Event 16, Anaphylactic and Anaphylactoid Reactions)
Transfusion reaction (see Event 50, Transfusion Reaction)
ACS (see Event 15, Acute Coronary Syndrome)

MANAGEMENT

Stop administration of protamine
Treat simple hypotension with rapid IV fluid administration
      Give CaCl$_2$ IV, 100 to 200 mg, repeat as necessary
Ensure adequate oxygenation and ventilation
      Administer 100% O$_2$
      Consider intubation in patients without definitive airway

Severe reactions may require crash onto CPB

Inform surgeons and perfusionist to prepare for crash onto CPB

True anaphylactic or anaphylactoid reactions will require aggressive resuscitation with fluids, vasopressors, and bronchodilators

Crystalloid bolus IV, 500 mL initially

May have very large ongoing fluid requirements (liters)

Consider placement of additional IV access

Epinephrine IV bolus, 10 to 50 μg; rapidly escalate the dose if no response; an infusion might be needed

Albuterol MDI, 5 to 10 puffs into breathing circuit

Diphenhydramine IV, 25 to 50 mg

Methylprednisolone IV, 100 mg

If pulmonary hypertension develops, begin inotropic support with epinephrine and/ or milrinone

Consider crash onto CPB, which will require anticoagulation with a full dose of heparin (see Event 76, Emergent "Crash" onto CPB)

After a severe reaction, protamine should not be readministered; the anticoagulant effect of heparin should be allowed to wear off

Consider inhaled nitric oxide therapy

Consider inhaled prostacyclin

COMPLICATIONS

Myocardial ischemia or infarction

Coagulopathy

ARDS

Renal failure

Cardiac arrest

Death

SUGGESTED READING

1. Shore-Lesserson L, Horrow JC, Gravlee GP. Coagulation management during and after cardiopulmonary bypass. In: Hensley FA, Martin DE, Gravlee GP, editors. The practical approach to cardiac anesthesia. Philadelphia: Lippincott Williams & Wilkins; 2008. p. 504.
2. DiNardo JA. Management of cardiopulmonary bypass. In: DiNardo JA, Zvara DA, editors. Anesthesia for cardiac surgery. Malden, Mass: Blackwell; 2008. p. 358.

Chapter 12
Obstetric Events
GILLIAN HILTON

81 Amniotic Fluid Embolism (Anaphylactoid Syndrome of Pregnancy)

DEFINITION

Amniotic fluid embolism (AFE) is thought to be an abnormal maternal immune response to fetal antigens when the maternal-fetal immunological barrier is breached during labor, pregnancy termination, or shortly after delivery. It results in a triad of hypoxemia, hypotension, and coagulopathy.

ETIOLOGY

The etiology of cardiovascular collapse is not clear but may result from activation of a cascade of immune mediators that causes a massive systemic reaction

TYPICAL SITUATIONS

Active labor
Pregnancy termination
Cesarean delivery
Induction of labor
Multiparity
Advanced maternal age
Ethnic minority groups
Placental abnormalities (placental abruption or placenta previa)
Operative delivery

PREVENTION

There are no known measures to prevent AFE
Create institutional plan for stat cesarean section of a parturient in cardiac arrest ("Code Blue Obstetrics")
Drill and practice the management of stat cesarean section during cardiac arrest (using simulation if available)

MANIFESTATIONS

Unexplained acute fetal distress may precede maternal deterioration in 20% of cases
Premonitory symptoms
　　Restlessness, agitation, paresthesia
Pulmonary symptoms
　　Acute onset of dyspnea, pleuritic chest pain, bronchospasm, coughing, or hemoptysis
　　Hypoxemia and cyanosis

CXR may initially be normal and later demonstrate ARDS
Respiratory arrest
Cardiovascular symptoms
Arrhythmias
Severe hypotension
Pulmonary hypertension with RV failure (early, first 30 minutes)
ECG signs of right heart strain
Left ventricular failure and pulmonary edema (following initial onset)
Cardiac arrest (PEA, asystole, VF, VT)
Neurologic symptoms
Hyperreflexia, seizure, coma
Acute severe consumptive coagulopathy
DIC
Massive hemorrhage
Obstetric complications
Uterine atony

SIMILAR EVENTS

Anaphylaxis (see Event 16, Anaphylactic and Anaphylactoid Reactions)
Pulmonary or venous air embolism (see Event 21, Pulmonary Embolism, and Event 24, Venous Gas Embolism)
Eclampsia (see Event 88, Preeclampsia and Eclampsia)
Sepsis (see Event 13, The Septic Patient)
Obstetric hemorrhage (see Event 87, Obstetric Hemorrhage)
Medication reaction (see Event 63, Drug Administration Error)
Local anesthetic overdose (see Event 52, Local Anesthetic Systemic Toxicity)
Total spinal anesthesia (see Event 89, Total Spinal Anesthesia)
Cardiac disease (MI or ischemia, aortic dissection, cardiomyopathy, Eisenmenger syndrome)
Seizures (see Event 57, Seizures, and Event 88, Preeclampsia and Eclampsia)

MANAGEMENT

Patients with AFE can rapidly deteriorate, are at high risk of maternal mortality, and have a high incidence of fetal distress. The key steps are early recognition, supportive management, prompt resuscitation, and delivery of the fetus.

Call for help
Labor and delivery team and additional anesthesia help
If the patient has arrested, start CPR immediately
Stat cesarean section may be necessary (if no return of spontaneous circulation after 4 minutes) with the goal of delivery within 5 minutes (see Event 82, Cardiac Arrest in the Parturient)
If the patient has NOT arrested, maintain left uterine displacement even if postpartum
Ensure adequate oxygenation and ventilation
Administer 100% O_2 by a nonrebreathing face mask
Patient may require urgent or emergent airway management

If urgent airway management is necessary, perform RSI with cricoid pressure
Etomidate IV, 0.2 to 0.3 mg/kg, or ketamine IV, 0.5 to 1.0 mg/kg
Succinylcholine IV, 1 to 2 mg/kg
Intubate the trachea if there is loss of consciousness, respiratory failure, or severe cardiovascular collapse
Stop $MgSO_4$ infusion, if running
If Mg^{2+} toxicity is suspected, administer $CaCl_2$ IV, 500 to 1000 mg
Initiate basic monitoring if not already present
ECG, NIBP, pulse oximeter, RR, level of consciousness, temperature, fetal monitoring
Support the circulation
Ensure adequate IV access above the diaphragm (2× large-bore IVs)
Rapidly infuse crystalloid and/or colloid
Treat hypotension with vasopressors, increasing doses as needed
Phenylephrine IV, 50 to 200 μg
Ephedrine IV, 5 to 10 mg
Epinephrine IV, 10 to 100 μg
Consider administering vasopressor infusions if the preceding measures are inadequate (see Event 9, Hypotension)
Place an arterial line and consider placement of CVP line for infusion of vasopressors
Prepare for massive transfusion and initiate MTP (if available)
Send for blood products if they are not already in the room
Inform the blood bank that more blood and blood products will be needed emergently
If crossmatched blood is not readily available, order uncrossmatched blood
Get help to set up a rapid infusor device
Transfuse blood products
Use a fluid warmer
Transfuse with an RBC:FFP ratio of 1:1 or 2:1
Transfuse RBCs to maintain hemoglobin >7 g/dL
Transfuse additional FFP if PT/aPTT is prolonged
Transfuse platelets if <50,000/μL
Transfuse cryoprecipitate if fibrinogen <200 mg/dL
Consult hematology and the critical care team
Maintain normothermia
Frequent lab draws (ABG/CBC/PT/aPTT/fibrinogen/metabolic panel/Ca^{2+})
At any time, if the patient has no pulse, start CPR immediately (C-A-B: compressions, airway, breathing)
Follow (ACLS) guidelines with modifications for the parturient (see Event 2, Cardiac Arrest, and Event 82, Cardiac Arrest in the Parturient)

COMPLICATIONS

Electrolyte abnormalities
Massive hemorrhage
ARDS
Aspiration pneumonitis
Cerebral hemorrhage

Cerebral anoxia
Cardiac arrest or death
Fetal distress or death

SUGGESTED READING

1. Kramer MS, Rouleau J, Liu S, et al. Health Study Group of the Canadian Perinatal Surveillance System: Amniotic fluid embolism: incidence, risk factors, and impact on perinatal outcome. Br J Obstet Gynaecol 2012;119:874-9.
2. Knight M, Tuffnell D, Brocklehurst P, Spark P, Kurinczuk JJ. On behalf of the UK Obstetric Surveillance System: incidence and risk factors for amniotic-fluid embolism. Obstet Gynecol 2010;115:910-7.
3. Clark SL. Amniotic fluid embolism. Clin Obstet Gynecol 2010;53:322-8.
4. Tuffnell D, Knight M, Plaat F. Amniotic fluid embolism: an update. Anaesthesia 2011;66:3-6.
5. Dedhia JD, Mushambi MC. Amniotic fluid embolism. Contin Educ Anaesth Crit Care Pain 2007;7:152-6.

82   Cardiac Arrest in the Parturient

DEFINITION

Cardiac arrest in the parturient is the absence of effective mechanical activity of the heart in the pregnant patient.

ETIOLOGY

Hypovolemia
Hypoxemia
PE, venous air embolism, or AFE
Toxins (e.g., LAST)
Anesthetic complications
Uterine atony
Hypertensive disease of pregnancy
Placental abnormalities (placental abruption or placenta previa)
Cardiac disease (MI or ischemia, aortic dissection, cardiomyopathy, Eisenmenger syndrome)
Sepsis
Tension pneumothorax
Cardiac tamponade

TYPICAL SITUATIONS

Anesthesia-related
    Failed or difficult tracheal intubation
    Unrecognized esophageal intubation
    Total spinal anesthesia
    LAST
Major hemorrhage
    Uterine atony
    Placental abnormalities

Placenta previa (placenta located in the lower uterine segment over the cervix)

Placenta accreta, increta, or percreta (placenta attaches to, into, or through the myometrium)

Placental abruption (premature separation of a normally implanted placenta after 20 weeks' gestation)

Preexisting medical condition

Acquired or congenital cardiovascular disease (e.g., peripartum cardiomyopathy, aortic dissection in presence of bicuspid aortic valve, coronary artery disease)

History of a PE

Other

Prostaglandin use in pregnancy

Mg^{2+} toxicity

AFE

PREVENTION

Create institutional plan for immediate cesarean section of a parturient in cardiac arrest ("Code Blue Obstetrics")

Drill and practice the management of immediate cesarean section during cardiac arrest (using simulation if available)

Immediate intervention at first signs of maternal or fetal instability

Manually perform left uterine displacement

Administer 100% O_2 through a nonrebreathing face mask

Ensure adequate IV access

Assess for and treat reversible causes (e.g., hypotension)

Anesthesia-related issues

Evaluate airway and prepare for a difficult intubation

Exclude intrathecal and intravascular placement of epidural catheters before administering incremental doses of local anesthetic

Manage preexisting medical issues in collaboration with specialists

In high-risk patients, consider placing invasive monitors

Carefully administer medications to parturients

Patients with a history of drug allergies

Patients with cardiac disease taking tocolytic agents (β-adrenergic agonists)

Administer potent drugs through infusion pumps (e.g., $MgSO_4$)

MANIFESTATIONS

Unresponsive to verbal commands

Absence of pulse oximeter waveform if present

Loss of consciousness or seizure-like activity

No palpable carotid pulse (palpation of peripheral pulses unreliable)

NIBP unmeasurable

Absence of heart tones on auscultation

Agonal or absent respirations

Arrhythmias

VT, VF, PEA, asystole

Rhythm in PEA may appear normal

Significant fall in ET CO_2 if present

Cyanosis

Regurgitation and aspiration of gastric contents
Lack of ventricular contraction on TEE or TTE

SIMILAR EVENTS

Anaphylaxis (see Event 16, Anaphylactic and Anaphylactoid Reactions)
PE, venous air embolism, or AFE (see Event 21, Pulmonary Embolism, Event 24, Venous Gas Embolism, and Event 81, Amniotic Fluid Embolism)
Eclampsia (see Event 88, Preeclampsia and Eclampsia)
Sepsis (see Event 13, The Septic Patient)
Obstetric hemorrhage (see Event 87, Obstetric Hemorrhage)
Medication reaction (see Event 63, Drug Administration Error)
Local anesthetic overdose (see Event 52, Local Anesthetic Systemic Toxicity)
Total spinal (see Event 89, Total Spinal Anesthesia)
Hypotension (see Event 9, Hypotension)
Seizures (see Event 57, Seizures, and Event 88, Preeclampsia and Eclampsia)
Artifacts on monitoring devices
    ECG artifact (always check the patient)
    Pulse oximeter
    NIBP or invasive BP

MANAGEMENT

The key steps are early recognition, prompt resuscitation, and delivery of the fetus. Attempts to transfer patients undergoing CPR to an OR for immediate cesarean section increase maternal and neonatal risk. Perimortem cesarean section should be performed at the site of the arrest to relieve aortocaval compression, increase maternal CO and allow more effective chest compressions.

Treat the patient, not the monitor
Verify that the patient is unresponsive and has no carotid pulse
    Other patient monitoring, if present, may confirm absence of circulation (e.g., pulse oximetry, ET CO_2, arterial line waveform)
Call a code
    Call for labor and delivery team and additional anesthesia help
    Prepare for stat cesarean section at the site of the arrest with the goal of delivery within 5 minutes
        A cesarean section will be necessary if no return of spontaneous circulation after 4 minutes
Call for the crash cart
    Apply defibrillation pads on chest
        Do not delay defibrillation for shockable rhythms
Start CPR immediately (C-A-B: compressions, airway, breathing)
    Chest compressions
        Place hands slightly higher on sternum
            Compressions should be at least **100 per minute** and at least **2 inches deep**
        Rotate compressors every 2 minutes
        Allow for complete recoil of the chest with each compression
        Interruptions in compressions should be less than 10 seconds

82

Adequate compressions should generate an ET CO_2 of at least 10 mm Hg and a diastolic pressure of greater than 20 mm Hg (if an arterial line is in place). You **MUST** improve CPR quality if above conditions are not met.

Airway/ventilation

Until the patient is intubated, establish bag mask ventilation with 100% O_2 at a compression to ventilation ratio of 30:2 and prepare for endotracheal intubation

Place ETT and then ventilate at a rate of 10 per minute with continuous compressions

Assign tasks to skilled responders

Ensure adequate IV access

If difficult IV access, place IO line

Place an arterial line

Call for TEE or TTE machine

Turn off ALL anesthetics if in use (including epidural infusions)

Follow BLS and ACLS guidelines (see Event 2, Cardiac Arrest) *but* **with modifications for the parturient (see the following)**

Employ cognitive aids (ACLS guidelines) to help determine diagnosis and treatment

Drug therapy, dosages, and defibrillation should follow standard ACLS guidelines

ACLS modifications in pregnant patients

Place hands slightly higher on sternum while performing chest compressions

Immediately intubate with an ETT and ventilate with 100% O_2

The routine use of cricoid pressure during cardiac arrest is not recommended, but if used, remove if impairing ventilation and/or intubation

Manual left uterine displacement to avoid aortocaval compression

Stop $MgSO_4$ infusion, if running

If Mg^{2+} toxicity is suspected, administer $CaCl_2$ IV, 500 to 1000 mg

Remove external fetal monitors prior to defibrillation

If an internal fetal monitor is present, disconnect from power supply prior to defibrillation

If parturient does not respond to resuscitation within 4 minutes, immediate perimortem cesarean section is indicated at the site of the arrest

Continue all maternal resuscitative interventions (CPR, positioning, defibrillation, drugs, and fluids) during and after perimortem cesarean section

Continually reassess patient without interrupting chest compressions

Resumption of spontaneous circulation

ECG and return of palpable pulse or BP

Pulse oximetry waveform

Consider postresuscitation hypothermia for brain protection

COMPLICATIONS

Aspiration of gastric contents
Laceration of liver
Pneumothorax or hemothorax
Rib fracture
Hypoxic brain injury
Multiorgan failure
Maternal death
Fetal death

SUGGESTED READING

1. Ramsay G, Paglia M, Bourjeily G. When the heart stops: a review of cardiac arrest in pregnancy. J Intensive Care Med 2012;28:204-14.
2. Jeejeebhoy FM, Zelop CM, Windrim R, et al. Management of cardiac arrest in pregnancy: a systematic review. Resuscitation 2011;82:801-9.
3. Hui D, Morrison LJ, Windrim R, et al. The American Heart Association 2010 guidelines for the management of cardiac arrest in pregnancy: consensus recommendations on implementation strategies. J Obstet Gynaecol Can 2011;33:858-63.
4. Neumar Robert W, Otto Charles W, Link Mark S, et al. Part 8: Adult Advanced Cardiovascular Life Support: 2010 American Heart Association guidelines for cardiopulmonary resuscitation and emergency cardiovascular care. Circulation 2010;122:S729-67.
5. Vanden Hoek TL, Morrison LJ, Shuster M, et al. Part 12: Cardiac Arrest in Special Situations: 2010 American Heart Association guidelines for cardiopulmonary resuscitation and emergency cardiovascular care. Circulation 2010;122:S829-61.
6. Lipman S, Daniels K, Cohen SE, Carvalho B. Labor room setting compared with the operating room for simulated perimortem cesarean delivery: a randomized controlled trial. Obstet Gynecol 2011;118:1090-4.

83   Difficult Airway in the Parturient

DEFINITION

Difficult airway in the parturient includes difficult mask ventilation, difficult placement of an SGA, or difficult tracheal intubation.

83

ETIOLOGY

Patient factors (specific to pregnancy)
    Airway edema
    Increased Mallampati score compared to nonpregnant state
    Breast engorgement
    High risk of regurgitation
    Decreased functional residual capacity
    Increased O_2 consumption
    Increased risk of bleeding from mucosal surface
Other anatomical causes of a difficult airway
    Full dentition
    Obesity/short neck
Physician factors
    Inexperience with airway management in the parturient
    Failure to respond effectively to a rapidly deteriorating situation
Equipment factors
    Inexperience with equipment
    Inadequate backup or alternative airway adjuncts or intubating devices

TYPICAL SITUATIONS

Cesarean section under general anesthesia
    Contraindication to neuraxial anesthesia

Failure of neuraxial technique
Insufficient time to place or dose neuraxial anesthetic
Maternal refusal to have neuraxial anesthesia
Maternal and preexisting anatomic abnormalities
Local anesthetic toxicity requiring airway management
Nonobstetric surgery during pregnancy

PREVENTION

Perform a complete airway assessment prior to inducing anesthesia (general or neuraxial)
In patients with known or anticipated difficult airway, perform awake fiberoptic intubation
Alert the obstetric team to the increased probability of difficult airway management during general anesthesia
Consider early placement of an epidural catheter in patients at risk of difficult intubation or stat/urgent cesarean section and ensure that the catheter is functional
Optimize patient positioning prior to induction of general anesthesia
Prepare for a difficult intubation and have contingency plans if you cannot ventilate and/or cannot intubate
Consider videolaryngoscope as primary choice for intubation
Review and practice difficult airway/failed intubation algorithm

MANIFESTATIONS

Failure to intubate the trachea after two attempts by an experienced anesthesia professional
Difficult insertion of laryngoscope
Small or restricted mouth opening
Masseter spasm secondary to succinylcholine
Difficult visualization of vocal cords
Difficult passage of ETT through vocal cords
Failure to successfully mask ventilate after induction of anesthesia
Failure to successfully place an SGA

SIMILAR EVENTS

Anesthesia workstation malfunction (e.g., bag/switch malposition)
Normal airway but unsuccessful intubation due to inexperience of the intubator
Functional airway obstruction
Laryngospasm (see Event 97, Laryngospasm)
Bronchospasm (see Event 29, Bronchospasm)
Gastric distention with air
Endobronchial intubation (see Event 30, Endobronchial Intubation)

MANAGEMENT

Obstetric patients have a higher risk of both difficult and failed intubation

If difficult airway is known or anticipated, perform an awake fiberoptic intubation since this may be the safest option
Prepare primary and backup airway equipment
Have contingency plans if primary plan fails

Before induction of general anesthesia
  Position patient appropriately (e.g., "ramp" patient for intubation, especially if obese)
  Maintain left uterine displacement
  Administer sodium citrate 0.3 M PO, 30 mL
  Administer ranitidine IV, 50 mg, and metoclopramide IV, 10 mg
  Preoxygenate with 100% O_2 with anesthesia breathing circuit
  Prep and drape the patient BEFORE general anesthesia is induced

If unanticipated difficult intubation after induction
  Call for additional anesthesia help stat if not already present (e.g., anesthesia professional, anesthesia tech)
  Call surgeon capable of establishing surgical airway and obtain equipment for surgical airway
  Call for difficult airway cart or supplies (including videolaryngoscope)
    Have help set up additional airway equipment
  Ensure adequate oxygenation and ventilation (may be difficult)
    Place an oral airway
    Consider two-person bag valve mask technique
    Apply continuous cricoid pressure
    Reposition the patient's head and neck
  Most experienced person should perform second laryngoscopy
    Use videolaryngoscope
    Use appropriately styleted ETT or bougie
    Adjust cricoid pressure if it is impairing ventilation or intubation
    Use smaller ETT

If intubation fails on second attempt
  Place an SGA (e.g., LMA) to maintain oxygenation and ventilation
    If SGA placement is successful, clinical situation will dictate whether or not to continue the anesthetic with this airway and deliver the fetus or awaken the patient
      Confirm ventilation with ET CO_2
      Maintain cricoid pressure after placement of SGA
    After delivery, consider whether to attempt tracheal intubation through the SGA (see Event 3, Difficult Tracheal Intubation)

If SGA placement is UNSUCCESSFUL, attempt face mask ventilation
If face mask ventilation is adequate, but intubation is not possible
  Wake the patient up and reevaluate for awake fiberoptic intubation
  Patient will be at increased risk of awareness with prolonged intubation attempts

If face mask ventilation is UNSUCCESSFUL, decide whether to awaken the patient or establish a surgical airway
  If muscle relaxation is wearing off, awaken the patient
  If the patient CANNOT BE INTUBATED OR VENTILATED
    Move early and aggressively to emergency cricothyrotomy or other emergency surgical airway. DO NOT WAIT for the O_2 saturation to fall precipitously
    Consider transtracheal jet ventilation, weighing the significant risk of the procedure

If surgical airway is established, consider whether to awaken the patient or proceed with cesarean section
Failed airway management may result in maternal cardiac arrest (see Event 82, Cardiac Arrest in the Parturient)

COMPLICATIONS

Hypoxemia
Aspiration of gastric contents
Esophageal intubation
Airway trauma/bleeding/swelling
Dental damage
Cerebral anoxia
Awareness
Fetal death
Maternal death

SUGGESTED READING

1. Berg CJ, Callaghan WM, Syverson C, Henderson Z. Pregnancy-related mortality in the United States, 1998 to 2005. Obstet Gynecol 2010;116:1302-9.
2. Hawkins JL, Chang J, Palmer SK, Gibbs CP, Callaghan WM. Anesthesia-related maternal mortality in the United States: 1979–2002. Obstet Gynecol 2011;117:69-74.
3. Quinn AC, Milne D, Columb M, Gorton H, Knight M. Failed tracheal intubation in obstetric anaesthesia: 2 yr national case–control study in the UK. Br J Anaesth 2013;110:74-80.
4. Rucklidge M, Hinton C. Difficult and failed intubation in obstetrics. Contin Educ Anaesth Crit Care Pain 2012;12:86-91.

84   Emergency Cesarean Section

DEFINITION

Emergency cesarean section is the urgent or stat operative delivery of the fetus through an abdominal incision.

ETIOLOGY

Maternal or fetal complication that, in the opinion of the obstetrician, requires an urgent or stat delivery of the neonate via cesarean section.

TYPICAL SITUATIONS

Stat cesarean section
  Severe fetal distress
  Prolapsed umbilical cord
  Massive hemorrhage
  Uterine rupture
  Maternal cardiac arrest unresponsive to immediate resuscitation
Urgent cesarean section
  Mild fetal distress (e.g., nonreassuring fetal trace, fetal intolerance of labor)
  Fetal malpresentation in labor
  Failed induction or trial of labor
  Failure to progress or descend in labor
  Abnormal placentation
  Failed forceps or vacuum delivery
  Previous hysterotomy (e.g., previous cesarean section, myomectomy, or other uterine surgery)

PREVENTION

Identify high-risk parturients
Maintain left uterine displacement to prevent aortocaval compression
Careful maternal and fetal monitoring during trial of labor
Care in the provision of neuraxial anesthesia
Reduce morbidity and mortality by having a written institutional plan for stat and urgent
   cesarean section
      Drill and practice management of stat and urgent cesarean sections (using simulation if
         available)

MANIFESTATIONS

Presence of maternal or fetal indications for emergency cesarean section

SIMILAR EVENTS

None

MANAGEMENT

*In patients presenting for stat cesarean section indicating an immediate threat to maternal or
fetal well-being, general anesthesia is the preferred technique. For urgent cesarean section,
when time permits and if there are no contraindications, regional anesthesia is the preferred
technique.*

**Determine the most appropriate anesthetic technique for the parturient after communi-
   cating with the obstetric team**
Intrauterine fetal resuscitation
      Optimize maternal position
      Administer 100% O_2 with nonrebreathing face mask
      Optimize maternal BP
      Discontinue oxytocin infusion
      Consider administration of a tocolytic
For a stat cesarean section or when regional anesthesia is contraindicated
General anesthesia
   Before induction of general anesthesia
      Call for anesthesia help
      Position patient appropriately (e.g., "ramp" patient for intubation if obese)
      Maintain left uterine displacement
      Check the fetal heart tones
            If the fetal HR is normal, emergency surgery may not be necessary or there may
               be time to institute a regional anesthetic
      Administer sodium citrate 0.3 M PO, 30 mL
      Administer ranitidine IV, 50 mg, and metoclopramide IV, 10 mg
      Preoxygenate with 100% O_2 with anesthesia breathing circuit
      Prep and drape the patient BEFORE general anesthesia is induced
      Administer prophylactic antibiotics as soon as possible for stat and urgent cesarean
         section

Induce general anesthesia
> Perform a RSI with cricoid pressure
>> Propofol IV, 2 to 2.5 mg/kg
>>> If the patient is hypotensive prior to induction
>>>> Etomidate IV, 0.2 mg/kg, or ketamine IV, 1 to 2 mg/kg
>>> Succinylcholine IV, 1 to 2 mg/kg
>>> Intubate the trachea and confirm placement with ET CO_2 and auscultation
>>> Proceed with surgery

Maintenance of general anesthesia before delivery
> Ventilate patient with 50% O_2/50% N_2O and 0.5 to 1.0 MAC of volatile anesthetic

Maintenance of general anesthesia after delivery
> Ventilate patient with 30% O_2/70% N_2O and 0.5 MAC of volatile anesthetic
> Administer opioids
>> Fentanyl IV, 100 to 250 μg
>> Morphine IV, 5 to 15 mg
>> Hydromorphone IV, 0.5 to 2 mg
> Consider midazolam IV, 1 to 2 mg for amnesia
> Consider bilateral transversus abdominis plane blocks prior to extubation
> Nondepolarizing muscle relaxants may not be required

After delivery of placenta
> Administer oxytocin IV, 1 to 2 U bolus followed by an infusion of 10 U/hr (e.g., 40 U of oxytocin/L at 250 mL/hr)
> Confirm adequate uterine tone (adjust oxytocin infusion rate as necessary)

Continue IV fluids to maintain circulating fluid volume

Extubation
> Suction the oropharynx
> Extubate the patient when fully conscious, in an upright or lateral position, NOT supine due to the risk of aspiration
> Transfer with 100% O_2 via a nonrebreathing face mask

For URGENT cesarean section (options include spinal, combined spinal-epidural [CSE], in situ epidural)

Prior to establishing regional anesthetic
> Infuse hetastarch IV, 500 mL
> Administer sodium citrate 0.3 M PO, 30 mL (if not NPO, otherwise it is not required routinely)
> Administer ranitidine IV, 50 mg, and metoclopramide IV, 10 mg
> Administer 100% O_2 via nonrebreathing face mask until delivery of the infant (or longer if required)

Spinal anesthetic
> Hyperbaric bupivacaine 0.75% (12 mg = 1.6 mL), fentanyl 10 μg, morphine 100 to 200 μg
> If patient is less than 5 feet, reduce bupivacaine dose to 10.5 mg

CSE anesthetic
> Hyperbaric bupivacaine 0.75% (12 mg = 1.6 mL), fentanyl 10 μg, morphine 100 to 200 μg
>> If parturient is less than 5 feet, or CSE is performed after an inadequate labor epidural top-up, reduce the bupivacaine dose to 10.5 mg (1.4 mL) and use the same dose of intrathecal fentanyl and morphine as previously stated. Use the epidural catheter for supplementation with local anesthetic if required.

Epidural in situ
> Administer local anesthetic via the epidural catheter

Lidocaine 2% with epinephrine (1:200,000) and $NaHCO_3$ (1 mL of 8.4% $NaHCO_3$ per 10 mL of lidocaine)

Administer lidocaine in 5 mL increments (usual dose required is 15 to 20 mL, with a maximum dose of 7 mg/kg)

Chloroprocaine 3% (usual volume 15 to 25 mL, maximum dose of 11 mg/kg)

Chloroprocaine has a shorter duration and less dense block compared to lidocaine, but should still be administered incrementally

Following placement of block

Ensure left uterine displacement

Measure NIBP every minute

Treat hypotension with increasing doses of vasopressor

Phenylephrine IV, 100 to 200 μg

Ephedrine IV, 5 to 10 mg

Check sensory level and motor block frequently prior to the start of surgery

Convert to general anesthetic if regional anesthetic is inadequate

COMPLICATIONS

Difficult intubation
Failed intubation
Awareness
Aspiration
Hypoxemia
Local anesthetic toxicity
Inadequate regional anesthetic
High or total spinal

SUGGESTED READING

1. American College of Obstetricians and Gynecologists and American Society of Anesthesiologists. Optimal goals for anesthesia in obstetric care. ACOG Committee Opinion No. 433. Obstet Gynecol 2009;113:1197-9.
2. Martin JA, Hamilton BE, Ventura SJ, et al. Births: final data for 2010. National vital statistics reports; vol 61 no 1. Hyattsville, Md: National Center for Health Statistics; 2012.
3. Rollins M, Lucero J. Overview of anesthetic considerations for cesarean delivery. Br Med Bull 2012;101:105-25.
4. American College of Obstetricians and Gynecologists. Antimicrobial prophylaxis for cesarean delivery: timing of administration. ACOG Committee Opinion No. 465. Obstet Gynecol 2010;116:791-2.

85 Hypotension Following Neuraxial Anesthesia

DEFINITION

Hypotension following neuraxial anesthesia is a decrease in arterial BP of 20% from baseline following neuraxial anesthesia or a systolic BP <90 mm Hg.

ETIOLOGY

Sympathetic blockade from neuraxial anesthesia in the parturient
Aortocaval compression

TYPICAL SITUATIONS

Spinal anesthesia
High dermatomal level of neuraxial anesthesia
Rapid induction of epidural anesthesia (e.g., not titrated)
Neuraxial anesthesia in the hypovolemic parturient
Parturient in the supine position without left uterine displacement

PREVENTION

Maintain left uterine displacement at all times
Ensure adequate IV access
Administer a 500 mL bolus of colloid as a preload or coload to spinal anesthesia for cesarean
    section
Use vasopressors to maintain normotension prior to delivery of the infant during a cesarean
    section
    Phenylephrine IV, 50 to 200 µg
    Ephedrine IV, 5 to 10 mg
Use thromboembolic stockings as aids to prevent hypotension
Use incremental doses of local anesthetic when dosing a labor epidural

MANIFESTATIONS

Nausea and/or vomiting (secondary to hypotension until proven otherwise)
Decrease in maternal BP from baseline
Diaphoresis
Weak or absent peripheral pulses
Inability of pulse oximeter or NIBP device to give a reading
Decreased O_2 saturation
Arrhythmias
Mental status changes
Fetal bradycardia or decelerations
Organ hypoperfusion
Decreased ET CO_2

SIMILAR EVENTS

Aortocaval compression
Hypotension from other causes (see Event 9, Hypotension)
Hemorrhage (see Event 1, Acute Hemorrhage, and Event 87, Obstetric Hemorrhage)
AFE (see Event 81, Amniotic Fluid Embolism)
PE (see Event 21, Pulmonary Embolism)
Venous air embolism (see Event 24, Venous Gas Embolism)
Total spinal anesthesia (see Event 89, Total Spinal Anesthesia)
Anaphylaxis (see Event 16, Anaphylactic and Anaphylactoid Reactions)
Artifact in BP measurement (see Event 9, Hypotension)
    Motion artifact with NIBP measurement (e.g., shivering)
    Incorrect NIBP cuff size
    Transducer height artifact

MANAGEMENT

Resuscitation equipment and medications should be immediately available at all sites where neuraxial anesthesia is performed.

Ensure left uterine displacement
Ensure adequate oxygenation and ventilation
Administer 100% O_2 by nonrebreathing face mask to the awake patient
Expand the circulating fluid volume
Infuse IV fluids
Hetastarch IV, 500 mL (more efficacious than crystalloid in preventing hypotension)
Monitor the parturient frequently after initiating neuraxial anesthesia
BP
Cesarean section: q1m intervals until delivery of the infant, then q2-3m thereafter if cardiovascularly stable
Labor epidural: q2m intervals for the first 20 minutes, then q15m for the duration of the epidural infusion
Assess level of sensory block frequently until stable
Monitor fetal HR
Immediately check the BP if
The parturient complains of nausea or feeling faint
The parturient is unresponsive to verbal stimuli
Fetal bradycardia or decelerations are observed
Persistent fetal distress will require stat or urgent cesarean section (see Event 84, Emergency Cesarean Section)
If patient is hypotensive, restore maternal BP to near-baseline values until delivery of the infant
Administer additional fluid rapidly
Administer vasopressor
Phenylephrine IV, 50 to 200 µg
Ephedrine IV, 5 to 10 mg
If patient is unresponsive and hypotension is profound, administer epinephrine IV, 10 to 100 µg
Reassess adequacy of IV access
Evaluate for other causes of hypotension (see Event 9, Hypotension)
If cardiac arrest occurs
Call for help and initiate CPR (see Event 2, Cardiac Arrest, and Event 82, Cardiac Arrest in the Parturient)

COMPLICATIONS

Hypoxemia
Hypoventilation
Aspiration of gastric contents
Organ hypoperfusion
Placental hypoperfusion and fetal acidosis
Acute renal failure
Cardiac arrest

SUGGESTED READING

1. Carvalho B, Mercier FJ, Riley ET, Brummel C, Cohen SE. Hetastarch co-loading is as effective as pre-loading for the prevention of hypotension following spinal anesthesia for cesarean delivery. Int J Obstet Anesth 2009;18:150-5.
2. Ngan Kee WD, Khaw KS, Ng FF. Comparison of phenylephrine infusion regimens for maintaining maternal blood pressure during spinal anaesthesia for Caesarean section. Br J Anaesth 2004;92:469-74.
3. Loubert C. Fluid and vasopressor management for Cesarean delivery under spinal anesthesia: continuing professional development. Can J Anaesth 2012;59:604-19.
4. American Society of Anesthesiologists Task Force on Obstetric Anesthesia. Practice guidelines for obstetric anesthesia: an updated report by the American Society of Anesthesiologists Task Force on Obstetric Anesthesia. Anesthesiology 2007;106:843-63.

86 Magnesium Toxicity

DEFINITION

Magnesium toxicity occurs with a serum Mg^{2+} level above the therapeutic range.

ETIOLOGY

Overdose of $MgSO_4$

Failure to monitor serum Mg^{2+} levels (especially in patients with oliguria and/or renal impairment)

TYPICAL SITUATIONS

Seizure prophylaxis in preeclampsia
Prophylaxis and seizure treatment in eclampsia
Fetal neuroprotection in preterm labor
Tocolysis in preterm labor
Renal insufficiency or failure

PREVENTION

Check baseline serum creatinine level before $MgSO_4$ administration or immediately after commencement
   Reduce $MgSO_4$ dose in patients with renal impairment
Administer $MgSO_4$ via an infusion pump
Monitor serum Mg^{2+} levels every 4 to 6 hours during infusions
Monitor BP, HR, O_2 saturation, RR, level of consciousness, deep tendon reflexes, urine output, and fetal HR during infusions

MANIFESTATIONS

General
   Warmth
   Flushing
   Nausea

Pulmonary
    Hypoventilation
    Pulmonary edema
Cardiovascular
    Palpitations
    Hypotension
    Chest pain and tightness
    ECG changes such as bradycardia, increased PR interval, increased QRS interval, increased QT interval, complete heart block
Neurologic
    Muscle weakness
    Double vision
    Slurred speech
    Sedation
    Confusion

SIMILAR EVENTS

Respiratory depression (see Event 56, Postoperative Failure to Breathe)
Cardiovascular collapse (see Event 82, Cardiac Arrest in the Parturient)
Adrenocortical insufficiency (see Event 38, Addisonian Crisis)
Hyperkalemia (see Event 40, Hyperkalemia)

MANAGEMENT

86

STOP and disconnect the MgSO$_4$ infusion
Assess patient
    Ensure adequate oxygenation and ventilation
        Administer 100% O_2 with a nonrebreathing face mask
        May require bag valve mask ventilation and/or RSI
            If advanced airway technique is required, **call for help**
    Maintain left uterine displacement
    Use fluids cautiously during magnesium infusion as pulmonary edema may occur
    Maintain BP with vasopressors
    Monitor ECG continuously
    Monitor neurological signs and symptoms, including level of consciousness and deep tendon reflexes
Check serum Mg^{2+} level
    1.7 to 2.4 mg/dL—normal serum concentration
    5.0 to 9.0 mg/dL—therapeutic serum concentration
    >12 mg/dL—deep tendon reflexes absent
    15 to 20 mg/dL—respiratory arrest
    >25 mg/dL—cardiac arrest
Administer calcium
    Calcium gluconate IV, 1000 mg over 3 minutes, repeat as necessary
    CaCl$_2$ 10% IV, 5 mL, may be given as an alternative
Promote Mg^{2+} excretion
    Administer small IV fluid boluses (250 to 500 mL)
    Furosemide IV, 20 mg

Consider hemofiltration
If ECG evidence of toxicity
    Consider insulin or dextrose infusion

COMPLICATIONS

Pulmonary edema
Respiratory depression/failure
Potentiation of nondepolarizing muscle relaxants
Hypotension
Bradycardia
Hypocalcemia
Hyperkalemia
Cardiac arrest

SUGGESTED READING

1. McDonnell NJ, Muchatuta NA, Paech MJ. Acute magnesium toxicity in an obstetric patient undergoing general anaesthesia for caesarean delivery. Int J Obstet Anesth 2010;19:226-31.
2. Altman D, Carroli G, Duley L, et al. Magpie Trial Collaboration Group. Do women with pre-eclampsia, and their babies, benefit from magnesium sulphate? The Magpie Trial: a randomised placebo-controlled trial. Lancet 2002;359:1877-90.
3. Belfort M, Saade G, Foley M, Phelan J, Dildy G. Critical care obstetrics. 5th ed. West Sussex, UK: Wiley Blackwell; 2010, p. 443.

87

87   Obstetric Hemorrhage

DEFINITION

Obstetric hemorrhage is peripartum blood loss of >500 mL for a vaginal delivery and >1000 mL for a cesarean delivery; these limits may or may not produce hemodynamic compromise in a particular patient.

ETIOLOGY

Uterine atony
Placental pathology
Obstetric trauma
Coagulopathy

TYPICAL SITUATIONS

Uterine atony (accounts for almost 80% of all causes of postpartum hemorrhage)
    Age <20 or >40 years
    Cesarean section
    Multiparous patients

Multiple gestation
Polyhydramnios
Macrosomia
Chorioamnionitis
Hypertensive disease of pregnancy
Prolonged labor
Retained placenta
Antepartum hemorrhage
Abnormal placentation
Placenta previa (placenta located in the lower uterine segment over the cervix)
Previous cesarean section or uterine surgery
Multiparity or advanced maternal age
Placenta accreta, increta, and percreta (placenta attaches to, into, or through the myometrium)
Other uterine surgery
Multiparity or advanced maternal age
Hypertensive disease of pregnancy
Smoking
Infection
Abruptio placentae (premature separation of a normally implanted placenta after 20 weeks' gestation)
Hypertensive disease of pregnancy
Premature rupture of membranes
Increased uterine size
Increasing parity
Previous history of placental abruption
Amniocentesis
Trauma
Maternal cocaine use
Uterine rupture
Previous cesarean section or uterine surgery
Vaginal birth after cesarean section
Dysfunctional labor
Augmented labor
Increasing parity
Uterine instrumentation either intrapartum or postpartum
Uterine inversion
Mismanaged third stage of labor
Precipitous labor
Retained placenta
Previous retained placenta
Scarred uterus
Preterm delivery
Induced labor
Increasing parity
Lacerations of the cervix or vagina during delivery
Instrumented delivery
Macrosomia
Acquired or congenital coagulopathy

PREVENTION

Create institutional MTP
> Will not prevent obstetric hemorrhage but may reduce morbidity

Identify parturients at risk of obstetric hemorrhage early
Treat coagulopathy early

MANIFESTATIONS

Abnormal bleeding from the vagina or surgical site
Tachycardia
Hypotension (may be a late sign in younger parturients)
Fetal bradycardia or decelerations
Acute anemia
Coagulopathy or DIC
> Oozing from puncture sites
> Abnormal coagulation profile

SIMILAR EVENTS

Anaphylaxis (see Event 16, Anaphylactic and Anaphylactoid Reactions)
Septic shock (see Event 13, The Septic Patient)
Hypotension from other causes (see Event 9, Hypotension)
> Occult bleeding from another site (e.g., gastrointestinal bleed)

Maternal dehydration
AFE (see Event 81, Amniotic Fluid Embolism)

MANAGEMENT

Management of obstetric hemorrhage requires a multidisciplinary team approach, including obstetric, anesthesiology, hematology, blood bank, critical care, and IR.

Check and verify maternal vital signs
Inform the obstetrician and call for help (see Event 1, Acute Hemorrhage)
Maintain left uterine displacement even if postpartum
> Enlarged uterus can cause aortocaval compression

Ensure adequate oxygenation and ventilation
> Administer 100% O_2 by a nonrebreathing face mask
>> Intubate the patient if there is loss of consciousness, respiratory failure, or severe cardiovascular collapse
>> Ventilate with 100% O_2 after intubation
> Patient may require urgent airway management
>> If urgent airway management is necessary and patient is conscious, perform RSI with cricoid pressure and intubate the trachea
>>> Etomidate IV, 0.2 to 0.3 mg/kg, or ketamine IV, 0.5 to 1.0 mg/kg
>>> Succinylcholine IV, 1 to 2 mg/kg

Identify and treat the cause of hemorrhage
For uterine atony
Surgical treatment
Bimanual uterine massage and/or uterine packing
Hold pressure on the bleeding site
Bakri balloon
B-Lynch suture
Vessel ligation (uterine or iliac vessels)
Hysterectomy
Pharmacological treatment
Administer oxytocin IV, 1 to 2 U bolus followed by an infusion at 10 U/hr (e.g., 40 U of oxytocin/L at 250 mL/hr [or greater if required]—may cause hypotension, nausea, vomiting)
Administer Methergine (methylergonovine) IM, 0.2 mg (may cause severe hypertension, palpitations, headache)
Administer Hemabate (carboprost) IM, 0.25 mg (may cause bronchospasm, hypertension, nausea, vomiting, diarrhea, flushing)
Administer Cytotec (misoprostol) buccal, 600 μg (may cause pyrexia, diarrhea)
IR
Emergency consultation for therapeutic options and possible uterine artery embolization
Support the circulation
Ensure adequate IV access (two large-bore IVs)
Rapidly infuse crystalloid and/or colloid
Treat hypotension with vasopressors, increasing doses as needed
Phenylephrine IV, 50 to 200 μg
Ephedrine IV, 5 to 10 mg
Epinephrine IV, 10 to 100 μg
Place an arterial line and consider placement of CVP line for infusion of vasopressors and monitoring of fluid status
Prepare for massive transfusion and initiate MTP
Inform the blood bank that more blood and blood products will be needed emergently
Get help to set up a rapid infusor device (and cell saver if appropriate)
Transfuse blood products
Use a fluid warmer
Transfuse an RBC:FFP ratio of 1:1 or 2:1
O-negative blood if crossmatched blood is not available
Transfuse RBCs to maintain hemoglobin >7 g/dL
Transfuse additional FFP if PT/aPTT is prolonged
Transfuse platelets if <50,000/μL
Transfuse cryoprecipitate if fibrinogen <200 mg/dL)
Consult hematology if necessary
Maintain normothermia
Frequent lab draws for ABG, CBC, PT/aPTT, fibrinogen, metabolic panel, and Ca^{2+}
If the patient is under general anesthesia
Use volatile anesthetic agents with caution (MAC <0.5) as they decrease uterine tone
Supplement anesthetic with IV agents (benzodiazepines and opioids)

COMPLICATIONS

Hypotension
Hypoxemia
ARDS or TRALI
Multiorgan failure
Coagulopathy
Hypothermia
Hypocalcemia
Hyperkalemia
Volume overload
Infection
Aspiration
Transfusion reaction

SUGGESTED READING

1. Bateman BT, Berman MF, Riley LE, Leffert LR. The epidemiology of postpartum hemorrhage in a large, nationwide sample of deliveries. Anesth Analg 2010;110:1368-73.
2. Pacheco LD, Saade GR, Gei AF, Hankins GD. Cutting-edge advances in the medical management of obstetrical hemorrhage. Am J Obstet Gynecol 2011;205:526-32.
3. Wise A, Clark V. Challenges of major obstetric haemorrhage. Best Pract Res Clin Obstet Gynaecol 2010;24:353-65.
4. Mayer DC, Smith KA. Antepartum and postpartum hemorrhage. In: Chestnut DH, Polley LS, Tsen LC, Wong CA, editors. Chestnut's obstetric anesthesia: principles and practice. 4th ed. Philadelphia: Mosby; 2009. p. 811-36.
5. Stafford I, Belfort MA, Dildy GA III. Etiology and management of hemorrhage. In: Belfort M, Saade G, Foley M, Phelan J, Dildy G, editors. Critical care obstetrics. 5th ed. West Sussex, UK: Wiley Blackwell; 2010. p. 308-26.

88 Preeclampsia and Eclampsia

DEFINITION

Preeclampsia is a multisystem disease characterized by hypertension, peripheral edema, proteinuria, and other organ involvement with onset of symptoms typically after 20 weeks' gestation. Eclampsia is the new onset of seizures in a woman with preeclampsia.

ETIOLOGY

Unknown

TYPICAL SITUATIONS

Primarily a disorder of first pregnancies
History of preeclampsia
Chronic hypertension
Multiple gestation
Diabetes
Obesity
Advanced maternal age

African American ethnicity
Vascular and connective tissue disease
Nephropathy
Asthma
Hydatidiform mole
Antiphospholipid antibody syndrome

PREVENTION

Identify patients at risk of preeclampsia
>   Low-dose aspirin has some benefit when used for prevention of preeclampsia in subsequent pregnancies

MANIFESTATIONS

Hypertension, defined as BP >140/90 mm Hg
Proteinuria, defined as >300 mg of protein/L of urine in a 24-hour period
Edema
>   Generalized facial and upper extremity edema as opposed to dependent edema of pregnancy
HELLP syndrome
>   Hemolysis, elevated liver enzymes, and low platelets (a variant of severe preeclampsia characterized by rapid clinical deterioration)
Airway edema
Pulmonary
>   Pulmonary edema, secondary to pulmonary capillary leak, which can be exacerbated by a decrease in colloid oncotic pressure
>   ARDS
Cardiovascular
>   Left ventricular function can be hyperdynamic or decreased
Renal
>   Decreased glomerular filtration rate
>   Elevated serum creatinine
>   Hyperuricemia
>   Oliguria
>   Acute renal failure
CNS
>   Hyperreflexia, clonus, headache, visual changes, somnolence, CNS irritability, cerebral edema, seizures (eclampsia), intracranial hemorrhage
Hematologic
>   Thrombocytopenia
>   HELLP syndrome
>   DIC
Hepatic
>   Epigastric pain
>   HELLP syndrome
>   Subcapsular bleeding
>   Hepatic rupture
Obstetric complications
>   Impaired uterine blood flow
>   Placental infarction

Intrauterine growth retardation
Oligohydramnios
Preterm labor
Placental abruption
Fetal distress

CLASSIFICATION OF HYPERTENSIVE DISORDERS IN PREGNANCY

Gestational hypertension
    No preexisting hypertension or other signs and symptoms of preeclampsia
Preeclampsia
    Mild preeclampsia
        Hypertension—BP $\geq$140/90 mm Hg
        Proteinuria—>300 mg/24 hr or 1+ on dipstick specimen
    Severe preeclampsia, one or more of the following criteria
        Hypertension—BP $\geq$160/110 mm Hg
        Proteinuria—>5 g/24 hr or 3+ on dipstick specimen
        Oliguria —<500 mL in 24 hours
        Cerebral or visual disturbance
        Pulmonary edema or cyanosis
        Epigastric or right upper quadrant pain
        Impaired liver function
        Thrombocytopenia
        Intrauterine growth retardation
    Chronic hypertension
        Preexisting hypertension without signs of preeclampsia
    Chronic hypertension with superimposed preeclampsia-eclampsia
        Preexisting hypertension with presence of signs of preeclampsia or eclampsia

SIMILAR EVENTS

Essential hypertension (see Event 8, Hypertension)
Preexisting congenital or acquired cardiac disease
Preexisting renal disease (see Event 48, Oliguria)
Seizures from other causes (see Event 57, Seizures)
Coagulopathy or DIC from other causes
Preexisting pulmonary disease
Acute surgical abdomen in parturient
Pain associated with placental abruption

MANAGEMENT

These patients are at higher risk of fetal distress and may require stat or urgent cesarean section. Early evaluation of the patient's airway, cardiac, pulmonary, and coagulation status will allow preparation for possible anesthetic intervention. Symptoms of preeclampsia usually resolve within 48 hours of delivery.

Control hypertension
    Pharmacologic treatment
        BP control prior to delivery is important. Lower BP to 140–160/90–100 mm Hg with carefully titrated medications

Labetalol IV, 20 mg, increase dose to 40 mg after 10 minutes if needed, then 80 mg after a further 10 minutes if needed

Hydralazine IV, 5 to 10 mg; then, after a 20-minute interval, repeat dose (10 mg) if BP remains elevated

Labetalol IV infusion

Nicardipine IV infusion

Extreme emergencies

Sodium nitroprusside IV, 0.2 to 2 μg/kg/min infusion (with invasive BP monitoring)

Regional anesthetic

Epidural analgesia will decrease catecholamine release and therefore decrease pain-mediated hypertensive responses

Check the platelet count and LFTs prior to placing epidural catheter. If platelet count <100,000/μL or LFTs are elevated, check the coagulation profile before proceeding with placement

Seizure prophylaxis and/or treatment

Administer MgSO$_4$ IV, 4 to 6 g loading dose over 20 minutes, followed by an infusion of 1 to 2 g/hr. Initiate at the onset of labor and continue for 24 hours postpartum

Monitor for signs of Mg^{2+} toxicity (see Event 86, Magnesium Toxicity)

Decreased patellar tendon reflexes

If seizures occur

Administer MgSO$_4$ IV, 2 g as a second bolus dose over 3 to 5 minutes

If seizures continue, administer midazolam IV, 1 to 2 mg, or clonazepam IV, 1 to 4 mg

Propofol IV, 20 to 40 mg, may also terminate the seizure (see Event 57, Seizures)

Ensure adequate oxygenation and ventilation

Patient may need to be intubated

Strict fluid balance

Limit fluid intake to 1 mL/kg/hr and continue for duration of MgSO$_4$ infusion

Measure hourly urine output with urinary catheter

Maintenance of urine output may require judicious use of fluid boluses, diuretics, and CVP monitoring in collaboration with obstetric and critical care teams

If signs of pulmonary edema or decreased O$_2$ saturation are observed, review fluid balance immediately

CVP monitoring and/or a PA catheter is recommended to guide further fluid management

Fetal assessment

Nonstress testing

Biophysical profile

Ultrasound to assess fetal weight and amniotic fluid volume

Doppler fetal blood flow studies

Severe preeclampsia is an indication for delivery

Vaginal delivery is the preferred route of delivery in preeclamptic women; however, the clinical situation may require cesarean section

Regional anesthesia is preferred for labor and delivery or delivery via cesarean section

If general anesthesia is indicated, consider arterial line monitoring

Standard induction agents should be supplemented with other agents to suppress the hypertensive response to laryngoscopy

Esmolol IV, 1 to 2 mg/kg

Lidocaine IV, 1 mg/kg

Remifentanil IV, 0.5 to 1 μg/kg

These drugs can also be used at extubation to blunt the hypertensive response to emergence

For the eclamptic patient

Treat the seizure (see previous)

Ensure adequate oxygenation and ventilation

Expeditious delivery of neonate is indicated

If fetal bradycardia persists after a seizure, immediate cesarean delivery is required

COMPLICATIONS

Fetal distress
Thrombocytopenia
DIC
Severe hemorrhage
Multisystem organ failure
Mg^{2+} toxicity (e.g., enhances effect of nondepolarizing muscle relaxants)
Subcapsular hematoma of the liver
Laryngeal edema
Difficult intubation
Hypoxemia
Aspiration
Intracranial hemorrhage
Cerebral edema
Maternal death
Fetal death

SUGGESTED READING

1. Polley LS. Hypertensive disorders. In: Chestnut DH, Polley LS, Tsen LC, Wong CA, editors. Chestnut's obstetric anesthesia: principles and practice. 4th ed. Philadelphia: Mosby; 2009. p. 975-1007.
2. Ramanathan J, Gill RS, Sibai B. Hypertensive disorders of pregnancy. In: Suresh MS, Segal BS, Preston RL, Fernando R, Mason CL, editors. Shnider and Levinson's anesthesia for obstetrics. 5th ed. Baltimore: Lippincott Williams & Wilkins; 2013. p. 437-61.
3. Dildy G, Belfort M. Complications of pre-eclampsia. In: Belfort M, Saade G, Foley M, Phelan J, Dildy G, editors. Critical care obstetrics. 5th ed. West Sussex, UK: Wiley Blackwell; 2010. p. 438-65.
4. American College of Obstetricians and Gynecologists. Emergent therapy for acute-onset, severe hypertension with preeclampsia or eclampsia. ACOG Committee Opinion No. 514. Obstet Gynecol 2011;118:1465-8.
5. Engelhardt T, MacLennan FM. Fluid management in pre-eclampsia. Int J Obstet Anesth 1999;8:253-9.
6. Dennis AT. Management of pre-eclampsia: issues for anaesthetists. Anaesthesia 2012;67:1009-20.
7. Altman D, Carroli G, Duley L, et al., for the Magpie Trial Collaboration Group. Do women with pre-eclampsia, and their babies, benefit from magnesium sulphate? The Magpie Trial: a randomised placebo-controlled trial. Lancet 2002;359:1877-90.

89   Total Spinal Anesthesia

DEFINITION

Total spinal anesthesia is caused by local anesthetic blockade of all spinal nerves, up to and possibly including the brainstem.

ETIOLOGY

Parturients are more sensitive to local anesthetics compared to nonpregnant women
Epidural
> Unintentional dural puncture during placement of epidural anesthetic
> Intrathecal placement or migration of the epidural catheter

Spinal
> Large spinal dose administered
> Excessive Trendelenburg position with hyperbaric solution
> Full spinal dose in short stature parturient
> Spinal anesthesia (normal dose) placed after labor epidural
> Repeat full spinal dose after initial failed spinal

CSE
> Excessive epidural bolus with a CSE

TYPICAL SITUATIONS

Difficult epidural placement leading to unintentional and/or unrecognized intrathecal catheter placement
Short stature parturients (<5 feet)
Intrathecal administration of local anesthetic after an epidural anesthetic

PREVENTION

Use the appropriate dose of local anesthetic during neuraxial blocks
In short stature parturients, place a CSE with a reduced intrathecal dose rather than a single shot spinal
Position the patient appropriately
Dose an epidural catheter or CSE incrementally and evaluate the patient for signs and symptoms of intrathecal/intravascular injection

MANIFESTATIONS

Signs and symptoms of a total spinal can develop very rapidly.
> Hypotension
> Nausea/vomiting
> Bradycardia
> Profound cardiovascular collapse
> Rapidly ascending loss of motor and sensory function
> Difficulty speaking
> Poor respiratory effort

Respiratory arrest
Loss of airway reflexes
Loss of consciousness
Patients may have fixed, dilated pupils

SIMILAR EVENTS

Hypotension from other causes (see Event 9, Hypotension)
Cardiac arrest (see Event 82, Cardiac Arrest in the Parturient)
Seizures (see Event 57, Seizures, and Event 88, Preeclampsia and Eclampsia)
Local anesthetic toxicity (see Event 52, Local Anesthetic Systemic Toxicity, and Event 85, Hypotension Following Neuraxial Anesthesia)
Vasovagal episode
Medication error (see Event 63, Drug Administration Error)

MANAGEMENT

Resuscitation equipment and medications should be immediately available at all sites where neuraxial anesthesia is performed.

Call for help
    Labor and delivery team and additional anesthesia help. If the patient arrests, immediate cesarean section may be necessary with the goal of delivery within 5 minutes (see Event 82, Cardiac Arrest in the Parturient)
Discontinue epidural bolus/infusion
Ensure left uterine displacement
Reassure the patient, as she may become acutely anxious
Ensure adequate oxygenation and ventilation
    Administer 100% O_2 by a nonrebreathing face mask
        Intubate the patient if there is loss of consciousness, respiratory failure, or severe cardiovascular collapse
        Ventilate with 100% O_2 after intubation
    Patient may require urgent airway management
        If urgent airway management is necessary and patient is conscious, perform RSI with cricoid pressure and intubation
            Etomidate IV, 0.2 to 0.3 mg/kg, or ketamine IV, 0.5 to 1.0 mg/kg
            Succinylcholine IV, 1 to 2 mg/kg
Check maternal vital signs continuously
Administer fluid bolus and increase IV fluid infusion rate
Administer a vasopressor, escalating doses as necessary
    Ephedrine IV, 5 to 10 mg
    Phenylephrine IV, 50 to 200 μg
    Epinephrine IV, 10 to 100 μg bolus and consider infusion if no response
Treat bradycardia
    Administer glycopyrrolate IV, 0.4 mg, or atropine IV, 0.4 to 1 mg
        Bradycardia can be profound and may require treatment with epinephrine IV, 10 to 100 μg
If maternal vital signs cannot be easily stabilized with IV fluids and vasopressors, consider cesarean section to aid maternal stability (i.e., relieve aortocaval compression and increase venous return)

Assess fetus

If there is no fetal compromise, immediate delivery is not indicated

If fetal compromise is identified, then stat cesarean section is required

Ventilate the patient until the effects of the local anesthetic have dissipated (usually 1 to 2 hours)

Administer IV sedation to prevent awareness

If cardiac arrest occurs, start CPR (see Event 82, Cardiac Arrest in the Parturient)

COMPLICATIONS

Hypoxemia

Cerebral or myocardial ischemia or injury

Aspiration of gastric contents

Awareness

Fetal death

Maternal death

SUGGESTED READING

1. Carvalho B. Failed epidural top-up for cesarean delivery for failure to progress in labor: the case against single-shot spinal anesthesia. Int J Obstet Anesth 2012;21:357-9.
2. Pan PH, Bogard TD, Owen MD. Incidence and characteristics of failures in obstetric neuraxial analgesia and anesthesia: a retrospective analysis of 19,259 deliveries. Int J Obstet Anesth 2004;13:227-33.
3. Wong CA. Epidural and spinal analgesia/anesthesia for labor and vaginal delivery. In: Chestnut DH, Polley LS, Tsen LC, Wong CA, editors. Chestnut's obstetric anesthesia: principles and practice. 4th ed. Philadelphia: Mosby; 2009. p. 462-3.

89

Chapter 13
Pediatric Events

CALVIN KUAN and ERIN WHITE PUKENAS

---

90 Acute Hemorrhage in the Pediatric Patient

DEFINITION

Acute hemorrhage in the pediatric patient is the acute loss of a large volume of blood and can be either overt or covert.

Overt
>   Can be visualized in the surgical field, on sponges, or in the suction containers

Covert
>   No outward sign of bleeding (e.g., retroperitoneal hemorrhage, blood loss hidden in the drapes)

ETIOLOGY

Bleeding from a large blood vessel (artery or vein) secondary to surgery, trauma, or disease
>   In pediatrics, massive blood loss is >2 to 3 mL/kg/min or 50% of blood volume over 3 hours

Underlying coagulopathy or therapeutic anticoagulation

Loose connection in the IV, central line, or arterial line, leading to potentially hidden blood loss

90

TYPICAL SITUATIONS

Major trauma
Procedural
>   Vascular, cardiac, thoracic, or major abdominal surgery
>   Major orthopedic surgery
>   Injury to fetus during delivery or cesarean section
>   Interventional radiologic or cardiac catheterization procedure
>   Covert hemorrhage is more likely where the surgical field is obscured by drapes or is distant from the anesthesia professional

Coagulopathy, either acquired or therapeutic
Occult blood loss (e.g., GI tract, long bone fractures, or into the retroperitoneal space)
Acute hemorrhage may be a delayed complication of an earlier injury or invasive procedure

PREVENTION

Identify and correct coagulopathy early
Identify, institute prophylaxis for, and treat other potential bleeding sites (e.g., GI ulcers, fractures in acute trauma)
In children, anticipate the need for massive transfusion and obtain adequate IV access prior to start of procedure
Establish an institutional MTP

MANIFESTATIONS

Overt
Blood in surgical field
Blood on surgical sponges, on the drapes, and on the floor
Increased suction noise
Accumulation of blood in suction containers
Surgeon comments or concerns about bleeding, volume status, or transfusion
Changes in vital signs (decreased BP, increased HR)
Covert
Changes in vital signs
Increased HR (or decreased HR if severe)
Decreased BP
Decreased CVP
Change in pulse oximeter reading due to poor perfusion
Physical examination if accessible
Increased RR if breathing spontaneously
Poor peripheral perfusion or capillary refill time
Poor pulses
Expanding soft tissue, abdomen, or thigh (i.e., retroperitoneal bleed, or long bone fracture)
Change in neurologic examination, bulging fontanelle, anisocoria (i.e., intracranial bleed)
Decreased NIRS monitor reading
Inadequate filling of ventricle on TEE or TTE
Decreased urine output
Increased fluid requirement above what is expected
Little or transient BP response to IV fluid bolus or vasopressor administration
Laboratory studies
Unexplained decreasing hematocrit
Increasing metabolic acidosis on ABG

SIMILAR EVENTS

Hypotension (see Event 96, Hypotension in the Pediatric Patient)
Anesthetic or vasodilator overdose (see Event 72, Volatile Anesthetic Overdose)
Any cause of shock (see Event 91, Anaphylaxis in the Pediatric Patient, and Event 13, The Septic Patient)
Cardiac failure
Cardiac tamponade (see Event 18, Cardiac Tamponade)
Pulmonary hypertension
PE (see Event 21, Pulmonary Embolism)
Arrhythmias
Progressively inadequate volume replacement due to bleeding, insensible losses (e.g., urine, evaporative losses), or third spacing
Occlusion of venous return by compression of IVC by surgical packing, pneumoperitoneum, or retraction
Tension pneumothorax (see Event 35, Pneumothorax)

MANAGEMENT

Special pediatric considerations

IV access may be challenging, especially in young infants

Small-gauge IV catheters (24 and 22 g) typically placed in infants and young children may not withstand infusions of large volumes

Anticipate the need for transfusion and obtain adequate IV access prior to the start of the procedure

CVP line or cut-down may be necessary, especially if rapid volume administration is anticipated

Ensure that air bubbles are not injected into the patient

These may result in paradoxical air emboli to the heart or brain

All IV tubing must be meticulously debubbled

Special care should be taken with pressurized rapid-infusion devices

Hyperkalemia

Children are at much greater risk of morbidity from hyperkalemia than adults

Arrhythmias and cardiac arrest can occur in young children, particularly those with congenital heart disease

Older blood and blood that has been irradiated may contain dangerously elevated levels of K^+

Employ strategies to minimize the risk of hyperkalemia from transfusion of RBCs

Use freshest RBCs

Use washed RBCs

Slow rate of RBC transfusion if possible

Monitor serum K^+ levels and ABGs frequently and initiate treatments if K^+ rises over 4.5

Diuretics, Ca^{2+}, $NaHCO_3$, Kayexalate, dialysis

Acidemia increases extracellular K^+ levels

Hypocalcemia

Secondary to transfusion of citrate-phosphate-dextrose-adenine (CPDA) blood products

CPDA present in higher levels in FFP than RBCs

Avoid hypothermia

Hypothermia will exacerbate coagulopathy and platelet dysfunction

Warm blood products

PREOPERATIVE

Send type and cross (especially if two samples are needed) before surgery as samples may be difficult to obtain in children without central venous or arterial access

Communicate the potential for significant bleeding and need for blood products with the blood bank

Extra time may be required to locate appropriately matched products for patients with antibodies

Determine acceptable values for HR and BP based on the child's age

Determine blood volume and "allowable" blood loss based on patient weight and hematocrit

INTRAOPERATIVE

Inform the surgeon of the problem

Initial treatment

Deliver 100% O_2

Consider reducing volatile anesthetic agents

Administer 10 to 20 ml/kg IV bolus of non–dextrose-containing isotonic fluid (e.g., saline, LR, 5% albumin, or blood) and watch for HR and BP response. Repeat as necessary to maintain adequate preload

Administer IV bolus of vasopressor (e.g., ephedrine, epinephrine, phenylephrine), carefully titrated to clinical effect

    Vasopressors temporize the situation while administering IV fluids

    Treatment of hypovolemic shock with vasopressors alone, without replacing volume, increases the risk of severe end organ damage

Additional monitoring data may help guide volume replacement

    Consider placement of an arterial line for ABG and BP monitoring

    Consider TEE or TTE examination for cardiac function and ventricular filling

    Consider placement of a CVP line

If patient is not responding to initial therapy, or major fluid resuscitation is necessary

Call for help

    Inform all team members of the situation and plans for resuscitation

Anesthesia professional's role

    Primary anesthesia professional should focus on leading and coordinating team members

    Obtain additional IV access if necessary

        Consider IO line early if IV access is difficult

    Place arterial line if appropriate

    Monitor patient hemodynamics and level of anesthesia

    Operate rapid transfusion devices or push blood

    Help to draw ABG and labs

Sugeon's role

    Identify and control source of bleeding

    Surgeons may have to pause surgery

        To allow anesthesia professional access to the patient to place an IV, CVP line, or arterial line

        To allow time for volume replacement

        To perform a necessary procedure (e.g., place a difficult CVP line or perform a cutdown for IV access)

Nurses' role

    Call for more nursing and tech help

        Charge nurse may help coordinate resources

    Order and arrange transport of blood products from blood bank

    Help to check and administer blood or blood products

    Ensure that a rapid infuser system is available

    Set up cell saver if indicated

    Consider activating MTP if available

Monitor venous access lines and sites

    Check all IV and central lines for loose connections and leaks

    Check IV site frequently for soft tissue infiltration, especially when fluid is being infused under pressure, as opposed to a drip IV set

For massive transfusion of blood or blood products

Activate MTP if available

    Notify blood bank of situation and anticipated needs as they may need to seek out additional sources of products

Order of preference for blood products
  Type-specific (or type-compatible) crossmatched unit
  Type-specific (or type-compatible) but not crossmatched unit (e.g., patient has been screened, but there is not enough time to complete crossmatching)
  Uncrossmatched, type-O, Rh-negative unit (O-neg RBCs)
If patient has received >1 blood volume of emergency release blood products (O-neg RBCs), keep transfusing O-neg RBCs. Testing for antibodies must be completed prior to switching back to patient's type-specific blood
Transfuse blood and blood products through fluid warmer to avoid hypothermia
  Washed PRBCs, platelets, FFP, and cryoprecipitate are usually at room temperature but also need to be warmed
Coagulopathy during massive transfusion is primarily due to dilution of clotting factors and/or platelets but may be due to fibrinolysis or DIC
Blood and blood product administration
  Platelets
    Monitor for thrombocytopenia and consider transfusion of platelets after 1 to 1.5 blood volumes have been lost
    Replacement should be 10 to 15 mL/kg of platelets for each blood volume replaced
    Hypothermia causes platelet dysfunction even with normal platelet counts
  Factors
    Initiate transfusion of FFP after 1 blood volume of RBCs has been transfused
    Transfusion of RBCs and FFP should be at a ratio of 2:1 (RBC:FFP)
Monitor labs and hemodynamics to guide therapy
  Hematocrit
  Platelets
  PT/aPTT
  Ca^{2+}
  K^+
  ECG tracing for evidence of electrolyte abnormalities
  HR and BP
  CVP
  TEE/TTE

COMPLICATIONS

Arrhythmias
Coagulopathy/DIC
Acidosis
Alkalosis
Hypocalcemia
Hyperglycemia
Hyperkalemia
Hypernatremia
Hypothermia
Transfusion-related infection
Transfusion reaction/ABO incompatibility
Transfusion-associated graft-versus-host disease
ARDS/TRALI
Volume overload and hypertension
Cardiac arrest

SUGGESTED READING

1. Chidester SJ, Williams N, Wang W, Groner JI. A pediatric massive transfusion protocol. J Trauma Acute Care Surg 2012;73:1273-7.
2. Cote CJ, Lerman J, Todres ID. A practice of anesthesia for infants and children. 4th ed. Philadelphia: Saunders; 2009, p. 313-4.
3. Davis PJ, Cladis FP, Motoyama EK, et al. Smith's anesthesia for infants and children. 8th ed. Philadelphia: Mosby; 2011, p. 1232-5.
4. Fuhrman BP, et al. Pediatric critical care. 4th ed. Philadelphia: Saunders; 2011, p. 338-63.

91   Anaphylaxis in the Pediatric Patient

DEFINITION

Anaphylaxis in the pediatric patient is an IgE-mediated response that is caused by exposure to an antigenic substance in a sensitized pediatric patient.

ETIOLOGY

Administration of, or exposure to, an agent that the patient has been previously sensitized to, with production of antigen-specific IgE

TYPICAL SITUATIONS

In patients with a known allergy or sensitivity to a specific agent or a history of atopy or allergy to nondrug allergens
After exposure to substances that can trigger anaphylaxis
  Neuromuscular blocking drugs
  Latex
  Antibiotics
  Opioids
  Protamine
  Amino-ester local anesthetic agents
  Blood and blood products
  Iodinated contrast material
  Chlorhexidine preparation solutions
  Sedative-hypnotics
  Colloid administration (e.g., dextrans, hydroxyethyl starch)
Patients with frequent latex exposure
  Patients requiring multiple reconstructive surgical procedures (e.g., myelomeningocele repair for spina bifida, patients with congenital genitourinary abnormalities)

PREVENTION

Avoid agents to which the patient has a documented allergy
Minimize the use of latex products in health care
  If there is a history of latex allergy, establish a latex-free environment

Avoid contact with, or manipulation, of latex devices
Use nonlatex surgical gloves
Use syringe/stopcock methods or unidirectional valves for injecting medications
Do not insert a needle through any multiple-dose vial with a natural rubber
stopper
Take the top of the vial completely off
Use the same medication from a glass ampule, if available
Use glass syringes as an alternative to plastic syringes with natural rubber seal on
plunger (plastic syringes may use nonlatex seals—check manufacturer's informa-
tion for syringe materials)
Obtain a careful history of previous allergic reactions, atopy, asthma, or significant latex
exposure
Avoid transfusion of blood or blood products whenever possible
If a specific drug must be administered to a patient known to be at risk of an allergic reaction,
administer prophylaxis
Corticosteroids, H_1 antagonists
Administer test dose of drug
Obtain consultation from an allergist if a critical allergy must be defined

MANIFESTATIONS

*Anaphylaxis has the potential for acute onset with catastrophic consequences. Severe hypo-
tension, increased peak airway pressure, and hypoxemia are the most common initial signs
but need not be present simultaneously.*

Cardiovascular
Severe hypotension
Tachycardia
Bradycardia may be initial sign
Arrythmias
Cardiac arrest
Respiratory
Hypoxemia
Decreased lung compliance
Severe bronchospasm
Cutaneous—may be obscured by surgical drapes
Flushing, hives, urticaria, pruritus
Swelling of mucosal membranes, angioedema, head and neck swelling

SIMILAR EVENTS

Medication causing direct histamine release (e.g., morphine)
Anesthetic overdose or medication error (see Event 72, Volatile Anesthetic Overdose, and
Event 63, Drug Administration Error)
Cutaneous allergy (rapid urticarial reactions)
Bronchospasm (see Event 29, Bronchospasm)
Hypotension from other causes (see Event 9, Hypotension)
Pulmonary edema from other causes (see Event 20, Pulmonary Edema)
Cutaneous manifestations of mastocytosis, carcinoid syndrome, hereditary angioedema

Transfusion reaction (see Event 50, Transfusion Reaction)
Cardiac tamponade (see Event 18, Cardiac Tamponade)
Stridor (see Event 97, Laryngospasm)
PE (see Event 21, Pulmonary Embolism)
Vasovagal reaction
Septic shock (see Event 13, The Septic Patient)
Aspiration of gastric contents (see Event 28, Aspiration of Gastric Contents)
Pneumothorax (see Event 35, Pneumothorax)
Esophageal intubation

MANAGEMENT

Stop administration of any possible antigen (e.g., discontinue antibiotics)
   Retain blood products for analysis
   Identify all latex products and remove from contact with the patient
Inform the surgeons and call for help
   Check to see whether they have injected or instilled a substance into a body cavity
   Consider aborting surgical procedure if severe or there is no response to initial treatment
      Anaphylaxis can be biphasic and can recur after successful initial treatment
Ensure adequate oxygenation and ventilation
   Administer 100% O_2
   Intubate the trachea if not already intubated
      The airway can rapidly become edematous, making intubation more difficult or
      impossible
Anaphylaxis is treated with epinephrine (the drug of CHOICE in anaphylaxis) and IV fluid
   Epinephrine dosing and route—drug calculations are CRITICAL
      For patients with profound hypotension or shock and a KNOWN working IV/IO
      line, administer epinephrine 0.5 to 1 µg/kg and increase rapidly up to 10 µg/kg as
      needed; maximum dose 1000 µg
      For patients in early phase without profound hypotension, shock or cardiac arrest, or
      for those patients in which IV/IO access HAS NOT BEEN OBTAINED, adminis-
      ter epinephrine IM, 10 µg/kg q5-15m; maximum 300 µg per dose
         Given difficulty in obtaining IV access in children, the IM dose is preferred
         by some anesthesia professionals and clinicians who deal with pediatric
         emergencies
      For cardiovascular collapse or cardiac arrest, give epinephrine IV, 10 µg/kg (see Event 94,
      Cardiac Arrest in the Pediatric Patient)
      Consider epinephrine infusion (20-200 ng/kg/min) with increasing dose to maintain BP
   Rapidly expand the circulating blood volume
      Administer 10-30 mL/kg NS or LR
      Immediate fluid needs may be massive
Decrease or stop the administration of anesthetic agents if hypotension is severe
If bronchospasm is present
   Administer bronchodilator
      Inhaled β-agonist (e.g., albuterol MDI)
      Volatile anesthetic agents may be administered for bronchodilation if the patient is
      normotensive
Administer H_1 and H_2 histamine antagonists
   Diphenhydramine IV, 1 mg/kg up to maximum of 50 mg
   Famotidine IV, 0.25 mg/kg, or ranitidine IV, 1 mg/kg IV

Administer corticosteroids

Methylprednisolone IV, 1 to 2 mg/kg, or dexamethasone IV, 0.2 mg/kg

In the absence of any other cause, consider latex allergy

Ensure all latex products in contact with the patient have been removed from the surgical field

Consider placement of an arterial line and urinary catheter to help guide vasopressor and fluid management

Obtain blood sample for mast cell tryptase levels within 2 hours to confirm the diagnosis of anaphylaxis

Arrange admission to ICU for continued postoperative management

Consider referring patient to an allergist on discharge from the hospital

COMPLICATIONS

Hypoxemia

Inability to intubate, ventilate, or oxygenate

Hypertension and tachycardia from vasopressors

ARDS

Renal failure

Cardiac arrest

DIC

Death

SUGGESTED READING

1. Ebo DG, Fisher MM, Hagendorens MM, et al. Anaphylaxis during anesthesia: diagnostic approach. Allergy 2007;62:471-87.
2. Hepner DL, Castells MC. Anaphylaxis during the perioperative period. Anesth Analg 2003;97:1381-95.
3. Karila C, Burnet-Langot D, Labbez F, et al. Anaphylaxis during anesthesia: results of a 12-year survey at a French Pediatric Center. Allergy 2005;60:828-34.
4. Lieberman PL, Nicklas RA, Oppenheimer J, et al. The diagnosis and management of anaphylaxis practice parameter: 2010 update. J Allergy Clin Immunol 2010;126:477-522.

92   Aspiration of a Foreign Body

DEFINITION

Aspiration of a foreign body into the respiratory tract

ETIOLOGY

Child placing a foreign body into the mouth

Tooth dislodged into the airway

Material left in the airway after a surgical procedure

TYPICAL SITUATIONS

Occurs in children between 7 months and 4 years of age with peak incidence at 1 to 2 years

Foreign body aspiration is a leading cause of death in children <1 year of age

Food is the most common foreign body in the infant/toddler age groups

Incomplete dentition and immature swallowing coordination increase susceptibility

Nonorganic material, such as disc batteries, beads, pins, tacks, coins, and parts of toys are common in older children

After a surgical procedure

PREVENTION

Encourage home-safety programs to keep food and small objects out of the reach of unsupervised toddlers

Perform laryngoscopy carefully

Consider extracting loose teeth prior to laryngoscopy

Double check that all materials placed in the airway are removed before extubation

MANIFESTATIONS

Cough

Dyspnea

Cyanosis

Decreased breath sounds

Tachypnea

Stridor

Wheezing

Hemoptysis

Hoarseness

Fever

Aphonia

Recurrent pneumonia

Physical examination may be normal

Radiographic visualization of the foreign body or of air trapping, infiltrates, or atelectasis

The right mainstem bronchus is the most common site for a foreign body to lodge

Organic material may be poorly visualized on CXR

High-resolution spiral CT scan can characterize disease severity distal to the foreign body

SIMILAR EVENTS

Recurrent pneumonia not related to aspiration of a foreign body

Foreign body in the esophagus

Laryngospasm (see Event 97, Laryngospasm)

Croup

Anaphylaxis (see Event 16, Anaphylactic and Anaphylactoid Reactions)

MANAGEMENT

Obtain history of onset of symptoms from witnesses

Check the O$_2$ saturation

Ensure adequate oxygenation and ventilation

This may not be possible until foreign body is removed emergently

Confirm the diagnosis of foreign body aspiration

Perform a physical examination of the airway and chest

Examine upper airway anatomy

Check for uniformity and symmetry of breath sounds and adventitious sounds (e.g., bronchospasm)

Obtain a CXR looking for the presence and location of a foreign body

Air trapping

Atelectasis

Pneumonia

Postobstructive airway collapse

Overexpansion

Anesthetic Induction for the Patient with a Foreign Body Aspiration

Discuss the surgical approach and method of ventilation with the team in advance

In addition to an ENT surgeon, consider consultation with a cardiothoracic or general surgeon depending on location and severity of foreign body obstruction

Obtain IV access

Cardiovascular collapse may occur in response to movement of the foreign body causing severe hypoxemia

Consider the potential need for ECMO or CPB

Plan for this early as it takes time to set up

Preoxygenate the lungs prior to induction of anesthesia

Complete airway obstruction may occur at any time, and rigid bronchoscopy must be performed immediately to remove the obstruction or dislodge it to another site that permits ventilation

Perform an inhalation induction with sevoflurane and 100% O_2

Controlled or spontaneous ventilation may be appropriate, depending on the location of the obstruction and the surgical approach

IV induction may be an acceptable alternative, depending on the clinical scenario

Following induction of anesthesia, the bronchoscopist should intubate the trachea with a ventilating bronchoscope in order to remove the foreign body

There may be increased resistance to ventilation when a telescopic lens is inserted through the bronchoscope

Ventilation may need to be alternated with attempts to locate and remove the foreign body

Facilitate passage of the foreign body through the laryngeal inlet

Maintain an adequate depth of anesthesia to prevent patient movement or coughing

Total IV anesthesia will maintain a consistent level of anesthesia during frequent circuit interruptions

Consider administering a small dose of a short-acting muscle relaxant just prior to removing the foreign body

If the foreign body cannot be removed through the bronchoscope and ventilation is inadequate, an emergency thoracotomy and bronchotomy may be necessary

Examine the tracheobronchial tree after removal of the foreign body

Following endoscopic examination, intubate the trachea with an ETT or allow the patient to awaken with a natural airway

The usual criteria for awake extubation should be applied

Allow the child with a natural airway to completely emerge prior to movement to the PACU

92

COMPLICATIONS

Hypoxemia
Hypercarbia
Laryngospasm
Pneumonia
    Chemical pneumonitis
    Bacterial infection
Hypotension
Massive hemoptysis
Severe bronchospasm
Pneumothorax
Airway rupture
Pneumomediastinum

SUGGESTED READING

1. Rimell FL, Thome Jr. A, Stool S, et al. Characteristics of objects that cause choking in children. JAMA 1995;274:1763-6.
2. Ciftci AO, Bingol-Kologlu M, Senocak ME, et al. Bronchoscopy for evaluation of foreign body aspiration in children. J Pediatr Surg 2003;38:1170-6.
3. Even L, Heno N, Talmon Y, et al. Diagnostic evaluation of foreign body aspiration in children: a prospective study. J Pediatr Surg 2005;40:1122-7.
4. Farrell PT. Rigid bronchoscopy for foreign body removal: anaesthesia and ventilation. Pediatr Anesth 2004;14:84-9.
5. Litman RS, Ponnuri J, Trogan I. Anesthesia for tracheal or bronchial foreign body removal in children: an analysis of ninety-four cases. Anesth Analg 2000;91:1389-91.
6. Metrangelo S, Monetti C, Meneghini L, et al. Eight years' experience with foreign-body aspiration in children: what is really important for a timely diagnosis? J Pediatr Surg 1999;34:1229-31.
7. Zur K, Litman RS. Pediatric airway foreign body retrieval: surgical and anesthetic perspectives. Pediatr Anesth 2009;19:109-17.

93 Bradycardia in the Pediatric Patient

DEFINITION

Bradycardia in the pediatric patient is a HR slower than the age-appropriate normal level.

ETIOLOGY

Hypoxemia is a common cause of bradycardia/cardiac arrest in pediatric patients
Decreased automaticity of sinus node
    Increased vagal tone
    Drug related
        Succinylcholine
        Digoxin
        Opioids
        Cholinesterase inhibitors
        Anesthetic agents
    Hypothermia

Reflex response to hypertension
    Treatment with phenylephrine
    CNS mass
    CNS conditions (e.g., autonomic dysreflexia)
Complication from congenital heart surgery or cardiac catheterization
    Caused by injury of the sinus node or the conduction pathway
Acquired heart disease
    Cardiomyopathies (e.g., dilated or hypertrophic)
    Inflammatory (e.g., rheumatic fever or post viral)
    Ischemic (e.g., Kawasaki disease)
    Right atrial thrombi or tumors
Congenital heart disease
    Certain forms of congenital heart disease (e.g., heterotaxy syndromes) are associated with bradycardia

TYPICAL SITUATIONS

Acute severe bradycardia from any etiology can be an indication of impending cardiac arrest in children. The most common cause of bradycardia is respiratory distress or failure.

Preoperative finding
    Isolated finding in asymptomatic patient
    Symptom of underlying medical condition
        Pacemaker malfunction
        Congenital or acquired heart disease
        OSA
        Side effect of medication
        Prematurity
        Increased ICP
Intraoperative finding
    Medications that can cause bradycardia
        Succinylcholine
        Volatile anesthetics
        Opioids (e.g., remifentanil)
        α_2-Agonists (e.g., clonidine, dexmedetomidine)
        Cholinesterase inhibitors (e.g., neostigmine)
        Cardiovascular agents (e.g., esmolol or phenylephrine)
    Increased vagal stimulation
        Mechanical/iatrogenic
            Laryngoscopy
            ETT too deep or pushing on carina
            Nasopharyngeal or oropharyngeal suctioning or tube placement
            Raised intraocular pressure or traction on eyeball
            Tracheal suctioning
            Traction on peritoneum
            Bladder catheterization
            Increased intrathoracic pressure or Valsalva maneuver
        Normal physiologic response
            Sleeping

93

> Breath holding
> Coughing
> Gagging or vomiting
Pathophysiologic
> Gastroesophageal reflux disease (GERD)
> Increased ICP
> Severe OSA
> Apnea and bradycardia of prematurity
Interruption of ongoing inotropic infusions (e.g., line disconnect or kinking)

PREVENTION

Maintain adequate oxygenation and ventilation
Ensure appropriate position of ETT
Premedicate children at risk of bradycardia with an anticholinergic agent
> Glycopyrrolate IV or IM, 10 to 20μg/kg
> Atropine IV or IM, 10 to 20μg/kg
Treat bradycardia early
Avoid excess vagal simulation
> External ocular pressure, traction on peritoneum, prolonged attempt at laryngoscopy

MANIFESTATIONS

Slow HR
> ECG
> Pulse oximeter
> Arterial line
> Peripheral pulses
> Junctional or ventricular escape beats
Hypotension
In the awake, nonanesthetized patient
> Dizziness
> Syncope
> Altered mental status
> Fatigue/lethargy
> Nausea/vomiting
Infants and nonverbal children
> Altered mental status
> Irritability
> Poor feeding

SIMILAR EVENTS

Monitor artifact
> ECG lead disconnection or failure
> Failure of monitor to count QRS or pulse
> Oximeter probe misplaced or failure
Heart block
> Second degree with intermittent dropped beats

Third-degree complete heart block with ventricular escape beats
Pacemaker malfunction or failure
Lead fracture
Lead disconnection
Inappropriate settings (e.g., output too low, sensitivity too high)
AF or flutter with poor perfusion

MANAGEMENT

Verify bradycardia and assess patient's hemodynamic status
ECG, pulse oximeter, arterial line
Check peripheral pulse
Check BP
Check ET CO_2 waveform for evidence of adequate CO
Ensure adequate oxygenation and ventilation
Bradycardia is a common sign of hypoxemia in small infants
Deliver 100% O_2 (except in certain forms of congenital heart disease)
Check position of ETT
Consider decreasing level of anesthesia
Decrease or turn off volatile anesthetics, propofol, and other infusions
Check surgical field for operative causes
Alert surgeon to stop the precipitating stimulus
Rule out intracranial hypertension as a possible treatable etiology
If bradycardia is mild-moderate but stable (e.g., HR is low but not dropping or is associated with mild-moderate symptoms such as modest decrease in BP and no change in ET CO_2)
Ensure adequate IV/IO access
Atropine IV, IO, or endotracheal
IV or IO dose: 20 µg/kg, NO minimum dose, maximum dose 0.5 mg
Endotracheal dose: 40 to 60 µg/kg
Glycopyrrolate IV, 10 to 20 µg/kg, maximum dose 0.4 mg
Ephedrine IV, 0.1 to 0.3 mg/kg
Not routinely used in young children
Consider isoproterenol IV infusion, 0.1 to 1 µg/kg/min
May result in vasodilation with inadequate coronary and cerebral perfusion
Anticipate and plan for deterioration in patient status
Consider obtaining crash cart and placing pediatric defibrillator/pacing pads
Continuously reassess for change in ECG or hemodynamic status
Be prepared to start CPR
Consider aborting procedure if problem persists
If bradycardia is unstable (e.g., dropping HR or associated with severe symptoms such as hypotension, loss of consciousness, or drop in ET CO_2) (see Event 94, Cardiac Arrest in the Pediatric Patient)
Administer epinephrine IV, IO, or endotracheal (SC/IM dosing is not appropriate treatment of bradycardia)
IV/IO dose: 10 µg/kg, maximum dose 1 mg
Endotracheal dose: 100 µg/kg, maximum dose 2.5 mg
Call for more help and notify surgeon

93

Start CPR
Call an OR or hospital code
Call for crash cart and defibrillator if not already done
> Place pediatric defibrillator/pacing pads on patient
>> Consider pacing the patient
>>> Transcutaneous pacemaker
>>> In situ pacer wires will be present in some postoperative patients
Search for and treat possible causes
Consider ECMO

COMPLICATIONS

Junctional or ventricular escape beats
Tachyarrhythmias or hypertension secondary to pharmacologic treatment of bradycardia
Inappropriate pacemaker firing
Pneumothorax from chest compression
Intracranial hemorrhage in premature infants
> Secondary to boluses of epinephrine or from acute hypertension
Cardiac arrest

SUGGESTED READING

1. Cote CJ, Lerman J, Todres ID. A practice of anesthesia for infants and children. 4th ed. Philadelphia: Saunders; 2009, p. 313-4.
2. Davis PJ, Cladis FP, Motoyama EK. Smith's anesthesia for infants and children. 8th ed. Philadelphia: Mosby; 2011 p. 1232-5.
3. Donoghue A, Berg RA, Hazinski MF, et al. Cardiopulmonary resuscitation for bradycardia with poor perfusion versus pulseless cardiac arrest. Pediatrics 2009;124:1541-8.
4. Fleming S, Thompson M, Stevens R, et al. Normal ranges of heart rate and respiratory rate in children from birth to 18 years of age: a systematic review of observational studies. Lancet 2011;377:1011-8.
5. Jones P, Dauger S, Peters MJ. Bradycardia during critical care intubation: mechanisms, significance and atropine. Arch Dis Child 2012;97:139-44.
6. Kleinman ME, Chameides L, Schexnayder SM, et al. Pediatric advanced life support: 2010 American Heart Association guidelines for cardiopulmonary resuscitation and emergency cardiovascular care. Circulation 2010;122: S876-908.

94   Cardiac Arrest in the Pediatric Patient

DEFINITION

Cardiac arrest is the absence of effective mechanical activity of the heart.

ETIOLOGY

The cause of cardiac arrest in children is different than in adults in that coronary artery disease is rare. Congenital or acquired heart disease accounts for one third of all pediatric cardiac arrests.

Hypoxemia
> Low FiO_2
>> Relative (inadequate for the patient's condition)
>> Absolute (problems delivering O_2 to the breathing circuit)

Inadequate alveolar ventilation
$\dot{V}/\dot{Q}$ mismatch
Anatomic shunt
Excessive metabolic O_2 demand
Low CO
Circulatory shock
Sepsis
Acidosis
Pulmonary or venous air embolism
Increased vagal tone (e.g., traction on extraocular muscles)
Toxins (e.g., LAST)
Hypovolemia
Electrolyte abnormalities
Hypothermia

TYPICAL SITUATIONS

Risk of cardiac arrest is inversely proportional to age and occurs more frequently in children than adults (children under 1 month of age are at greatest risk).

Inadequate oxygenation or ventilation
Oversedation
Inability to secure difficult airway
Accidental extubation
Infection (e.g., pneumonia or sepsis)
Neurologic condition (e.g., seizure)
Patients who are currently receiving mechanical ventilatory support
Patients who have already had a cardiac arrest or are currently receiving inotropic
support
Arrhythmias
Pulmonary hypertensive crisis
Acute myocardial depression
Anesthetic agents
Hypoxemia (e.g., from cyanosis or "Tet" spell)
Hypovolemia
Hemorrhage
Inadequate volume administration
Electrolyte abnormalities
Hyperkalemia
Hypocalcemia
Hypomagnesemia
Coronary thromboemboli or air emboli
Insufficient coronary perfusion
Unbalanced systemic versus pulmonary circulation in single-ventricle patient
Surgery
Vagal response secondary to surgical traction or pressure
Iatrogenic causes
Accidental interruption of inotropic infusions
R on T phenomenon with unsynchronized cardioversion
CVP line related dysrhythmia or tamponade

Other
  Trauma (nearly half of all pediatric deaths are motor vehicle related)
  Anaphylaxis
  LAST
  MH
  Emergency department consults (e.g., aspiration of foreign body, poisoning)
Preexisting severe or systemic diseases
  Congenital or acquired cardiac disease
    Single ventricle physiology, especially prior to SVC anastomosis, or Glenn
      procedure
    Aortic stenosis
    Cardiomyopathies
    Severe cyanotic lesions
    History of life-threatening arrhythmias
  Pulmonary hypertension
  Multisystem organ failure
  Metabolic disease or derangement (i.e., diabetic ketoacidosis)
Emergency cases
Any case performed without a full preoperative evaluation

PREVENTION

Discuss the risks and benefits of any planned procedure or care plan with the surgeon, medical team, and family.

Ensure adequate oxygenation and ventilation
Perioperative care of the complex pediatric patient requires clinicians experienced in managing pediatric patients
  Knowledge of normal age-related vital signs in pediatric patients
  Appropriate use of monitoring
  Early recognition of patients with impending respiratory or cardiac arrest
  Careful use of medications (e.g., local and general anesthetics)
Consider consulting cardiologist for pediatric patients with unrepaired or complex congenital heart disease
  Understanding complex physiology and anatomy of congenital heart disease and surgical repair is essential to proper care
    Single ventricle anatomy (e.g., hypoplastic left heart syndrome or tricuspid atresia)
    Patients after cavo pulmonary anastomoses, or Glenn or Fontan procedure
    Pulmonary hypertension
    Cardiomyopathies

MANIFESTATIONS

Patient becomes limp and unresponsive
Absence of pulse oximeter waveform
No palpable pulse (carotid, femoral, brachial)
  NIBP unmeasurable
  Invasive arterial pressure without pulsations

Absence of heart tones on auscultation
Apnea
Significant fall in ET CO_2
Poor skin perfusion, cyanosis
Regurgitation and possible aspiration of gastric contents
Arrhythmias (VT, VF, asystole)
PEA (rhythm in PEA may appear normal)
Lack of ventricular contraction on TEE or TTE

SIMILAR EVENTS

Hypotension (see Event 96, Hypotension in the Pediatric Patient)
Anaphylaxis (see Event 91, Anaphylaxis in the Pediatric Patient, and Event 16, Anaphylactic and Anaphylactoid Reactions)
Pulmonary or venous air embolism (see Event 21, Pulmonary Embolism, and Event 24, Venous Gas Embolism)
Sepsis (see Event 13, The Septic Patient)
Acute hemorrhage (see Event 1, Acute Hemorrhage, and Event 90, Acute Hemorrhage in the Pediatric Patient)
Medication reaction (see Event 63, Drug Administration Error)
Local anesthetic overdose (see Event 52, Local Anesthetic Systemic Toxicity)
Total spinal (see Event 89, Total Spinal Anesthesia)
Seizures (see Event 57, Seizures)
Artifacts on monitoring devices
    ECG
    Pulse oximeter
    BP measurement systems (NIBP or invasive)
Pacemaker malfunction or inappropriate settings
    Pacemaker causing electrical activity on monitor without actual CO
In children with shunt-dependent pulmonary blood flow (Blalock-Taussig shunt, central shunt, or aorto pulmonary window), occlusion of the shunt may result in severe decrease in measured ET CO_2, severe hypoxemia, and cardiac arrest.

MANAGEMENT

Treat the patient, not the monitor
Verify that there is no pulse or if the patient is bradycardic with signs of poor perfusion
    Check the pulse, which can be difficult in children
    Do NOT spend more than 10 seconds searching for a pulse
        Umbilical or femoral arteries in the newborn
        Brachial or femoral arteries in the infant
        Carotid or femoral arteries in the older child
            Surgeon may have better access to palpable pulses
    Check pulse oximeter and ET CO_2 waveforms
    Check NIBP and ECG monitors and leads
    Auscultate chest for heart sounds
    Check arterial line waveform

Immediately notify surgeons and other OR personnel of the cardiac arrest
> Call for help
> Call for hospital or OR "code"
> Call for crash cart and defibrillator
>> Apply pediatric defibrillation pads to the chest

Start CPR immediately (C-A-B: compressions, airway, breathing)

Turn off all anesthetics

Administer 100% O_2 at high flows to flush circuit of inhaled anesthetics and verify change
> **If intubated, set ventilator to age-appropriate rate and tidal volume. Avoid hyperventilation**

Begin BLS/PALS
> **Assign someone to start chest compressions**
>> Compressions should be at least 100 per minute and depth should be one third to one half the anterior-posterior diameter of the chest; release completely to allow chest to fully recoil
>>> **Neonate or Infant:** two thumbs encircling hands technique (place thumbs together over lower sternum and forcefully squeeze the thorax)
>>> **Child:** compress the lower half of sternum with heel of one or two hands, avoiding compression on ribs or xiphoid process
>> Two or more compressors are optimal for the older child or for adult CPR
>> Minimize interruptions in compressions and keep interruptions brief (less than 10 seconds)
>> Monitor for fatigue of the person performing chest compressions (rotate every 2 minutes)
>> Adequate compressions should generate an ET CO_2 of at least 10 to 15 mm Hg. **You MUST improve CPR quality if ET CO_2 is less than 10 mm Hg**

> **Airway**
>> Mask ventilate with 100% O_2 at high flow
>> Intubation **should not** delay defibrillation in children with VF or pulseless VT
>> Secure airway with an ETT as soon as possible
>> Consider an SGA if unable to intubate

> **Breathing**
>> **Neonate:** There should be a 3:1 ratio of compressions to ventilations, with 90 compressions and 30 breaths to achieve approximately 120 events per minute
>>> 3:1 compression-to-ventilation ratio should be used for neonatal resuscitation where compromise of ventilation is nearly always the primary cause of arrest
>> Consider using higher compression:ventilation ratios (e.g., 15:2) if the arrest is believed to be of cardiac origin
>> **Infant and child:** If the infant or child is not intubated and there is one rescuer, compression-to-ventilation ratio is 30:2, and for two rescuers the compression-to-ventilation ratio is 15:2
>> Once the infant or child is intubated, ventilate 8 to 10 times per minute without interrupting chest compressions
> After advanced airway is established, mechanically ventilate to free up hands and resources
> Avoid hyperventilation

Employ cognitive aids (neonatal resuscitation and PALS algorithms) to help determine diagnosis and treatment

Assign tasks to skilled responders, BUT make sure that C-A-B continues

94

Ensure adequate IV access
> Ensure patency of the IV
> Consider placement of an IO line early
> Consider central venous line or a venous cut-down if having difficulty with peripheral access
> Consider placing an arterial line for monitoring and ABGs

Diagnose and Treat Arrythmias
> Determine whether patient is in a shockable (VT or VF) or nonshockable rhythm (PEA or asystole)
>> Analyze rhythm during very short breaks in CPR
>>> CPR artifact can appear as a shockable rhythm

VT/VF (shockable pathway)
> **Continue high-quality CPR** between defibrillations
> **Administer 1 shock at 2 J/kg**
> Resume five cycles of CPR (about 2 minutes) and quickly recheck rhythm
> **If a shockable rhythm persists, give a second shock at 4 J/kg**
> **Administer epinephrine IV or IO**, 10 µg/kg and immediately resume five cycles of CPR
> Repeat epinephrine dose every 3 to 5 minutes
>> **Consider endotracheal administration of epinephrine if IV or IO access is not available**
>>> Endotracheal epinephrine dose: 100 µg/kg
>>>> The total volume of drug and flush should not exceed 5 mL in infants
> DEFIBRILLATE EVERY 2 MINUTES (4 J/kg) IF A SHOCKABLE RHYTHM PERSISTS
> Consider amiodarone IV or IO, 5 mg/kg, or lidocaine IV or IO, 1 mg/kg

Torsades de pointes
> Therapy as mentioned previously for VT/VF
> Administer $MgSO_4$ IV or IO, 25 to 50 mg/kg

Search for treatable cause of VT/VF
> Hyperkalemia (see Event 40, Hyperkalemia)
>> Stop fluids containing K^+ (LR and PRBCs)
>> Administer $CaCl_2$ 10% IV, 10 mg/kg
>> Administer dextrose 50% IV, 0.25 to 1 g/kg, and regular insulin IV, 0.1 U/kg
>> $NaHCO_3$ IV, 1 to 2 mEq/kg
>> If patient is successfully resuscitated from a hyperkalemic arrest, consider furosemide or dialysis
> Local anesthetic toxicity (see Event 52, Local Anesthetic Systemic Toxicity)
>> Administer 20% lipid emulsion (Intralipid), IV bolus 1.5 mL/kg over 1 minute and start infusion at 0.25 mL/kg/min
>> Repeat Intralipid boluses every 2 to 5 minutes until circulation is restored
>> Maximum total Intralipid dose is 10 mL/kg over first 30 minutes

IF SHOCKABLE RHYTHM CHANGES TO A NONSHOCKABLE RHYTHM—SWITCH TO PEA/ASYSTOLE PATHWAY

PEA/Asystole (nonshockable pathway)
> **Continue high-quality CPR**
> **Administer epinephrine IV or IO**, 10 µg/kg q3-5m

Search for treatable causes of PEA/asystole
> **Hypovolemia** (see Event 90, Acute Hemorrhage in the Pediatric Patient, and Event 96, Hypotension in the Pediatric Patient)

Administer fluid bolus, rule out occult bleeding, administer blood for massive hemorrhage or severe anemia

Rule out inadequate preload from compression of the great vessels

Surgical retraction or pneumoperitoneum

Consider using TEE or TTE for diagnosis and response to therapy

Hypoxemia (see Event 10, Hypoxemia)

Ventilate and oxygenate with 100% O_2

Auscultate breath sounds

Suction ETT

Reconfirm presence of ET CO_2

Tension pneumothorax (see Event 35, Pneumothorax)

Auscultate for unilateral breath sounds

Look for distended neck veins or deviated trachea

Perform emergent needle decompression at second intercostal space at the midclavicular line

Patient will require pleural drainage after needle decompression

Toxins (including infusions)

Confirm that IV and volatile anesthetics are off

Check all infusions and confirm they are correct

Discontinue if they are not indicated

If a large dose of local anesthetic has been administered, treat as local anesthetic toxicity (see Event 52, Local Anesthetic Systemic Toxicity)

Send toxicology screen

Cardiac tamponade

Use TEE or TTE to rule out pericardial effusion

If present, perform emergent pericardiocentesis

Electrolyte and acid/base abnormalities

Send stat labs (ABG and metabolic panel)

Evaluate for acidosis, hyperkalemia, hypokalemia, hypoglycemia, hypocalcemia

Treat hyperkalemia as previously stated

VGE (see Event 24, Venous Gas Embolism)

Acute hypotension with drop in ET CO_2

Flood surgical field with saline

Aspirate CVP catheter if present

PE (see Event 21, Pulmonary Embolism)

Pulmonary hypertension

Use TTE or TEE to assess RV function

Hyperthermia

Rule out MH (see Event 45, Malignant Hyperthermia)

Hypothermia (see Event 44, Hypothermia)

Continually reassess patient without interrupting chest compressions

Look for return of spontaneous circulation

ECG for return of electrical activity

Correlate with return of palpable pulse or BP

Pulse oximetry

Consider post-resuscitation hypothermia for brain protection

Echocardiography may be employed to assess heart function and rule out correctable pathology

Other therapeutic options
  Open chest cardiac massage
  Open chest defibrillation
  Automated external defibrillation
  Pacing
    Transcutaneous pacing
    Transvenous pacing
    Epicardial pacing
Consider extracorporeal cardiopulmonary resuscitation (ECPR)/ECMO if available
  Call ECMO code or obtain ECMO/ECPR consult from ICU
  Determine whether cause may be reversible or heart may be transplantable
  This is only successful if rapid deployment ECMO/ECPR protocols are already established in your institution

COMPLICATIONS

Rib fracture and pneumothorax from chest compression
Skin burns from defibrillation
Hypotension or hypertension from treatment of the arrest
Death

SUGGESTED READING

1. Cote CJ, Lerman J, Todres ID. A practice of anesthesia for infants and children. 4th ed. Philadelphia: Saunders; 2009, p. 313-4.
2. Davis PJ, Cladis FP, Motoyama EK. Smith's anesthesia for infants and children. 8th ed. Philadelphia: Mosby; 2011, p. 1232-5.
3. Fuhrman BP, Zimmerman JJ, Carcillo JA, et al. Pediatric critical care. 4th ed. Philadelphia: Saunders; 2011, p. 338–63.
4. Kleinman ME, Chameides L, Schexnayder SM, et al. Pediatric advanced life support: 2010 American Heart Association guidelines for cardiopulmonary resuscitation and emergency cardiovascular care. Circulation 2010;122:S876-908.
5. Morray JP. Cardiac arrest in anesthetized children: recent advances and challenges for the future. Pediatr Anesth 2011;21:722-9.
6. Nadkarni VM, Larkin GL, Peberdy MA, et al. First documented rhythm and clinical outcome from in-hospital cardiac arrest among children and adults. JAMA 2006;295:50-7.

95   Difficult Airway Management in the Pediatric Patient

DEFINITION

Difficult airway management in the pediatric patient includes difficult mask ventilation, difficult placement of an SGA or difficult tracheal intubation.

ETIOLOGY

Patient factors (specific to pediatrics)
  Increased O_2 consumption leading to rapid desaturation
  Decreased functional residual capacity
  History of respiratory problems (e.g., snoring, recurrent croup, sleep apnea)

Possible anatomical causes of a difficult airway (specific to pediatrics)
  Tongues are large relative to the oropharyngeal cavity
  Tonsillar hypertrophy
  Subglottic stenosis
  Infection (e.g., retropharyngeal abscess)
  Foreign body aspiration
  Trauma
  Craniofacial abnormalities (e.g., Pierre-Robin syndrome, Treacher-Collins syndrome)
Physician factors
  Inexperience with airway management in the pediatric patient
  Failure to respond effectively to a rapidly deteriorating situation
Equipment factors
  Inexperience with equipment
  Inadequate backup or alternative airway adjuncts or intubating devices

TYPICAL SITUATIONS

Difficulty with intubation is thought to occur less frequently in children compared with adults and to be inversely dependent on age (incidence of 0.57% in newborns and toddlers, 0.12% in preschoolers, and 0.05% in school-age children)

Variations of normal anatomy not associated with a congenital syndrome
  Limited mouth opening restricting visualization and/or insertion of laryngoscope
  Larynx may be more anterior or superior, limiting visualization on direct laryngoscopy
  Small larynx or trachea may not permit passage of an ETT
Extreme prematurity or small for gestational age
Obesity
Tonsillar or adenoid hypertrophy
Congenital malformations or conditions
  Craniofacial syndromes
  Musculoskeletal syndromes
  Mucopolysaccharidosis
Acquired conditions
  Trauma to face, head, or neck
  Burns (especially inhalational injuries)
  Presence of a foreign body
  Infections
  Tumors
  Following radiation therapy to head/neck
  History of tracheostomy or tracheal reconstruction
  Anaphylaxis
  Fluid overload
  Barotrauma
  SVC syndrome
MMR
Postoperative conditions
  Prone or Trendelenburg positioning leading to airway edema
  Head/neck surgery
  Massive fluid shifts and third spacing

PREVENTION

Careful assessment of airway anatomy, which may be difficult in young and uncooperative children
> Use the classification schemes of Mallampati or Samsoon and Young for older children and teenagers, but they may not be reliable in younger children

Prepare a wide range of age-appropriate sizes of airway equipment

Preoxygenate all patients prior to intubation

If there is any concern that mask ventilation or insertion of an SGA may be difficult (e.g., obstruction in lower airway or restricted mouth opening), then proceed with caution
> Contingency plans should include fiberoptic intubation, surgical airway, CPB or ECMO standby

Limit the number of attempts at direct laryngoscopy

Have the most experienced clinician intubate

Avoid causing airway trauma, which may result in edema and/or bleeding
> Narrowing of the airway in smaller patients may result in hypoventilation

Create a difficult airway cart with necessary supplies and equipment

Drill and practice management of difficult airway/failed intubation (using simulation if available)

MANIFESTATIONS

Expected or known difficult pediatric airway or tracheal intubation
> Previous history of difficult airway or tracheal intubation
> An airway examination reveals a Samsoon and Young's class III or IV airway
> Presence of anatomic features that make the patient difficult to intubate
> Congenital syndromes associated with difficult intubation

Unexpected difficult pediatric airway or tracheal intubation
> Failure to intubate the trachea by an experienced anesthesia professional
>> Difficult insertion of laryngoscope
>>> Small or restricted mouth opening
>>> MMR after succinylcholine administration
>> Difficult visualization of vocal cords
>> Difficult passage of ETT through vocal cords

Inability to mask ventilate after induction of anesthesia

Inability to place, and ventilate through, a SGA

Multiple failed attempts to intubate the trachea

SIMILAR EVENTS

Anesthesia workstation malfunction (e.g., bag/ventilator switch malposition)

Normal airway but unsuccessful intubation due to inexperience of the intubator

Functional airway obstruction
> Laryngospasm (see Event 97, Laryngospasm)
> Laryngomalacia
> Bronchospasm (see Event 29, Bronchospasm)
> Chest wall rigidity
> Gastric distention with air
> Aspiration of gastric contents (see Event 28, Aspiration of Gastric Contents)
> Endobronchial intubation (see Event 30, Endobronchial Intubation)

MANAGEMENT

Special considerations for pediatric patients

Less time to secure the airway compared to adults

O_2 consumption in children is significantly higher

Faster onset of hypoxemia during periods of hypoventilation or apnea (especially for younger and/or sicker children)

IV access may be difficult or impossible

For expected or known difficult airway, consider placing IV prior to induction

Have experienced help available at induction to place IV

Consider IO access or CVP line placement

Options for airway management

Awake oral or nasal intubation is the safest option in neonates

Most children will not be able to cooperate with awake intubation

Some level of anesthesia (from sedation to general anesthesia) will be required

Emergent surgical airway (cricothyrotomy, tracheostomy) or transtracheal jet ventilation are not recommended in smaller children (e.g., <5 years old) because of difficult anatomy, the time needed to establish a surgical airway, the low success rate, and the high complication rate

For the child with an expected or known difficult airway

Consider transfer of care to a tertiary pediatric hospital with subspecialists (pediatric anesthesiologists and pediatric ENT surgeons) experienced in the management of children with difficult airways and the capability for pediatric ECMO. Do not proceed with anesthesia unless fully prepared for management of potential loss of airway.

Preoperative or preinduction assessment

Carefully assess airway anatomy

Mouth opening

Size of tongue in relation to oropharynx

Neck range of motion (extension and flexion)

Size and shape of mandible

Thyromental distance

Special attention to dysmorphic or asymmetric facial features

Physical examination

Paradoxical chest movement with respirations

Stridor

Wheezing

Cyanosis

Obtain history from parents, focusing on airway symptoms

Snoring

Obstructed breathing patterns

Cyanosis with feeding or when asleep

Problems with airway management in the past

Review old anesthetic records for history of prior airway management

Assess baseline cardiopulmonary status

Preoperative or preinduction preparation

Err on the side of caution

Devise primary and contingency plans

Discuss plans with team

Have experienced help present

95

Consider alternatives to general endotracheal anesthesia, but recognize that emergency airway management will be difficult if a major complication occurs

Obtain difficult airway cart if available

Prepare all equipment, drugs, and resources

Multiple laryngoscope blades

Multiple ETT sizes

Consider using a cuffed ETT (vs. uncuffed ETT), which will avoid having a large leak

Appropriately sized SGAs

Appropriately sized video laryngoscope

Appropriately sized fiberoptic bronchoscope

Emergency drugs

Cricothyrotomy kit (only for older children)

Have experienced surgeon present for rigid bronchoscopy or emergent surgical airway

Consider CPB or ECMO standby

Set up PRIOR to induction because this requires considerable time and resources

Induction

Preoxygenation

Ensure adequate oxygenation throughout induction

Increased FiO_2 may be contraindicated in children with unrepaired cyanotic heart disease

Maintain spontaneous ventilation if possible

For the child with an unexpected difficult airway

Call for help stat if not already present (e.g., anesthesia professional, anesthesia tech)

Call for difficult airway cart

Once help arrives, have them set up airway equipment and ensure IV/IO access, or consider having them take over airway management if they are more experienced

Assess adequacy of oxygenation and ventilation

Place an oral or nasopharyngeal airway

Consider two-person bag valve mask

If mask ventilation is possible, determine whether to place an SGA or to intubate the trachea

Placement of an SGA

Use age- and size-appropriate SGA as the primary airway device or as a conduit for endotracheal intubation

Consider allowing spontaneous ventilation to occur if possible, and awaken the patient; convert to an awake intubation

Intubation of the trachea

Optimize patient position for intubation

Limit intubation attempts by inexperienced anesthesia professionals

Most experienced person should perform subsequent laryngoscopies

Consider intubation with video-assisted laryngoscope

Use a stylet or bougie

Use smaller ETT if difficulty in passing ETT through cords

If mask ventilation or intubation is impossible

Attempt to place an SGA

If successful, consider whether to wake the patient, to continue the case with the SGA or to attempt to intubate the trachea through the device

95

If SGA is unsuccessful, consider moving early to emergency cricothyrotomy, tracheostomy, or emergency CPB or ECMO

These options take time and resources and should be set up in advance if they are to be effective

General Considerations

Adult techniques and equipment can generally be used for children >40 kg or >10 to 12 years of age

Many different techniques to secure a difficult pediatric airway have been reported but are not applicable for all ages or situations

Clinicians should use techniques with which they have experience and expertise

COMPLICATIONS

Airway trauma
Airway edema from multiple laryngoscopies
Endobronchial intubation
Hypoxemia
Hypercarbia
Regurgitation or aspiration of gastric contents
Dental trauma
Hyperextension or damage to cervical spine
Complications of surgical airway or tracheostomy
Cardiac arrest
Death

SUGGESTED READING

1. Updated report by the American Society of Anesthesiologists Task Force on Management of the Difficult Airway. Practice guidelines for management of the difficult airway. Anesthesiology 2013;118:251-70.
2. Cote CJ, Lerman J, Todres ID. The pediatric airway in a practice of anesthesia for infants and children. 4th ed. Philadelphia: Saunders; 2009.
3. Engelhard T, Weiss M. A child with a difficult airway: what do I do next? Curr Opin Anesthesiol 2012;25:326-32.
4. Gregory GA, Riazi J. Classification and assessment of the difficult pediatric airway. Anesthesiol Clin North America 1998;16:729-41.
5. Heinrich S, Birkholz T, Ihmsen H, et al. Incidence and predictors of difficult laryngoscopy in 11219 pediatric anesthesia procedures. Pediatr Anesth 2012;22:729-36.
6. Holzman RS. Airway management. In: Davis PJ, Cladis FP, Motoyama EK, editors. Smith's anesthesia for infants and children. 8th ed. Philadelpha: Mosby; 2011.
7. Weiss M, Engelhardt T. Proposal for the management of the unexpected & difficult pediatric airway. Paediatr Anaesth 2010;20:454-64.

96 Hypotension in the Pediatric Patient

DEFINITION

Hypotension in the pediatric patient is a systolic BP less than the 5th percentile of the normal range for age.

<60 mm Hg in term neonates (0 to 28 days)
<70 mm Hg in infants (1 to 12 months)
<70 mm Hg + (2×age in years) in children 1 to 10 years old
<90 mm Hg in children more than 10 years old

ETIOLOGY

Decreased preload
> Hypovolemia (e.g., hemorrhage, including occult blood loss)
> Vasodilation
> Impaired venous return
> Elevated intrathoracic pressure (e.g., pneumothorax)
> Cardiac tamponade
> PE

Decreased contractility
> Negative inotropic drugs (e.g., anesthetic agents)
> Arrhythmias
> Congenital cardiac lesions
> Cardiomyopathy
> Hypoxemia
> Heart failure
> Abrupt increase in afterload

Decreased SVR
> Drug-induced vasodilation (e.g., anesthetics, ACEI)
> Shock (e.g., sepsis, anaphylaxis)
> Endocrine abnormalities (e.g., hypoglycemia, Addisonian crisis, hypothyroidism)

Arrythmias
> Tachycardia or irregular rhythm (loss of ventricular filling)
> Bradycardia

TYPICAL SITUATIONS

96

After anesthetic induction and before surgical incision
> More common after IV induction or combined IV/inhalation induction and in adolescents

Hypovolemia
> Inadequate replacement of fluids and blood loss from ongoing losses during the surgical procedure
> Surgery with major fluid shifts or occult blood loss
> Preexisting hypovolemia (e.g., trauma, burns, vomiting)

Preexisting hypotension
Neuraxial anesthesia
Children with high body mass index, especially in positions other than supine
Congenital heart disease
Prolonged NPO status
Peritoneal insufflation
During arrhythmias

PREVENTION

*Hypotension is a **late** sign of cardiovascular compromise in the pediatric patient, and the symptoms may be masked by anesthesia. Up to 35% of blood volume may be lost before hypotension becomes manifest.*

Carefully assess cardiovascular status preoperatively, checking for
> Patient history and fluid status (e.g., vomiting, diarrhea)
> Capillary refill

SECTION II — Catalog of Critical Events in Anesthesiology

Peripheral pulses and increased HR

Urine output

Skin turgor and mottling

Central filling pressures when available

Avoid excessive NPO times

Ensure adequate intravascular volume and correct electrolyte abnormalities before induction of anesthesia

Obtain preoperative ECG and/or TEE/TTE in patients with structural cardiac lesions and arrhythmias

Optimize preoperative medical status of patients with congenital heart disease

Avoid high doses of anesthetic agents

Administer drugs by slow IV infusion if hypotension is a known side effect (e.g., vancomycin)

Use appropriate doses of local anesthetic when performing regional anesthesia techniques

Monitor surgical activities and track blood loss carefully

MANIFESTATIONS

Systolic BP less than the 5th percentile of the normal range for age

NIBP cuff with low value or continuously cycling

Dampened or low arterial line waveform

Tachycardia

Decreased or absent pulse oximetry value

Decreased ET CO_2

Delayed capillary refill

Weakened or absent peripheral pulses

Decreased urine output

Decreased skin turgor and temperature

Skin mottling

Altered level of consciousness

Arrhythmias, including compensatory sinus tachycardia

SIMILAR EVENTS

Artifact

Motion artifact (surgeon leaning on cuff)

Incorrect size of BP cuff

Faulty or improperly positioned transducer

Vasospasm of artery with indwelling catheter

BP measurement in extremity with decreased perfusion (e.g., coarctation of aorta)

MANAGEMENT

Rule out rapidly lethal, often missed, causes of severe hypotension: hemorrhage, anesthetic overdose, pneumothorax, anaphylaxis, congenital heart disease, and surgical causes.

Ensure adequate oxygenation and ventilation

Check the O_2 saturation

Auscultate breath sounds (see Event 35, Pneumothorax, Event 91, Anaphylaxis in the Pediatric Patient, and Event 29, Bronchospasm)

Check airway pressure (see Event 7, High Peak Inspiratory Pressure)

Increase the FiO_2 if O_2 saturation is low or if hypotension is severe

Verify the patient is hypotensive

Repeat NIBP measurement once

Appropriate BP cuff size is two-thirds of the length of the upper arm

Flush arterial line if present

Palpate peripheral pulse (brachial artery) and check capnograph

If no pulse, start CPR (see Event 94, Cardiac Arrest in the Pediatric Patient)

Call for help and get crash cart/defibrillator

If pulse is strong and other vital signs stable, consider artifact or transient

Repeat NIBP measurement, ensuring nobody is leaning on cuff

Measure at a different site (e.g., leg)

Measure BP manually

Re-zero the arterial line transducer

Check that the transducer is at the desired level

Ensure that the transducer is connected to the appropriate monitoring cable of the physiologic monitor

Check the arterial line for any open or loose stopcocks or connections

Discontinue anesthetic and vasodilating drugs

Inform team and ask surgeon to visually inspect field, sponges, and suction canister

Call for help if additional vascular access and immediate volume resuscitation is needed

Ask the surgeon to pause the operation to assist in diagnosis and allow time to treat hypotension

Check for retractors causing venous compression

Check for ongoing or occult blood loss

Discuss the need for additional expert surgical help or whether the surgical procedure should be terminated

Identify cause of hypotension and treat

Decreased preload

Expand circulating volume by administration of IV fluid boluses (20 mL/kg IV LR or NS)

Consider colloid/blood administration

Place patient in Trendelenburg position

Place another large-bore IV if continued volume replacement is anticipated

Consider placement of IO line if peripheral access is difficult or not possible

Decreased contractility

Consider inotropic infusions (e.g., dopamine, epinephrine)

Review ECG for arrhythmia or ischemia

Consider TEE/TTE to evaluate myocardial function

Decreased afterload

Start vasopressor therapy (phenylephrine, norepinephrine)

If anaphylaxis is suspected, administer epinephrine and IV fluids (see Event 91, Anaphylaxis in the Pediatric Patient)

Consider administration of corticosteroid (hydrocortisone IV) to treat Addisonian crisis (see Event 38, Addisonian Crisis)

Consider placement of an arterial line and urinary catheter if not present

Check ABG and labs including CBC, electrolytes, Ca^{2+}, lactate, and type and crossmatch (see Event 13, The Septic Patient, and Event 46, Metabolic Acidosis)

Consider use of CVP monitoring

COMPLICATIONS

CHF or pulmonary edema from excessive fluid administration
Hypertension from treatment of artifact or transient
Cerebral ischemia
Acute renal failure
Cardiac arrest

SUGGESTED READING

1. Kleinman M, Chameides L, Schexnayder S, et al. Pediatric advanced life support. 2010 guidelines for cardiopulmonary resuscitation and emergency cardiovascular care. Circulation 2010;122:S876-908.
2. Nafiu OO, Kheterpal S, Morris M, et al. Incidence and risk factors for preincision hypotension in a noncardiac pediatric surgical population. Paediatr Anaesth 2009;19:232-9.
3. Nafiu OO, Voepel-Lewis T, Morris M, et al. How do pediatric anesthesiologists define intraoperative hypotension? Paediatr Anaesth 2009;19:1048-53.
4. Nafiu OO, Maclean S, Blum J, et al. High BMI in children as a risk factor for intraoperative hypotension. Eur J Anaesthesiol 2010;27:1065-8.

97 Laryngospasm

DEFINITION

Laryngospasm is occlusion of the glottis and laryngeal inlet by action of the laryngeal muscles.

ETIOLOGY

Laryngospasm is the result of a prolonged LCR
    Triggered by mechanical stimuli (e.g., laryngeal or pharyngeal manipulation) or chemical stimuli (e.g., gastric contents)
    Exaggerated by pathologic alteration in pharyngolaryngeal sensation (e.g., GERD, URI, and neurologic disorders) and other physiologic factors (e.g., age)

TYPICAL SITUATIONS

During the excitement phase of anesthetic induction or emergence
During light anesthesia relative to the surgical stimulus
When there are mechanical irritants in the airway
    Blood or secretions
    Airway instrumentation
    Oro/nasopharyngeal suction catheter
During surgical procedures involving the airway
In patients with GERD
In patients with onset of URI in the last 2 weeks
During anesthesia administration by an inexperienced provider

PREVENTION

Identify risk factors for laryngospasm
    Young age (<5 years)
    Male

Recent URI (symptoms day of surgery or within preceding 2 weeks)
Emergency procedure
Airway surgery
Wheezing at exercise more than three times in past year
History of eczema
Nocturnal dry cough
Family history of asthma or atopy
Exposure to second-hand smoke
Postpone elective procedures 2 to 3 weeks after URI
Seek supervision by an experienced pediatric anesthesia professional
Choose induction of anesthesia via the IV route if possible
Provide anesthesia via face mask when feasible (e.g., short cases requiring general anesthesia)
Ensure an adequate depth of anesthesia prior to laryngeal manipulation or surgical stimulation
Use muscle relaxants to facilitate tracheal intubation
Provide an adequate level of anesthesia during maintenance
Extubate the trachea when the patient is either deeply anesthetized or is fully awake
Clear all secretions from the airway prior to and after extubation
Consider topical or IV lidocaine

MANIFESTATIONS

Sudden onset
Retractions (sternal, intercostal)
Paradoxical chest and abdominal movements
Inability to phonate
No airflow despite ventilatory efforts
Inability to mask ventilate
Stridor (if vocal cords are not completely closed)
Hypoxemia
Tachypnea
Tachycardia
Increase in pharyngeal secretions
Inability to intubate or pass ETT
Loss of ET CO_2
High PIP if trying to provide positive pressure ventilation
Bradycardia
Cyanosis
Cardiac arrest

97

SIMILAR EVENTS

Extrathoracic respiratory tract obstruction from other causes
Intratracheal foreign bodies (see Event 92, Aspiration of a Foreign Body)
Infectious croup
Subglottic hemangioma
Glottic web
Vocal cord dysfunction or tumor
Arytenoid dislocation from traumatic instrumentation of the larynx
Pharyngeal edema or abscess
Angioneurotic edema
Pneumothorax or pneumomediastinum (see Event 35, Pneumothorax)

MANAGEMENT

Call for help

Institute 5 to 10 cm H_2O CPAP with an FiO_2 of 100% using an anesthesia breathing circuit or bag valve mask

Use maximum efforts to open the airway

Jaw thrust, head tilt, oral or nasal airway

CPAP may break laryngospasm by lowering the pressure gradient across the obstructed segment and possibly by pneumatically stenting the pharyngeal and laryngeal muscles

Remove the offending stimulus

Suction the oropharynx

Deepen the anesthetic and prepare for the administration of muscle relaxant

Monitor oxygenation carefully

If laryngospasm does not break

Administer atropine IV 20 μg/kg and succinylcholine IV, 0.5 to 2 mg/kg

Or propofol IV, 1 mg/kg (data limited in patients <3 years)

Or rocuronium IV, 0.9 to 1.2 mg/kg (if succinylcholine is contraindicated)

If no IV access, administer succinylcholine IM, 1.5 to 4 mg/kg, or IO, 0.5 to 1 mg/kg

Continue to provide positive pressure ventilation with CPAP

Maintain a patent airway

Consider spontaneous ventilation after muscle relaxation resolves

Prepare for more invasive airway maneuvers if oxygenation cannot be maintained

Intubation/reintubation (see Event 95, Difficult Airway Management in the Pediatric Patient)

Cricothyrotomy

Tracheostomy

If the child manifests bradycardia that is profound or unresponsive to treatment, begin CPR (see Event 93, Bradycardia in the Pediatric Patient, and Event 94, Cardiac Arrest in the Pediatric Patient)

COMPLICATIONS

Hypoxemia

Hypercarbia

Bradycardia

Arrhythmias

Negative pressure pulmonary edema

Cardiac arrest

SUGGESTED READING

1. Alalami AA, Ayoub CM, Baraka AS. Laryngospasm: review of different prevention and treatment modalities. Paediatr Anaesth 2008;18:281-8.
2. Alalami AA, Zestos MM, Baraka AS. Pediatric laryngospasm: prevention and treatment. Curr Opin Anaesth 2009;22:388-95.
3. Burgoyne LL, Anghelescu DL. Intervention steps for treating laryngospasm in pediatric patients. Paediatr Anaesth 2008;18:297-302.
4. Flick RP, Wilder RT, Pieper SF, et al. Risk factors for laryngospasm in children during general anesthesia. Paediatr Anaesth 2008;18:289-96.
5. Hamilton ND, Hegarty M, Calder A, Erb TO, von Ungern-Sternberg BS. Does topical lidocaine before tracheal intubation attenuate airway responses in children? An observational audit. Paediatr Anaesth 2012;22:345-50.
6. Mc Donnell C. Interventions guided by analysis of quality indicators decrease the frequency of laryngospasm during pediatric anesthesia. Paediatr Anaesth 2013;23:579-87.
7. Orestes MI, Lander L, Verghese S, Shah RK. Incidence of laryngospasm and bronchospasm in pediatric adenotonsillectomy. Laryngoscope 2012;122:425-8.

8. Orliaguet GA, Gall O, Savoldelli GL, Couloigner V. Case scenario: perianesthetic management of laryngospasm in children. Anesthesiology 2012;116:458-71.
9. von Ungern-Sternberg BS, Boda K, Chambers NA, et al. Risk assessment for respiratory complications in paediatric anaesthesia: a prospective cohort study. Lancet 2010;376:773-83.

98   Masseter Muscle Rigidity

DEFINITION

Masseter muscle rigidity (MMR) is a contracture of the masseter muscle following administration of succinylcholine, and ranges from mild (limited ability to open the mouth) to severe ("jaws of steel").

ETIOLOGY

The etiology is uncertain
  An abnormal or exaggerated response at the neuromuscular junction to succinylcholine administration
    Involves stimulation of the deep layers of the masseter muscles

TYPICAL SITUATIONS

Following administration of succinylcholine during induction of anesthesia
  Highest incidence when used with volatile anesthetics in children
  Occurs less commonly when IV induction agents are used
Following administration of succinylcholine for emergency securing of airway outside of OR

PREVENTION

Avoid using succinylcholine during anesthesia with a volatile anesthetic
Avoid succinylcholine and volatile anesthetics in patients with prior history of MMR
Consider alternatives to succinylcholine for RSI
Administer the correct dose of succinylcholine and wait a sufficient time for it to produce muscle relaxation prior to attempting laryngoscopy

MANIFESTATIONS

Subjective difficulty in opening the mouth
  This can range from a slight increase in masseter muscle resistance to apparent active tetany
  Other skeletal muscles are typically relaxed
  If generalized rigidity in the presence of MMR occurs, MH is likely to follow
Administration of additional succinylcholine does not result in relaxation of the masseter muscles
MMR persists until neuromuscular function begins to return in the peripheral musculature
  Increased tension of the masseter muscle may last as long as 30 minutes
Ventilation is usually possible, as other airway muscles remain relaxed
Myalgia and weakness may be present for as long as 36 hours following the acute episode
All patients with significant MMR develop rhabdomyolysis over the ensuing 24 hours
  Elevation of CK and presence of myoglobinemia and myoglobinuria

SIMILAR EVENTS

Congenital or acquired anatomic abnormalities that restrict mouth opening
> Hemifacial microsomia, diseases of the temporomandibular joint, prior surgical procedures producing contractures

Myotonic syndromes

Light anesthesia

Normal increase in masseter muscle tension during induction of anesthesia and administration of succinylcholine

MH (see Event 45, Malignant Hyperthermia)

Inadequate level of neuromuscular blockade

Failure to wait until the maximal effect of succinylcholine occurs

MANAGEMENT

If generalized rigidity is present or if signs of MH develop, declare an MH emergency and immediately administer dantrolene (see Event 45, Malignant Hyperthermia).

Maintain positive pressure ventilation with bag valve mask until the masseter muscles relax
> Even though it is difficult to open the mouth, positive pressure ventilation is typically not a problem

Intubate the trachea whenever it becomes feasible to do so
> Consider administration of an intubating dose of nondepolarizing muscle relaxant to facilitate intubation
> If ventilation and intubation are not possible, prepare for surgical airway (see Event 95, Difficult Airway Management in the Pediatric Patient)

Inform surgical team of MMR and discuss plans for surgery
> **Consider continuing with surgery if**
>> MMR is mild/transient (mouth can eventually be opened with increased effort)
>> No generalized rigidity is present
>> Patient is hemodynamically stable
>
> **Consider terminating surgery if**
>> MMR is severe (mouth cannot be opened)
>> Peripheral muscle rigidity is present
>
> **Terminate the surgery if**
>> Signs of increasing metabolic rate begin to appear
>>> Immediately commence treatment of MH

If the surgery is emergent
> Change the anesthetic to nontriggering agents
> Consider administration of dantrolene
> Consider placement of an arterial line
> Assess adequacy of IV access

Observe the patient carefully for signs of MH
> Skeletal muscle rigidity
> Increased CO_2 production and O_2 consumption
> Metabolic acidosis and hyperkalemia (check blood gas)
> Tachycardia or arrhythmias
> Increase in body temperature
> Myoglobinuria

All patients with significant MMR will develop rhabdomyolysis and should be observed for 24 hours in the hospital
> Send blood to lab for CK and presence of myoglobinemia q6h until trending downward
> Observe for dark urine
>> Test for myoglobinuria
> Monitor for signs of MH
> Consider IV hydration to promote diuresis

Evaluate the patient for an undiagnosed muscular disorder
Counsel parents to consult an expert regarding MH susceptibility

COMPLICATIONS

Inability to intubate the trachea
Difficulty maintaining ventilation by mask
Hypoxemia

SUGGESTED READING

1. Brandom BW. Malignant hyperthermia. In: Motoyama EK, Davis PJ, editors. Smith's anesthesia for infants and children. 6th ed. St. Louis: Mosby; 2006. p. 1018.
2. Dexter F, Epstein RH, Wachtel RE, Rosenberg H. Estimate of the relative risk of succinylcholine for triggering malignant hyperthermia. Anesth Analg 2013;116:118-22.
3. Glahn KP, Ellis FR, Halsall PJ, et al. Recognizing and managing a malignant hyperthermia crisis: guidelines from the European Malignant Hyperthermia Group. Br J Anaesth 2010;105:417-20.
4. Rawicz M, Brandom BW, Wolf A. The place of suxamethonium in pediatric anesthesia. Paediatr Anaesth 2009;19:561-70.

99   Sinus Tachycardia in the Pediatric Patient

DEFINITION

Sinus tachycardia in the pediatric patient is a HR faster than the age-appropriate normal value (see Table, next page).

ETIOLOGY

Enhanced automaticity of sinus node for any reason

TYPICAL SITUATIONS

Isolated finding in an asymptomatic patient
Response to anxiety or pain
Inadequate anesthesia during surgery
Compensatory mechanism to maintain adequate CO and O_2 delivery
> Hypovolemia
> Anemia
> Hypoxemia
> Shock states

Other physiologic responses
    Infection/sepsis
    Hypercarbia
    Fever
    Hypoglycemia
    Electrolyte abnormalities
    Endocrine conditions (e.g., hyperthyroidism, pheochromocytoma)
    CNS conditions (e.g., seizures)
Side effect of medication
    Ketamine
    β_2-Agonists
    Anticholinergics
    Inotropic agents
    Sympathomimetics (e.g., caffeine, over-the-counter cold remedies)
Iatrogenic
    During central line placement
    During or after cardiac surgery (e.g., surgical manipulation of the right atrium)
    Pacemaker malfunction
    Bladder distention (e.g., from blocked urinary catheter)
    ETT resting on carina
Acquired heart disease
    Congestive heart failure, cardiomyopathy, or myocarditis
    Cardiac tumors

99

PEDIATRIC RESPIRATORY RATE AND HEART RATE BY AGE*

Age Group	Respiratory Rate Median (1st-99th Percentile)	Heart Rate Median (1st-99th Percentile)
0-3 mo	43 (25-66)	143 (107-181); term newborn at birth: 127 (90-164)
3-6 mo	41 (24-64)	140 (104-175)
6-9 mo	39 (23-61)	134 (98-168)
9-12 mo	37 (22-58)	128 (93-161)
12-18 mo	35 (21-53)	123 (88-156)
18-24 mo	31 (19-46)	116 (82-149)
2-3 yr	28 (18-38)	110 (76-142)
3-4 yr	25 (17-33)	104 (70-136)
4-6 yr	23 (17-29)	98 (65-131)
6-8 yr	21 (16-27)	91 (59-123)
8-12 yr	19 (14-25)	84 (52-115)
12-15 yr	18 (12-23)	78 (47-108)
15-18 yr	16 (11-22)	73 (43-104)

Data from Fleming S, Thompson M, Stevens R, et al. Normal ranges of heart rate and respiratory rate in children from birth to 18 years of age: a systematic review of observational studies. Lancet 2011;377:1011.
*The RR and HR provided are based upon measurement in awake, healthy infants and children at rest. Many clinical findings besides the actual vital sign measurement must be taken into account when determining whether a specific vital sign is normal in an individual patient. Values for HR or RR that fall within normal limits for age may still represent abnormal findings that are caused by underlying disease in a particular infant or child.

PREVENTION

Maintain adequate oxygenation and ventilation
Ensure adequate depth of anesthesia
Verify correct position of ETT
Minimize use of medications that may increase HR
Maintain adequate volume status
Maintain adequate hematocrit
Verify appropriate serum glucose level
Maintain normothermia

MANIFESTATIONS

Tachycardia
    Older children may report fast heartbeats, or "heart jumping out of chest"
    Chest pain or discomfort
    Dizziness
    Syncope
    Altered mental status
    Shortness of breath
    Poor perfusion
    Fatigue/lethargy
    Nausea/vomiting
Infants and nonverbal children
    Irritability
    Poor feeding
Cardiac manifestations of prolonged tachycardia
    Impaired diastolic filling
    Decreased ventricular preload
    Compromised CO
Monitors
    Fast HR on ECG
    Hypotension
    Poor perfusion on pulse oximeter
    Decreased ET CO_2 waveform

99

SIMILAR EVENTS

Monitor artifact
    ECG "double counting"
    Electrocautery interference
Pacemaker malfunction or inappropriate settings
Other tachyarrhythmias
Denervated heart status post-transplantation
Congenital heart conditions
    Wolff-Parkinson-White syndrome
    Other conduction system disorders

MANAGEMENT

Pathologic tachyarrhythmias are rare in children without underlying cardiac disease. Sinus tachycardia is much more common in everyday practice, and this section focuses on the evaluation and treatment of sinus tachycardia in the pediatric patient.

Determine whether HR is too high for the patient's age

Use age-appropriate normal value chart

Rates greater than 170 beats per minute in infants, and greater than 140 beats per minute in children, require further investigation

HRs >200 beats per minute are unlikely to be sinus tachycardia

Assess the clinical situation (e.g., presence of hyperthermia or infusion of inotropes)

Verify HR and assess patient's hemodynamic status

Check monitors of HR (e.g., ECG, pulse oximeter, arterial line)

Check BP

Check peripheral pulse

Check ET CO_2 waveform for evidence of adequate CO

Check TEE or TTE for cardiac function and filling

Ensure adequate oxygenation and ventilation

Consider increasing FiO_2

Obtain 12-lead ECG or print rhythm strip

Check presence of P waves and P wave axis before each QRS complex and QRS morphology to determine whether the rhythm is sinus

Assess the clinical situation to determine whether the tachycardia is a compensatory response to another problem

Treat potential causes of sinus tachycardia

Ensure adequate level of anesthesia

Verify that anesthetic agents (inhaled or IV) are being administered to the patient

Ensure patency of IV access

Verify that patient is not paralyzed without adequate anesthesia

Check ALL infusions (see Event 63, Drug Administration Error)

Check the patient's temperature

Check the surgical field for operative causes

Consider possibility of occult hemorrhage

Look for increased level of surgical stimulation

Evaluate the patient's volume status

Assess response to IV fluid bolus, Trendelenburg positioning, or leg raising

CVP

TEE or TTE for ventricular filling

Liver size

Drug treatment of tachycardia in pediatric patients

Many of the drugs used can depress myocardial function and lower CO

β-blockers and calcium channel blockers are negative inotropes and depress the myocardium

CO is rate-dependent in pediatric patients

Specialist consultation is recommended prior to treatment with these drugs

Anticipate and plan for deterioration in patient status

Consider obtaining crash cart and placing pediatric defibrillator pads

Obtain 12-lead ECG if not already done

Call for pediatric cardiology consult

Continuously reassess for change in ECG or hemodynamic status

Be prepared to start CPR

Consider aborting procedure if problem persists

If the patient becomes unstable or has no pulse (see Event 94, Cardiac Arrest in the Pediatric Patient)

  Call for more help and notify surgeon

  Start CPR

  Call an OR or hospital code

  Call for crash cart and defibrillator

    Place pediatric defibrillator pads on patient

  Synchronized cardioversion or defibrillation if patient is in a shockable rhythm

COMPLICATIONS

Hypotension

Hypervolemia

Cardiac arrest

SUGGESTED READING

1. Cote CJ, Lerman J, Todres ID. A practice of anesthesia for infants and children. 4th ed. Philadelphia: Saunders; 2009 p. 313-4.
2. Davis PJ, Cladis FP, Motoyama EK. Smith's anesthesia for infants and children. 8th ed. Philadelphia: Mosby; 2011 p. 1232-5.
3. Fleming S, Thompson M, Stevens R, et al. Normal ranges of heart rate and respiratory rate in children from birth to 18 years of age: a systematic review of observational studies. Lancet 2011;377:1011-8.
4. Fuhrman BP, Zimmerman JJ, Carcillo JA, et al. Pediatric critical care. 4th ed. Philadelphia: Saunders; 2011, p. 338-63.
5. Kleinman ME, Chameides L, Schexnayder SM, et al. Pediatric advanced life support: 2010 American Heart Association guidelines for cardiopulmonary resuscitation and emergency cardiovascular care. Circulation 2010;122:S876-908.
6. Park MK. Pediatric cardiology for practitioners. 5th ed. Philadelphia: Mosby; 2008, p. 417-8.

Index

Note: Page numbers followed by *f* indicate figures and *t* indicate tables.

Faulty oxygen supply
  complications of, 281
  definition of, 279
  etiology of, 279
  management of, 281
  manifestations of, 280
  prevention of, 280
  similar events to, 280–281
  in typical situations, 279
Feedback, *vs.* debriefing, 66
Fire, in operating room, 122
First responder, in ACRM simulation, 62
Fixation errors, 46
  ways to break, 46–47
Focused assessment with sonography in trauma
    (FAST), 88
Follow-up protocol, of Harvard Medical School's
    Department of Anesthesia, 48
Followership, 40
Foreign body aspiration
  complications of, 364
  definition of, 361
  etiology of, 361
  management of, 362–363
  manifestations of, 362
  prevention of, 362
  similar events to, 362
  in typical situations, 361–362
Fraction of inspired oxygen (FiO$_2$), 90

G

Gas embolism, 171
Gas flow control malfunction
  complications of, 283
  definition of, 282
  in electrical power failure, 278
  etiology of, 282
  management of, 283
  manifestations of, 282–283
  prevention of, 282
  similar events to, 283
  in typical situations, 282
Gastric contents, aspiration of, 181
General anesthesia
  and hypoglycemia, 218
  pulmonary embolism and, 158
Generalization phase, of debriefing, 71
Generalized emergency procedures, 35
Generalized seizure, 262
Generic events, 88–136
Glucose control, of septic patient, 131
Glycopyrrolate, 205
Good judgment, debriefing with, 73–74
Green herring, category of additional information in
    scenarios, in crisis resource management, 61*t*

H

Haste, 10
Hazardous attitudes, 27–28, 28*t*

Heart rate, pediatric, 390*t*
Hemodynamic abnormalities, in acute coronary
    syndrome, 138
Hemodynamic changes, 170
Hemodynamic goals, 150
Hemoglobinuria, frank, transfusion
    reaction and, 241
Hemoptysis, massive, 197
Hemorrhage
  acute, 88
    complications of, 357
    definition of, 353
    etiology of, 353
    intraoperative assessment of, 355–357
    management of, 355
    manifestations of, 354
    preoperative assessment of, 355
    prevention of, 353
    similar events to, 354
    in typical situations, 353
  obstetric
    complications of, 345
    definition of, 341
    etiology of, 341
    management of, 343–344
    manifestations of, 343
    prevention of, 343
    similar events to, 343
    in typical situations, 341–342
Heuristics, 19–20
High inspired CO$_2$
  complications of, 107
  definition of, 105
  etiology of, 105
  management of, 106–107
  manifestations of, 106
  prevention of, 106
  similar events to, 106
  in typical situations, 106
High peak inspiratory pressure
  complications of, 110
  definition of, 107
  etiology of, 107–108
  management of, 109–110
  manifestations of, 109
  similar events to, 109
  in typical situations, 108
High reliability organizations (HROs), 9
Hindsight bias
  in debriefing, 70
  in trigger videos, 55
Histamine antagonists, for anaphylaxis, 360
Hydrocortisone, for Addisonian crisis, 210
Hypercarbia
  complications of, 195
  definition of, 193
  etiology of, 193
  management of, 194–195
  manifestations of, 194
  prevention of, 193